INFECTIOUS DISEASES OF THE SKIN

Dirk M Elston, MD
Director, Department of Dermatology
Geisinger Medical Center
Danville, Pennsylvania, USA

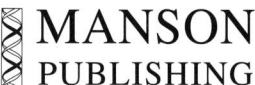

DEDICATION

To my wife, Kathy, and my children, Carly and Nate. You are my source of inspiration.

Dirk M Elston, MD

Softcover edition 2011

Copyright © 2009 Manson Publishing Ltd

ISBN: 978-1-84076-177-1

All rights reserved. No part of this publication may be reproduced, stored in a retrieval system or transmitted in any form or by any means without the written permission of the copyright holder or in accordance with the provisions of the Copyright Act 1956 (as amended), or under the terms of any licence permitting limited copying issued by the Copyright Licensing Agency, 33–34 Alfred Place, London WC1E 7DP, UK.

Any person who does any unauthorized act in relation to this publication may be liable to criminal prosecution and civil claims for damages.

A CIP catalogue record for this book is available from the British Library.

For full details of all Manson Publishing Ltd titles please write to:
Manson Publishing Ltd, 73 Corringham Road, London NW11 7DL, UK.
Tel: +44(0)20 8905 5150
Fax: +44(0)20 8201 9233
Website: www.mansonpublishing.com

Commissioning editor: Jill Northcott
Project manager: Paul Bennett
Copy-editor: Ruth Maxwell
Design and layout: Cathy Martin, Presspack Computing Ltd
Colour reproduction: Tenon & Polert Colour Scanning Ltd, Hong Kong
Printed by: Grafos SA, Barcelona, Spain

CONTENTS

PREFACE	6
CONTRIBUTORS	7
CHAPTER 1 BACTERIAL INFECTIONS	8
Introduction	8
Impetigo	8
Folliculitis	10
Furuncle/carbuncle	11
Abscess	12
Staphylococcal scalded skin syndrome	12
Scarlet fever	14
Erysipelas	14
Cellulitis	16
Necrotizing fasciitis	17
Peri-anal streptococcal disease	18
Cutaneous anthrax	19
Pitted keratolysis	19
Trichomycosis axillaris	20
Erythrasma	20
Ecthyma	20
Ecthyma gangrenosum	22
Meningococcemia	23
Cat-scratch disease	24
Chancroid	24
Granuloma inguinale (Donovanosis)	24
Gonorrhea	26
Typhus	27
Rocky Mountain spotted fever	28
Fish tank granuloma	29
Lyme disease	30
Syphilis (Lues)	30

CHAPTER 2 FUNGAL INFECTIONS — 34
　Introduction — 34
SUPERFICIAL FUNGAL INFECTIONS — 34
　Dermatophytosis — 34
　Onychomycosis — 44
　Candidiasis — 46
　Pityriasis versicolor — 48
　Tinea nigra — 48
DEEP FUNGAL INFECTIONS — 50
　Chromoblastomycosis — 50
　Sporotrichosis — 50
　Histoplasmosis — 50
　North American blastomycosis — 52
　Paracoccidioidomycosis (South American blastomycosis) — 52
　Coccidioidomycosis — 52
　Cryptococcosis — 54
　Lobomycosis — 55
　Hyalohyphomycosis (aspergillosis and fusariosis) — 55
　Mucormycosis — 56
RELATED INFECTIONS — 58
　Rhinosporidiosis — 58
　Protothecosis — 59

CHAPTER 3 VIRAL DISEASES — 60
　Introduction — 60
　Herpes simplex infection — 60
　Varicella zoster virus infection — 65
　Epstein–Barr virus infection — 68
　Gianotti–Crosti syndrome (papular acrodermatitis of childhood) — 69
　Unilateral laterothoracic exanthem — 69
　Cytomegalovirus infection — 70
　Exanthem subitum infection — 71
　Kaposi's sarcoma infection — 71
　Erythema infectiosum (fifth disease) infection — 73
　Human papillomavirus infection — 74
　Measles infection — 78
　Rubella infection — 80
　Poxvirus infection — 80

CHAPTER 4 TROPICAL AND EXOTIC INFECTIOUS DISEASES   84
   Introduction   84
   Rhinoscleroma   84
   Bacillary angiomatosis   85
   Cutaneous tuberculosis   86
   Leprosy   88
MYCETOMA   90
   Chromoblastomycosis   91
   Lobomycosis   92
   Paracoccidioidomycosis   93
   Acanthamebiasis   94
   Amebiasis   94
   Leishmaniasis   96
   Onchocerciasis   98
   Schistosomiasis   99
   Strongyloidiasis   100
   Cutaneous larva migrans   101

CHAPTER 5 ARTHROPODS AND INFESTATIONS   102
   Introduction   102
INSECTS   102
   Pediculosis   102
   Insect bites   104
   Hymenopterids   106
   Hemipterids   108
   Lepidopterids   109
   Coleopterids   110
   Siphonapterids   110
ARACHNIDS   112
   Mites   112
   Ticks   116
   Spiders   118
   Scorpions   121
CENTIPEDES AND MILLIPEDES   123

REFERENCES   124

ILLUSTRATED GLOSSARY   136

INDEX   141

PREFACE

Despite the rise of modern medicine, infections remain the leading cause of death worldwide. As we develop new antibiotics, organisms develop mechanisms of resistance. The battle rages on. In this battle, the most critical determinant of successful treatment remains an accurate diagnosis. This atlas will serve as a pictorial guide to the diagnosis of common bacterial, fungal, and viral skin infections, as well as recognition of arthropods of medical importance. Drug names are used as they are licensed in the United States.

The text is divided into chapters by class of organism, and in each chapter by clinical entity. We have found this approach to be the most useful for those using the text. It can serve as both a tutorial and a handy clinical reference in the daily practice of medicine.

The skin is readily visible, and therefore visual inspection remains the most important means of accurate dermatologic diagnosis. Skin infections are no exception. Morphology, symptoms, exposure, and time course generally establish the diagnosis. Laboratory tests can provide confirmation, but therapy must usually be initiated based on the initial clinical assessment. This text will provide many images to assist you in recognizing skin infections. We hope we have provided you with a reference that will become one of your favorites and will be useful in your daily practice.

Dirk M Elston

CONTRIBUTORS

CHAPTER 1
Tammie Ferringer, MD
Department of Dermatology and Pathology
Geisinger Medical Center
Danville, Pennsylvania, USA

CHAPTER 2
Whitney A High, MD
Assistant Professor, Departments of Dermatology
& Dermatopathology
University of Colorado School of Medicine
Denver, Colorado, USA

CHAPTER 3
Anita Arora, MD
Center for Clinical Studies
Houston School of Medicine, University of Texas
Houston, Texas, USA

Natalia Mendoza, MSc
Center for Clinical Studies
Houston School of Medicine, University of Texas
Houston, Texas, USA
and Universidad El Bosque
Bogotá, Colombia

Adriana Motta
Department of Dermatology
Universidad El Bosque
Bogotá, Colombia

Vandana Madkan, MD
Center for Clinical Studies
Houston School of Medicine, University of Texas
Houston, Texas, USA

Stephen K Tyring, MD, PhD, MBA
Department of Dermatology
Center for Clinical Studies
Houston School of Medicine, University of Texas
Houston, Texas, USA

CHAPTER 4
Omar P Sangüeza, MD
Professor, Departments of Pathology and
Dermatology
Wake Forest University School of Medicine
Winston-Salem, North Carolina, USA

Daniel J Sheehan, MD
Department of Pathology
Wake Forest University School of Medicine
Winston-Salem, North Carolina, USA

Gary Goldenberg, MD
Department of Dermatology
Wake Forest University School of Medicine
Winston-Salem, North Carolina, USA

CHAPTER 5
Dirk M Elston, MD
Director, Department of Dermatology
Geisinger Medical Center
Danville, Pennsylvania, USA

CHAPTER 1

BACTERIAL INFECTIONS

Tammie Ferringer

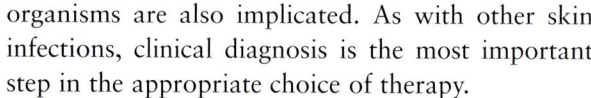

INTRODUCTION
Bacterial infections remain the most common infectious cause of visits to a physician. Most cutaneous infections are caused by staphylococci and streptococci, but a wide range of other organisms are also implicated. As with other skin infections, clinical diagnosis is the most important step in the appropriate choice of therapy.

IMPETIGO
Impetigo may be staphylococcal or streptococcal in origin. In either case, it is a contagious, superficial skin infection that occurs most frequently in early childhood but all ages may be affected. Transmission is by direct contact or fomites.

The non-bullous form of impetigo presents as transient vesicles or pustules that rupture with resultant erosions surmounted by a golden-yellow crust (**1–6**). The crust can usually be removed easily, leaving an eroded surface. The infection spreads to contiguous and distal areas through inoculation from scratching. Lesions tend to resolve within days to weeks without scarring. The face (around the mouth and the nose) and sites with an impaired cutaneous barrier (e.g. insect bites, abrasions, burns, eczema) are most frequently involved (**7–9**).

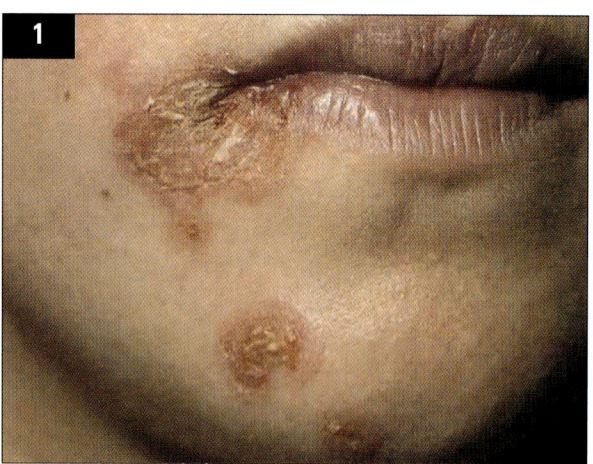

1 Honey-colored crust of impetigo in a common anatomic location.

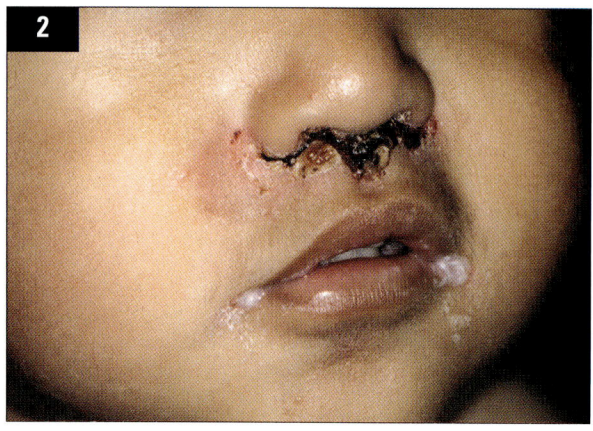

2 Crusted impetigo in a patient with nasal staphylococcal carriage.

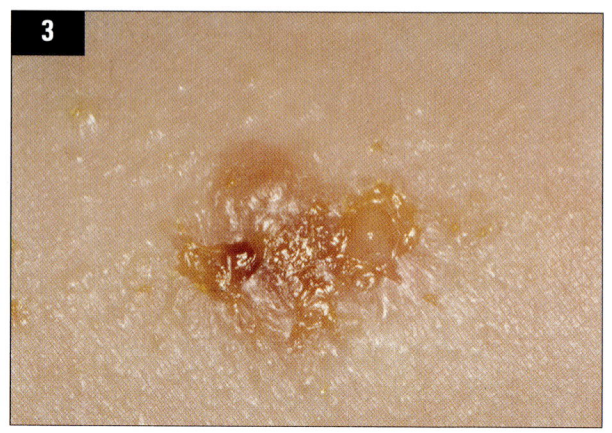

3 Honey-colored crusts in impetigo represent coagulated serum.

Bacterial Infections

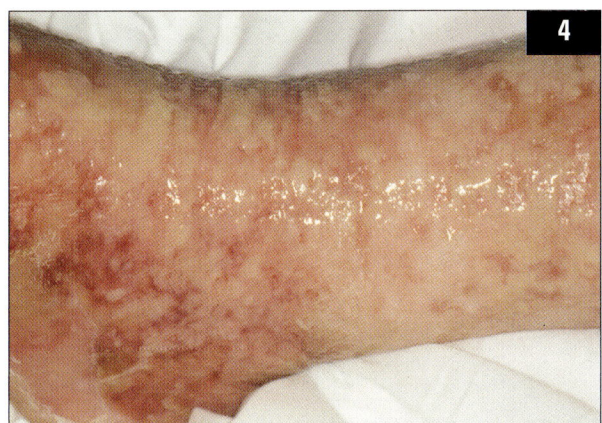

4 Secondary impetiginization in an area of impaired cutaneous barrier.

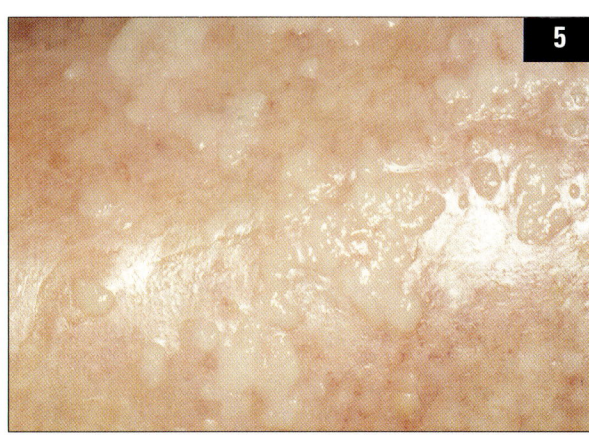

5 Close-up demonstrates soft adherent fibrinous material that is secondarily impetiginized.

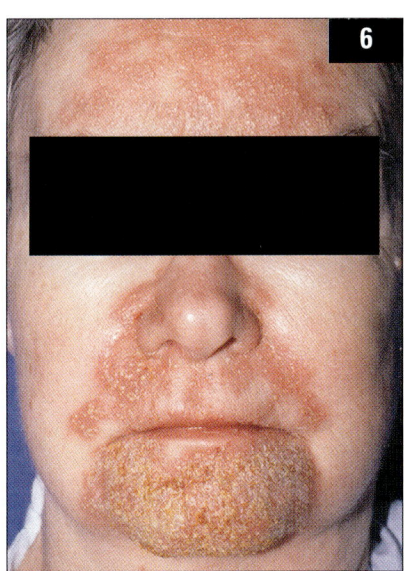

6 Impetiginized dermatitis on the face. Both anti-staphylococcal therapy and a topical corticosteroid will be needed.

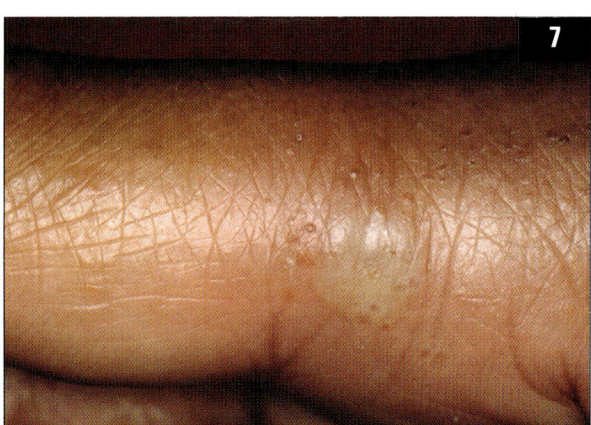

7 Impetiginized eczema overlying a joint presents a risk of septic arthritis.

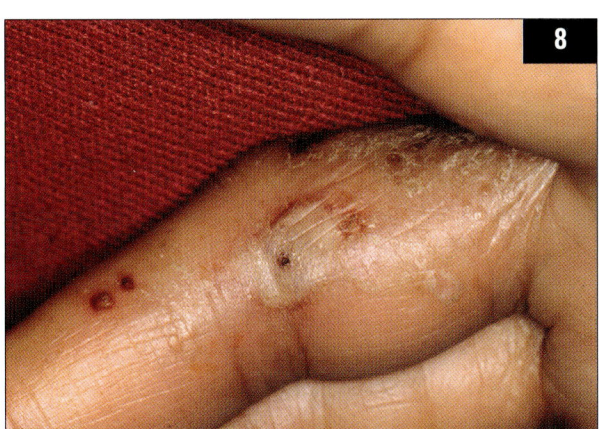

8 Impetiginized eczema evolves from vesicles to pustules.

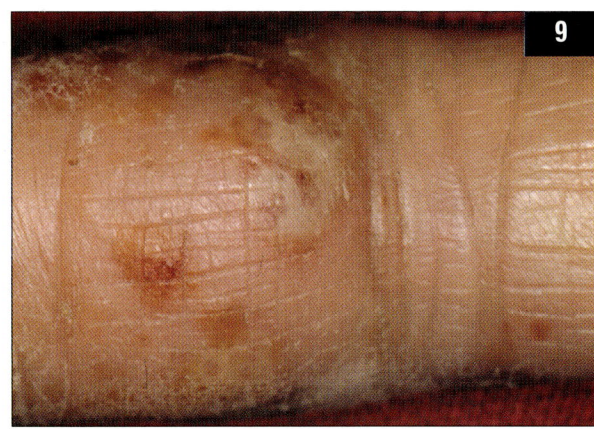

9 Impetiginized eczema. The image demonstrates multilocular vesicles of dyshidrotic eczema with superimposed impetiginized pustules.

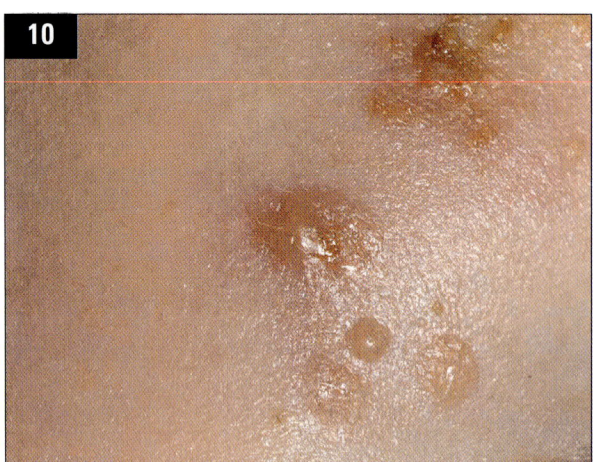

10 The bullae in bullous impetigo are superficial and fragile.

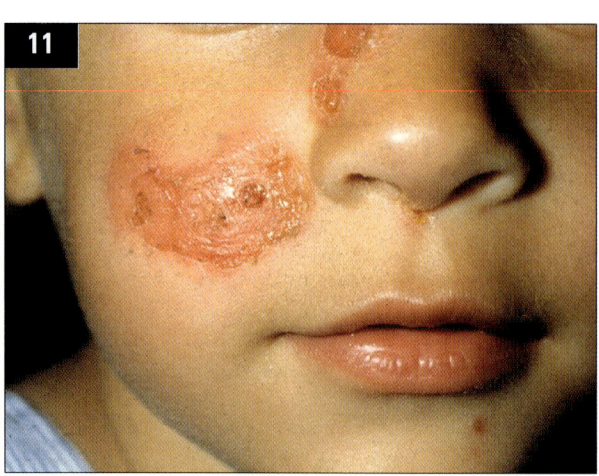

11 Bullous impetigo: intact bullae are still visible on the lateral cheek and nose. The majority of the lesion typically demonstrates denuded skin resulting from ruptured bullae.

Bullous impetigo (**10–12**) most commonly occurs in the neonate as vesicles that rapidly enlarge into fragile bullae that rupture leaving an erosion with a surrounding crust. Adults are rarely affected.

Staphylococcus aureus is the cause of all cases of bullous impetigo and most cases of non-bullous impetigo. The remainder are due to *Streptococcus pyogenes* or a combination of both organisms. Although rare, glomerulonephritis may follow impetigo caused by certain strains of *S. pyogenes* and treatment will not prevent or halt the nephritis (Weinstein & Le Frock, 1971). Gram stain and/or culture of exudate from the base of the erosion or the bullae fluid may be indicated for diagnosis.

Topical mupirocin can be effective for localized disease, although resistance is emerging (Perez-Roth *et al*., 2006). Newer topical antibiotics, such as retapamulin are valuable additions to our armamentarium (Rittenhouse *et al*., 2006). Widespread disease requires oral beta-lactamase-resistant antibiotics, a first-generation cephalosporin, such as cephalexin, or an extended-spectrum cephalosporin such as cefdinir (Giordano *et al*., 2006). Failure of oral antibiotics may be an indication of infection by methicillin-resistant *S. aureus* (MRSA), but it may also be an indication that there is an abscess cavity that must be drained. Patients with recurrent infections may require evaluation and treatment of nasal, axillary, and/or perineal carriage of *S. aureus* (Elston, 2007).

FOLLICULITIS

Folliculitis (**13, 14**) is an inflammation of the hair follicles caused by infection or physical or chemical irritation. The primary lesion is an erythematous papule or pustule with a central hair, occurring on hair-bearing areas of the body. The majority of bacterial folliculitis is due to *Staphylococcus aureus*. Predisposing factors include friction, hyperhydration, occlusion, shaving, pre-existing dermatitis, reduced host resistance, nasal carriage, wounds, application of corticosteroids, and exposure to oils and certain chemicals. 'Hot tub' folliculitis is a *Pseudomonas* infection acquired from exposure to contaminated heated water (hot tubs, heated swimming pools). This results in a pruritic, truncal eruption 1–4 days after exposure, characterized by erythematous follicular papules and pustules.

The diagnosis of folliculitis is typically based on the history and clinical findings; however, bacterial culture from the pustules is routinely collected. In resistant cases, non-bacterial etiologies may be elucidated by viral culture, fungal culture, or punch biopsy.

Each lesion of folliculitis represents a small abscess, and each will resolve as it drains. Washing with antibacterial agents can control some mild cases of folliculitis. If topical therapy fails, a first-generation or extended-spectrum cephalosporin or a pencillinase-resistant penicillin such as dicloxacillin is indicated unless MRSA is suspected. Chronic bacterial colonization should be considered in

Bacterial Infections

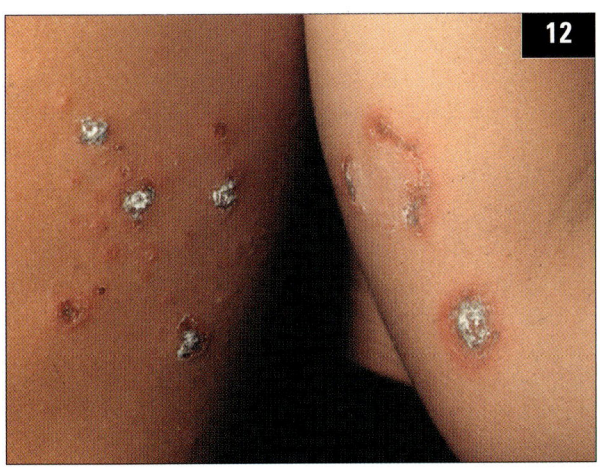

12 Kissing lesions, late stage of bullous impetigo. Bullae have resolved and hyperkeratosis is present.

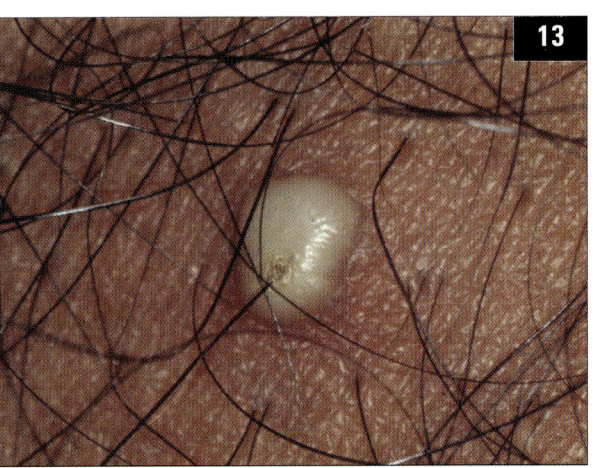

13 Folliculitis due to *Staphylococcus aureus*. A solitary lesion will respond to drainage alone.

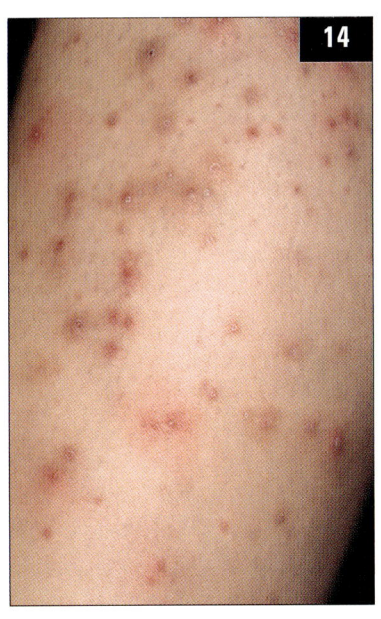

14 Folliculitis due to *Staphylococcus aureus*. Multiple lesions will need an antibiotic in addition to drainage of individual lesions. Most cases are still caused by methicillin-sensitive staphylococci, although the prevalence of methicillin-resistant strains is increasing.

15 Furuncle. Staphylococcal axillary furuncles are extremely tender. Those caused by pseudomonas tend to itch.

recurrent and recalcitrant folliculitis. Good hygiene with frequent bathing and laundering of separate towels, washcloths, and bed linens reduce the risk of folliculitis. Loose clothing and daily changing of disposable razors also lessen the risk.

Treatment of 'hot tub' folliculitis is usually not necessary, as spontaneous resolution occurs in 1–2 weeks. In the case of an immunosuppressed host or a persistent infection, a course of ciprofloxacin would be advised. The best prevention is attention to the water conditions to eliminate pseudomonal colonization (Bhatia & Brodell, 1999).

FURUNCLE/CARBUNCLE

A furuncle (boil) is an acute, tender, red nodule that generally ends in suppuration (**15**). They occur as a result of the spread of infection (usually staphylococcal) in folliculitis beneath the infundibulum. Carbuncles are collections of furuncles which extend deep into the subcutaneous tissue and usually display multiple draining sinus tracts. Unlike furuncles, systemic symptoms are usually present with carbuncles. Sites of predilection include the nape of the neck, axilla, thigh, perineum, and buttocks but they can occur anywhere on hairy skin.

Furuncles are more common in young adults, especially males. Predisposing factors include chronic staphylococcal carriage, diabetes, malnutrition, and immunosuppression.

As noted, staphylococci are the most common causative organism. Streptococci and coliform bacteria are less frequently identified. Multiple or recurrent furuncles can be associated with personal or familial chronic *S. aureus* carriage. Small furuncles may simply require warm compresses to promote spontaneous drainage. Fluctuant lesions require incision and drainage. Systemic antibiotics with *S. aureus* coverage should be used empirically for large and recurrent lesions, those with surrounding cellulitis, and in immunosuppressed patients. In cases unresponsive to the usual measures, antibiotic-resistant strains should be suspected and antibiotics should be adjusted based on sensitivities.

Control of recurrent furuncles requires daily bathing with an antibacterial wash such as chlorhexidine. For patients or family members with nasal colonization, application of mupirocin ointment twice a day to the anterior nares for the first 5 days each month has been used, but resistance is emerging (Raz et al., 1996). Topical retapamulin may play a role in this setting. Few systemic antibiotics attain adequate levels in the nasal secretions to achieve long-term clearance of staphylococci. Clindamycin, 150 mg daily for 3 months decreases recurrent infections in patients with methicillin-sensitive *Staphyloccus aureus* (MSSA) colonization by 82% (Klempner & Styrt, 1988). Rifampin with dicloxacillin for MSSA (or with minocycline or trimethoprim-sulfamethoxazole for MRSA), is another approach for eradication of the carrier state (Falagas et al., 2007). Complex regimens may be required for the eradication of MRSA carriage.

ABSCESS

An abscess is a walled off collection of pus that presents as a painful, fluctuant mass often with a rim of erythema (**16, 17**). Lesions are typically polymicrobial, reflecting the normal regional skin flora. In only 25% of cases is *S. aureus* isolated as the sole pathogen. Approximately 5% of abscesses are sterile (Meislin et al., 1977). Community strains of MRSA are an important cause of large and rapidly evolving abscesses. Abscesses adjacent to the gastrointestinal tract commonly contain anaerobes.

Incision and drainage is sufficient alone in most cases, regardless of the causative organism (Macfie & Harvey, 1977). Antibiotics are only necessary with lesions with surrounding cellulitis, multiple and recurrent lesions, lesions not responding to local care, severe systemic manifestations such as high fever, immunocompromised patients, in patients with abscesses of the central face, and in those with abscesses containing gas or that involve muscle or fascia.

STAPHYLOCOCCAL SCALDED SKIN SYNDROME

Staphylococcal scalded skin syndrome (SSSS), also known as Ritter's disease, begins abruptly with fever, skin tenderness, and erythema especially involving the face, axilla, neck, and groin. The erythema evolves to generalized sloughing in hours to days, resembling scalding (**18, 19**). The palms, soles, and mucous membranes are spared. Gentle lateral pressure causes shearing off of the superficial epidermis (Nikolsky's sign). The sloughing is due to an exfoliative exotoxin produced by group II *Staphylococcus aureus*, most commonly phage type 71. The toxin is renally excreted and this may be why infants (who naturally have immature kidneys), and adults with chronic renal insufficiency are most commonly affected. The exfoliative toxin acts at the granular layer of the epidermis. Identification of this cleavage plane on frozen section differentiates SSSS from toxic epidermal necrolysis where the split is at the dermal–epidermal junction. Unlike bullous impetigo, Gram-positive cocci are cultured only at the site of colonization, typically the conjunctiva, nasopharynx, feces, or pyogenic foci of the skin, not in areas of epidermolysis.

The treatment of choice is a penicillinase-resistant penicillin, such as dicloxacillin or a cephalosporin, in addition to supportive measures. The prognosis is good in children; however, the mortality rate in adults can reach 60% (Ladhani, 2001).

Bacterial Infections

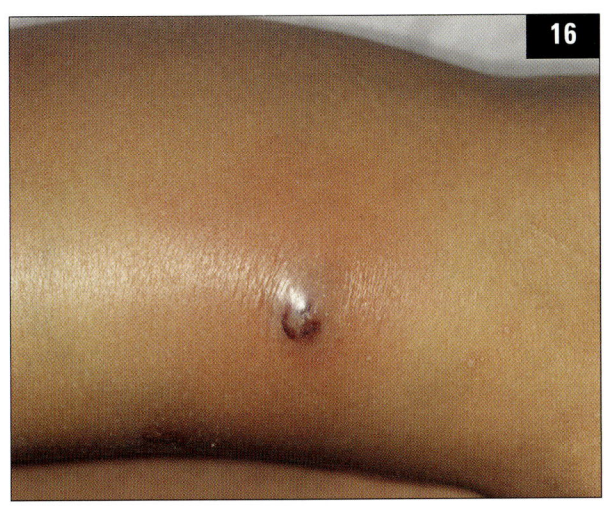

16 MRSA infections often begin as a furuncle with pain out of proportion to physical findings. MRSA infections typically evolve rapidly from furuncles to fluctuant abscesses.

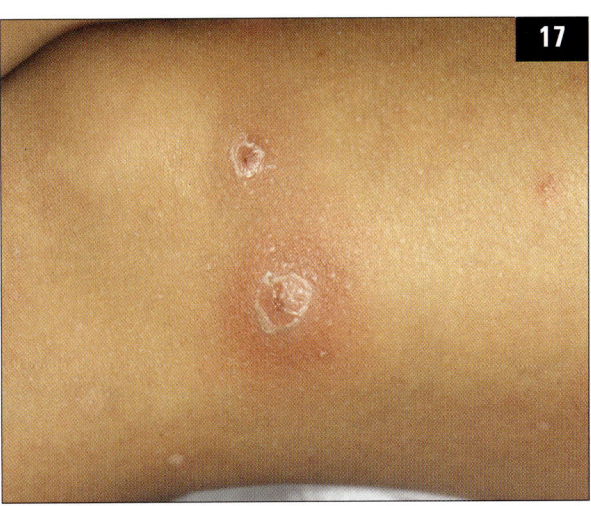

17 Abscesses will feel fluctuant and often extend much deeper than what is apparent on the surface.

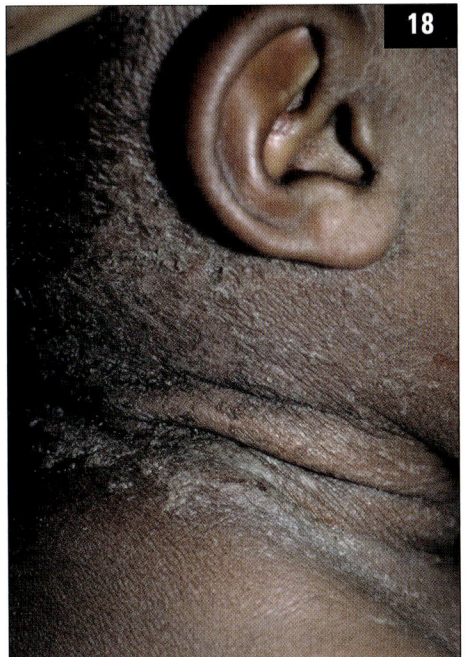

18 Staphylococcal scalded skin syndrome. Desquamation commonly begins on the neck and other intertriginous sites.

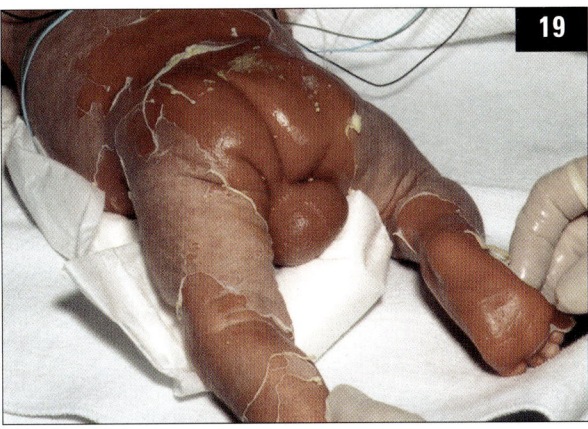

19 Staphylococcal scalded skin syndrome. Erythema and generalized sloughing resembling scalding gives the syndrome its name.

SCARLET FEVER

Scarlet fever (20, 21) is due to infection with an erythrogenic exotoxin-producing group A beta-hemolytic streptococcus (*Streptococcus pyogenes*). The condition is typically seen in children shortly after the onset of streptococcal pharyngitis but rarely occurs after streptococcal wound infection. The erythematous rash appears on the neck and trunk with extension to the extremities. A papular component can give the skin a sandpaper feel. Facial flushing with perioral pallor is often seen. The tongue becomes red with swollen papillae giving the so-called strawberry tongue appearance (20). Pastia's lines are linear petechial streaks in the antecubital, inguinal, and axillary folds (21). After 7–10 days desquamation, especially of the palms and soles, occurs as the eruption fades. In some cases, the exanthem and primary site of infection go unnoticed and the palmoplantar exfoliation may be the first and only sign. Throat culture or, rarely, culture of a surgical wound or burn will recover the organism. An elevated antistreptolysin O titer may provide evidence of recent infection.

As with other Group A streptococcal infections, penicillin, erythromycin, and dicloxacillin are curative and the prognosis is excellent. Rare complications include otitis, mastoiditis, sinusitis, pneumonia, myocarditis, meningitis, arthritis, hepatitis, acute glomerulonephritis, and rheumatic fever.

ERYSIPELAS

Unlike cellulitis, which involves the deep dermis and subcutaneous tissue, erysipelas (22–25) is a streptococcal infection that primarily involves the superficial dermis and lymphatics. The well demarcated edge and elevation of the involved area above the surrounding skin distinguish erysipelas from other cutaneous infections. The lesions are characterized by fiery red, warm, tender, indurated plaques with progressive spread. Vesicles or bullae occur in some cases. Historically the face is involved, but currently the lower extremities are more commonly affected. Hours to days before the plaque develops, there is a prodrome of fever, chills, malaise, and nausea. Infants, the elderly, and those with lymphedema or chronic cutaneous ulcers are most commonly affected.

The diagnosis can be made clinically in most cases, but serologic testing for antistreptolysin (ASO), streptozyme, specific IgG, and anti-DNAase titers may be used for confirmation (Akesson *et al.*, 2006). There is an elevated leukocyte count with a left shift. Gram stain and culture of tissue are generally not helpful.

Penicillin, given orally or parenterally depending on the clinical severity, is the treatment of choice. Third-generation cephalosporins, clindamycin, and macrolides are options for penicillin-allergic patients.

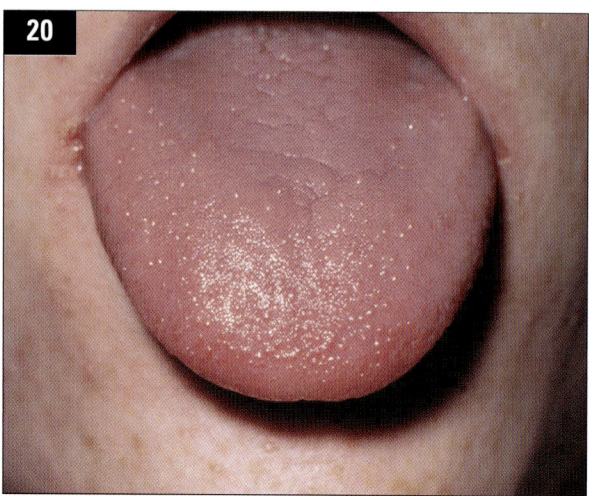

20 Tongue in scarlet fever. The prominent papillae contribute to the 'strawberry tongue' appearance.

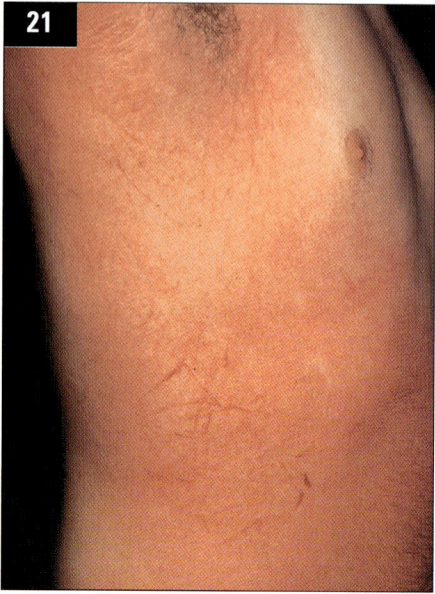

21 Linear petechial streaks known as Pastia's lines of scarlet fever.

Bacterial Infections

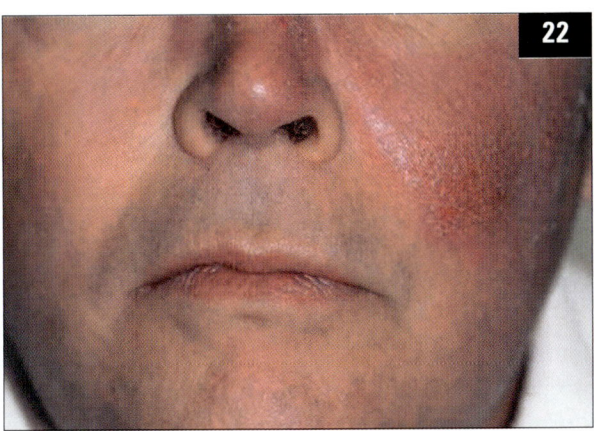

22 Early well demarcated red, indurated plaque of erysipelas.

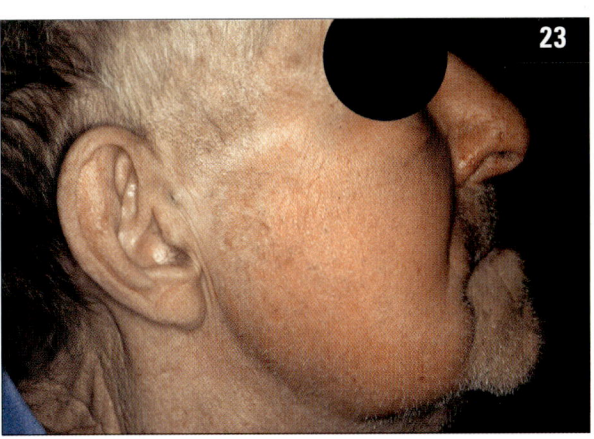

23 Erysipelas. Fully evolved well demarcated red, indurated plaque.

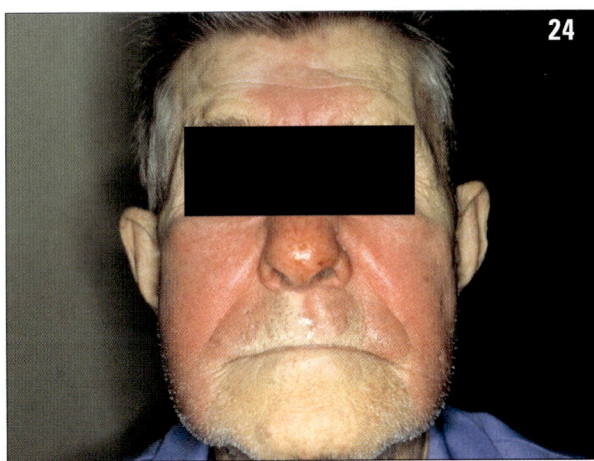

24 Erysipelas. Note the sharp demarcation at the philtrum.

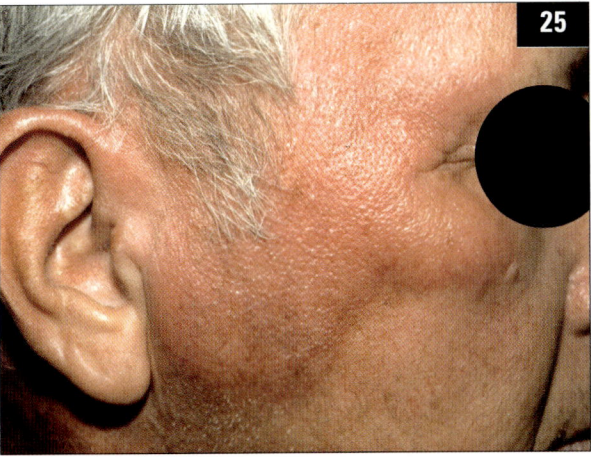

25 Erysipelas. Characteristic 'cliff-drop' border on the cheek.

CELLULITIS

Cellulitis (26–30) presents with rapidly spreading areas of pain, erythema, edema, and warmth. The erythema is not as well defined as in erysipelas, but the cause is generally *Streptococcus pyogenes*. Vesicles, bullae, abscesses, hemorrhage, and necrosis may form on the plaque in severe cases. Streaks of lymphangitis may extend from the area to the draining lymph nodes. Malaise, fever, and chills can develop before the cellulitis. The head and neck are most commonly affected in children. The lower extremity is a common site in adults and the portal of entry may be a clinically unapparent crack on the foot or between the toes due to tinea pedis. The upper extremity is typically involved in IV drug abusers and follows axillary node dissection in patients with breast cancer (Simon & Cody, 1992). Surgical or traumatic wounds, IV catheters, orthopedic pins, and pre-existing dermatitis can be portals of entry. Predisposing factors include peripheral vascular disease, diabetes, alcoholism, malignancy, IV drug abuse, chronic lymphedema, prior episodes of cellulitis, immunosuppression, and malnutrition.

Haemophilus influenzae cellulitis has a distinct blue-red color and occurs in children under 5 years of age. It typically occurs on the face following an upper respiratory tract infection but is rarely seen in countries with vaccinations.

The white blood cell count is usually normal or only slightly elevated in streptococcal cellulitis and

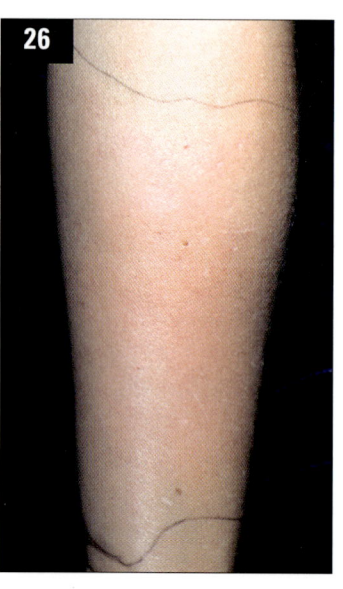

26 Cellulitis. In contrast to erysipelas, the erythema gradually fades into the surrounding skin.

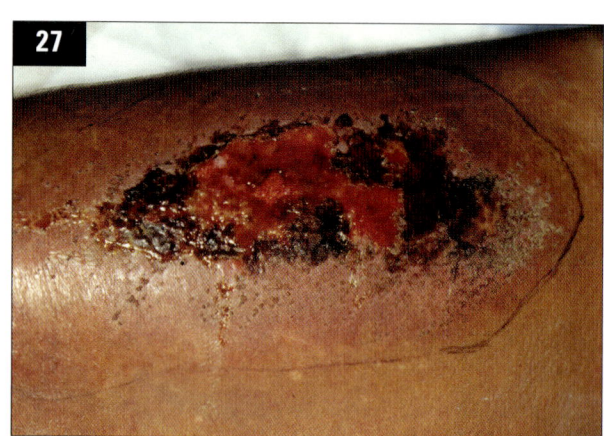

27 Cellulitis extending from the area of an abrasion.

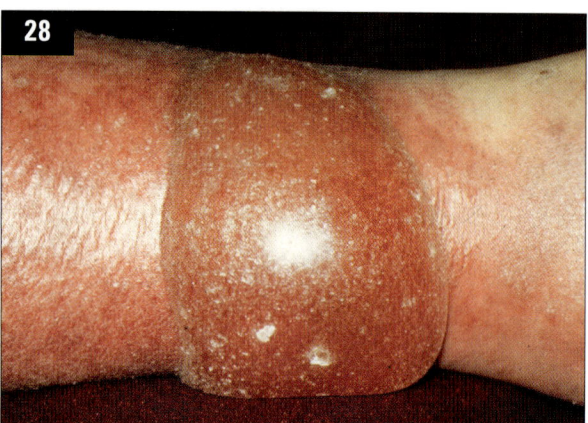

28 Bullae are common in severe cellulitis.

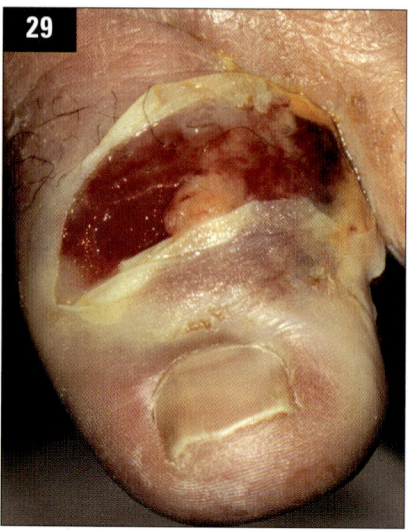

29 Cellulitis with surrounding necrosis. The underlying joint space was involved.

blood cultures are nearly always negative. *H. influenzae* cellulitis in pediatric patients is an exception: the white blood cell count is greater than 15,000 (Fleisher *et al.*, 1983) and blood cultures are positive in more than two-thirds of cases (Meislin, 1986). Aspiration or punch biopsy for culture is of limited use. The yield is positive in less than one-third of cases (Sigurdsson & Gudmundsson, 1989). Cultures from areas of abscess or bullae have a high yield and may be helpful if present.

For most forms of cellulitis, empiric therapy should cover both staphylococci and streptococci. Penicillinase-resistant penicillins and first-generation or extended-spectrum cephalosporins are reasonable choices. Mild cases require 5–10 days of oral antibiotic. Intravenous antibiotics are reserved for facial cellulitis and the seriously ill. Cefotaxime or ceftriazone provide coverage for *H. influenzae*. If there is a lack of response, resistant strains should be considered. Recurrent cellulitis may require long-term antibiotics and skin care to avoid entry portals such as tinea pedis and stasis dermatitis.

NECROTIZING FASCIITIS

Necrotizing fasciitis (31–33), is a deep, rapidly progressing infection involving the subcutaneous tissue and fascia, generally due to streptococci. The majority of cases occur on the lower extremities following surgery, perforating trauma, minor skin abrasions, or bites. There is often a predisposing

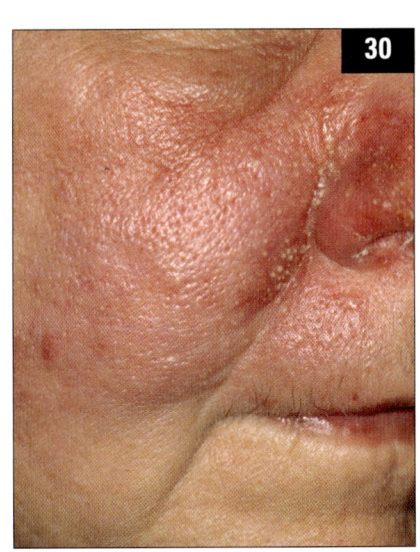

30 Facial cellulitis. The nasal crusting and small pustules are features of staphylococcal cellulitis.

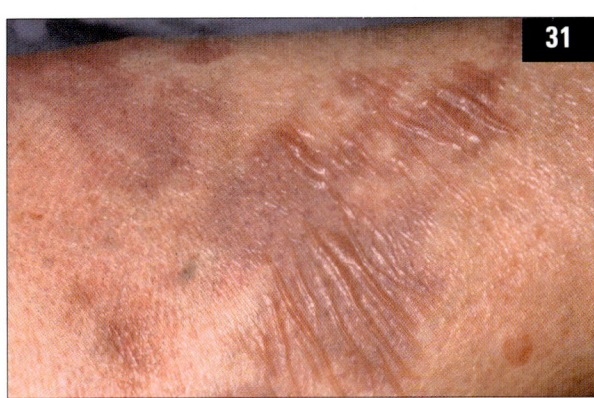

31 Necrotizing fasciitis with overlying skin necrosis.

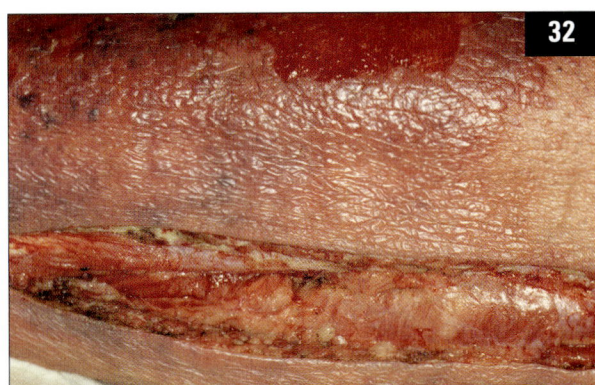

32 Necrotizing fasciitis. A foul odor is present when the tissue is incised. The depth and extent of necrosis are typically not evident on initial physical examination.

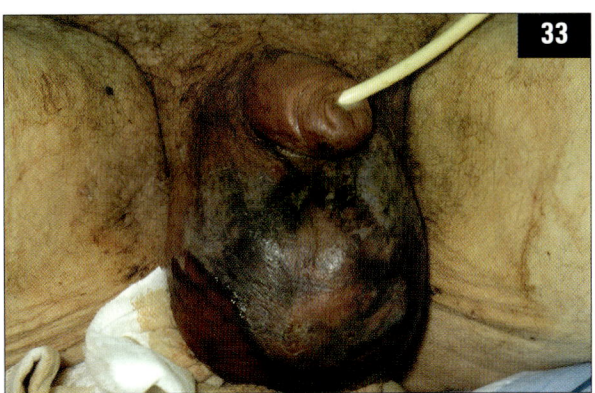

33 Scrotal necrosis in Fournier's gangrene.

condition, such as diabetes, atherosclerosis, or venous insufficiency. The disease progresses rapidly with a change from erythema, pain, and edema to a central dusky violaceous discoloration with cutaneous anesthesia and hemorrhagic blisters by 36 hours from onset.

Features that distinguish necrotizing fasciitis from cellulitis include severe constant pain, necrosis, crepitus, edema extending beyond the erythema, cutaneous anesthesia, rapid spread despite antibiotics, woody hard feel, and systemic toxicity, manifested by fever, leukocytosis, change in mental status, and renal failure.

Fournier's gangrene is considered a form of necrotizing fasciitis, as it spreads along fascial planes. However, this variant is localized to the scrotum and perineal area. Infection can spread anteriorly up the abdominal wall. Most patients have predisposing trauma which may be peri-anal suppuration, local trauma, or recent perineal surgery. A discernible cause may not be identified in some. Diabetes is a comorbid factor in the great majority.

Imaging studies may be valuable in evaluating the extent of disease. Computed tomography (CT) scan or magnetic resonance imaging (MRI) may show edema extending along fascial planes, but the most important diagnostic test is the appearance of the subcutaneous tissue and fascia during surgical exploration. Gram stain and both aerobic and anaerobic cultures should be taken from deep tissue at the time of emergent surgical debridement. The bacteriology of the surface wound or ulcer (if present) may not be indicative of that in the deep infection.

Although the condition is typically caused by *Streptococcus pyogenes*, it may be polymicrobial or caused by *S. aureus*, *Vibrio vulnificus*, *Aeromonous hydrophila*, or anaerobic streptococci such as *Peptostreptococcus*. Community-acquired MRSA strains have also been implicated. Polymicrobial cases typically originate from bowel flora (involving mixed aerobic and anaerobic flora) in the setting of penetrating surgery involving the bowel and peri-anal abscesses or decubitus ulcers.

Urgent surgical debridement is essential in conjunction with parenteral antibiotics, empirically covering aerobes and anaerobes, and supportive care. The mortality rate ranges from 20% to 40% (Byrnes, 2006; Golger *et al.*, 2007).

PERI-ANAL STREPTOCOCCAL DISEASE

Peri-anal streptococcal disease (34, 35) predominantly affects children under the age of 8 years with rare exceptions in adulthood. Fecal hoarding behavior can occur from painful defecation. Pruritus and blood-streaked stool are also reported. Although sometimes referred to as peri-anal cellulitis, peri-anal streptococcal disease may present as a dermatitis with well demarcated erythema that mimics seborrheic dermatitis, psoriasis, and candidiasis.

Oral penicillin or erythromycin for 14–21 days until clinical and microbiological cure are obtained is recommended. Topical antibiotics may be adjunctive. Urinalysis should be monitored for post-streptococcal glomerulonephritis.

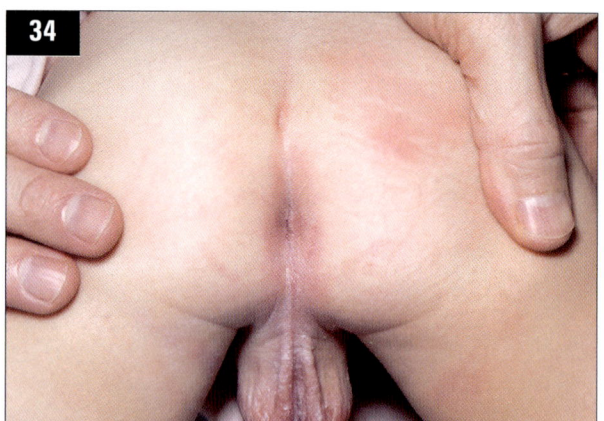

34 Peri-anal streptococcal disease. The skin may be brightly erythematous, or symptoms may be prominent and out of proportion to the degree of erythema.

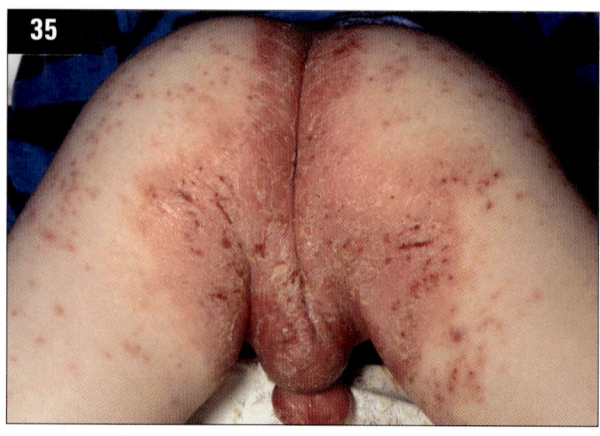

35 Peri-anal streptococcal disease may accompany eczematous changes.

CUTANEOUS ANTHRAX

Three forms of anthrax occur: cutaneous (36), which accounts for 95% of cases worldwide and nearly all United States cases, inhalational, and gastrointestinal (Friedlander, 1999). *Bacillus anthracis*, the causative organism, is a large, aerobic, spore-forming, Gram-positive rod. Humans can acquire the disease if they are exposed to infected animals or handle their infected hides or other animal products (woolsorter's disease). Bioterrorism has led to renewed interest in this condition.

One to 12 days after exposure, pruritus begins at the entry site, followed by a papule, development of superimposed vesicles and, finally a painless ulcer with a black eschar that separates in 12–14 days. The absence of pain is of diagnostic importance. Mild to moderate fever, headache, and malaise often accompany the infection. Suppurative regional adenopathy is common. In severe cases, extensive edema and necrosis develop with high temperatures and potential death.

The vesicle fluid or ulcer base, which may require unroofing of the eschar, can be cultured. Histology (with tissue Gram stain and possible polymerase chain reaction [PCR]) of a biopsy specimen, direct fluid antibody test or enzyme-linked immunosorbent assay (ELISA) of serum, can help make the diagnosis. The treatment of choice is ciprofloxacin or doxycycline (Wenner & Kenner, 2004). A vaccine exists that is used in the military and for workers at a high risk of infection.

PITTED KERATOLYSIS

Pitted keratolysis (37) is characterized by shallow pits on the weight-bearing plantar surface and, rarely, the palms. The pits may become confluent and result in erosions. Odor is the most common complaint; however, soreness and itching uncommonly occur. Hyperhidrosis and occlusive footwear predispose to pitted keratolysis. Proteases from a bacterial proliferation destroy the stratum corneum and cause the pits. *Micrococcus sedentarius* (renamed *Kytococcus sedentarius*), *Dermatophilus congolensis*, species of *Corynebacterium*, and species of *Actinomyces* have been identified etiologies (Nordstrom *et al.*, 1987; Longshaw *et al.*, 2002).

Reducing the predisposing hyperhidrosis with frequent sock changes and 25% aluminum chloride is helpful. Topical clindamycin or erythromycin is effective. Topical mupirocin, benzoyl peroxide, miconazole, and clotrimazole have also been used. Oral erythromycin is another option.

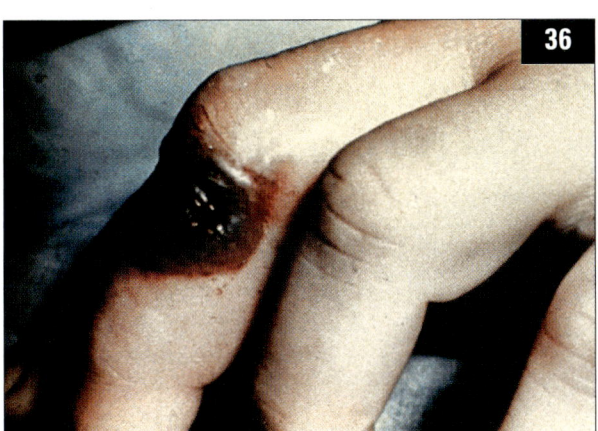

36 Painless black eschar of cutaneous anthrax.

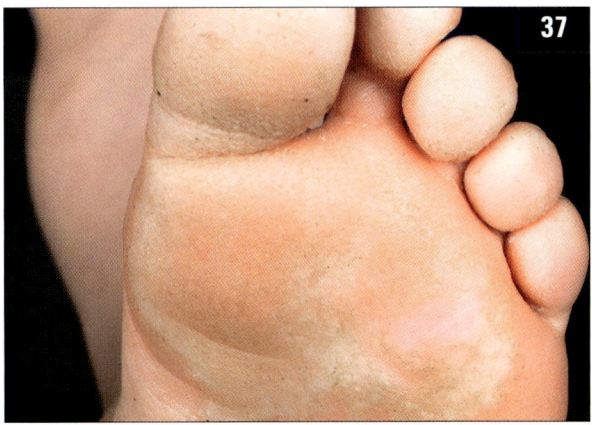

37 Malodorous shallow pits on the weight-bearing plantar surface characterize pitted keratolysis.

TRICHOMYCOSIS AXILLARIS

Trichomycosis axillaris (38) is a superficial bacterial infection of the axillary hair, and to a lesser extent, pubic hair (trichomycosis pubis) caused by several species of the Gram-positive diphtheroid *Corynebacterium*. The hair shafts develop firmly adherent yellow, red, or black nodules or sheaths. Occasionally, the disorder may result in stained clothing and patients may complain of malodorous sweat. Diagnosis is clinical, based on identification of the hair shaft nodules. Gram stain of these concretions reveals the coryneform morphology, which can be distinguished from the fungal organisms of piedra. Hair casts are easily distinguished by their mobility along the hair shaft.

Shaving is the quickest cure. Bathing with antibacterial soaps or benzoyl peroxide aids in treatment and inhibits future infection. Oral erythromycin, bacitracin ointment, and clindamycin lotion or gel are also effective. Antiperspirant reduces the predisposing axillary hyperhidrosis.

ERYTHRASMA

Erythrasma (39, 40) is caused by *Corynebacterium minutissimum*, a lipophilic, Gram-positive, diphtheroid. It typically presents as a well demarcated, brown–red macular patch with fine scale. It is commonly asymptomatic, but can be pruritic. This superficial infection commonly is located in the occluded intertriginous areas such as the axilla, submammary area, intergluteal fold, over the inner thighs, crural region, and the interdigital spaces of the toes. The web space between the fourth and fifth toes is the most common and presents with chronic maceration and fissuring. Predisposing factors include a warm, humid environment, hyperhidrosis, obesity, and diabetes.

The differential diagnosis includes psoriasis, dermatophytosis, candidiasis, and intertrigo, and methods for differentiating include mycologic examination and Wood's light examination. The lesions of erythrasma fluoresce coral-red with Wood's light due to porphyrin produced by the bacteria. However, recent bathing may result in a false negative result.

Oral erythromycin 250 mg four times a day or 500 mg twice a day for 7–14 days is the treatment of choice. A one-time oral dose of 1 g of clarithromycin has been reported. Topical clindamycin, erythromycin, Whitfield's ointment (benzoic acid 6%, salicylic acid 3%), fusidic acid cream, miconazole cream, and antibacterial soaps may be required for treatment and can be used prophylactically once the infection has cleared (Holdiness, 2002). Erythrasma tends to recur if the predisposing factors are not eliminated and the area kept dry. Concurrent dermatophyte or *Candida albicans* infection should also be treated with antifungal agents. Diabetes should be suspected in recurrent or extensive erythrasma.

ECTHYMA

Ecthyma (41–43) presents with a thick oyster shell-like crust and an underlying ulcer. It may be caused by *Streptococcus pyogenes* or *Staphylococcus aureus*. Treatment requires removal of the crust together with topical or oral antimicrobial therapy. Topical mupirocin or retapamulin, and beta-lactam drugs are commonly used.

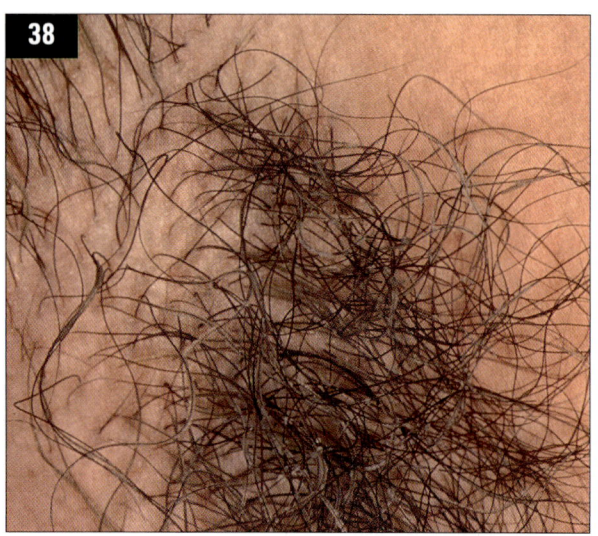

38 Adherent yellow concretions on hair shafts in trichomycosis axillaris.

Bacterial Infections

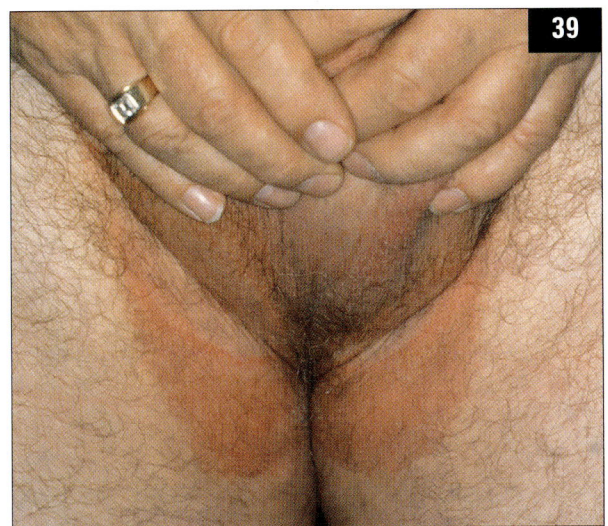

39 Well demarcated brown-red macular patch with minimal scale characterize erythrasma.

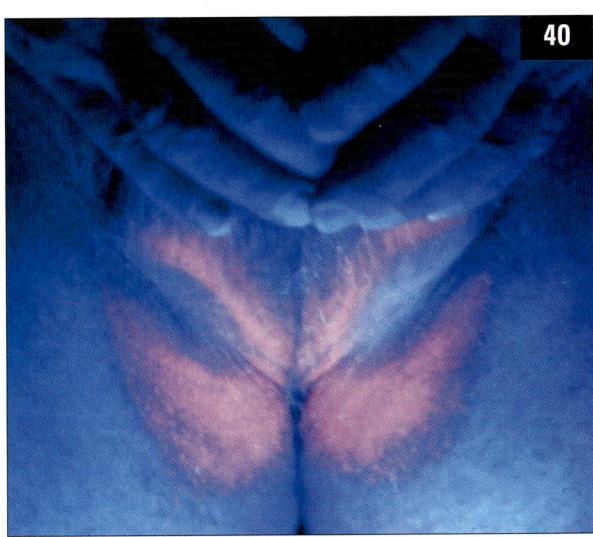

40 Coral-red fluorescence of erythrasma under Wood's light due to porphyrins produced by the bacteria.

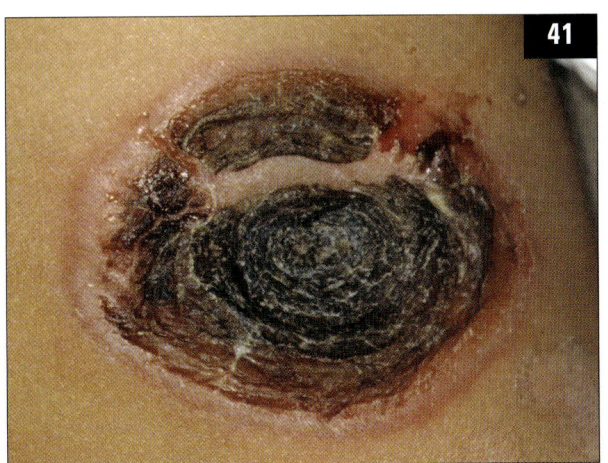

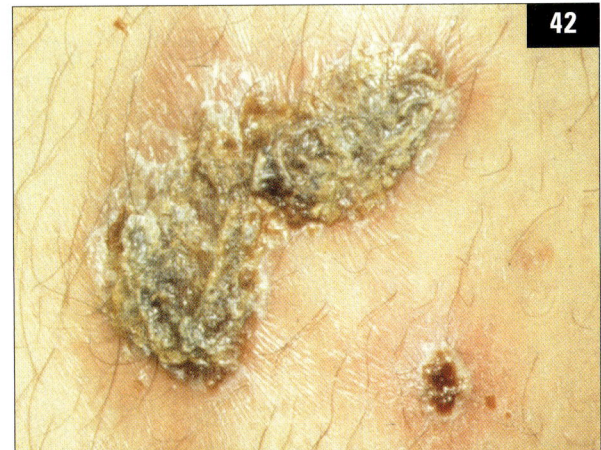

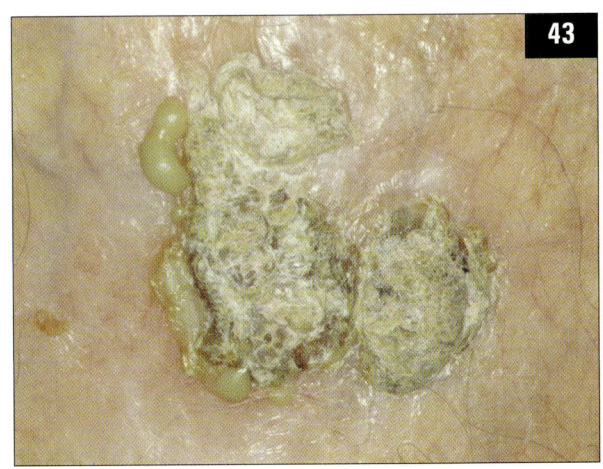

41 Streptococcal ecthyma. The thick crust forms a hard shell over a cutaneous ulcer.

42 Streptococcal ecthyma. Thick 'oyster shell' crust and surrounding erythema.

43 Staphylococcal ecthyma with characteristic gold pus.

ECTHYMA GANGRENOSUM

Ecthyma gangrenosum (44–46) is generally a sign of *Pseudomonas aeruginosa* septicemia. Predisposing causes include neutropenia, hematologic malignancies, immunodeficiency syndromes, chemotherapy, burns, or indwelling catheters. Occasionally, identical lesions can present as a localized cutaneous infection, not accompanied by systemic infection. Erythematous or purpuric macules, most in the anogenital region or on the extremity, develop into a hemorrhagic bullae which rupture and become ulcers with eschar. Skin biopsy and tissue or exudate culture for bacteria, fungus, yeast, and mycobacteria should be performed at the first clinical suspicion of ecthyma gangrenosum. As this is usually a manifestation of sepsis, blood culture will be positive in most cases.

Although ecthyma gangrenosum is most commonly associated with *Pseudomonas* infection, similar lesions have been observed in patients with other bacterial and fungal infections including *Escherichia coli*, *Aeromonas hydrophila*, *Staphylococcus aureus*, *Serratia marcescens*, *Neisseria meningitidis*, *Candida*, *Fusarium*, and *Aspergillus* species (Gucluer et al., 1999).

Immediate empiric institution of an IV aminoglycoside (gentamicin) and an antipseudomonal penicillin (piperacillin) is appropriate while the causative agent is being established. Treatment should be adjusted according to sensitivities and results of culture when they become available. There is a high mortality rate with delayed diagnosis and therapy. In the absence of bacteremia, prognosis is more favorable.

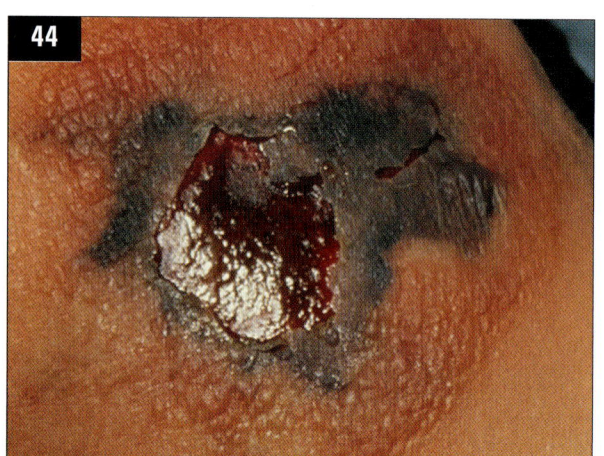

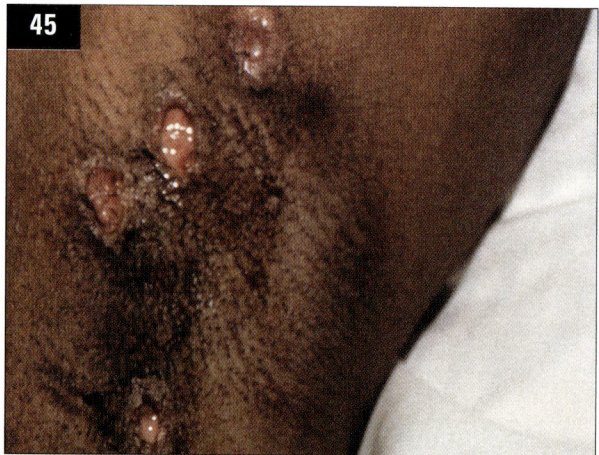

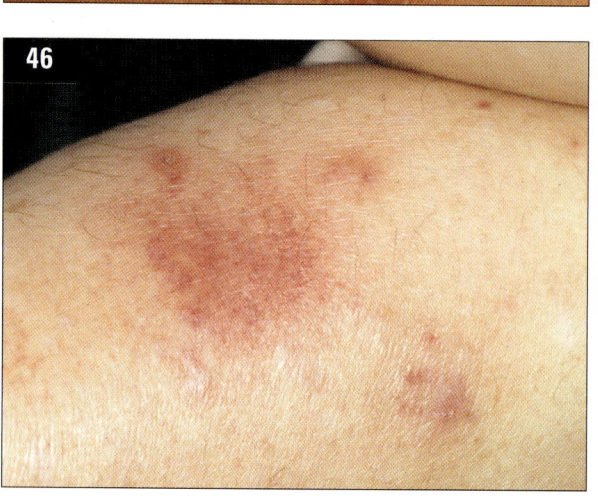

44 Ecthyma gangrenosum. Note the erythematous rim and violaceous necrotic center.

45 Ecthyma gangrenosum. A Gram stain from the undermined edge of the ulcer will demonstrate sheets of Gram negative rods.

46 Ecthyma gangrenosum in a patient who developed pseudomonas sepsis after using contaminated eyedrops.

MENINGOCOCCEMIA

Meningococcemia (47, 48) is an acute or chronic disease caused by the Gram-negative diplococcus *Neisseria meningitidis*. It most commonly affects children and young adults. Patients with asplenia, immunoglobulin deficiencies, or deficiencies of the terminal complement components are at increased risk. Acute meningococcemia presents with fever, chills, hypotension, and meningitis. Approximately half of patients develop a petechial eruption, most evident on the trunk and lower extremities, that may progress to ecchymoses, bullae, and necrosis. Acral petechiae are common. Gray infarctive lesions with an erythematous rim are characteristic. Rarely, infection is chronic with recurrent episodes of fever, headache, arthralgias, and erythematous macules that may evolve to central hemorrhage.

Cultures of blood, cerebrospinal fluid, and skin lesions are often positive in acute meningococcemia. However, due to the rapid progression, the initial diagnosis often must be clinical. Chronic disease is diagnosed through blood culture during a febrile episode. Skin lesions of chronic disease typically fail to reveal bacteria. The only known reservoir is the human nasopharynx. Transmission is by the respiratory route.

Acute infection is rapidly progressive and can be fatal if antibiotics are not instituted emergently (Ramos-e-Silva & Pereira, 2005). Intravenous penicillin is the treatment of choice for acute disease. Chloramphenicol is the alternative for penicillin-allergic patients. A third-generation cephalosporin should be considered in areas of penicillin resistance. Chronic meningococcemia is treated with similar antibiotics. Household members, exposed hospital personnel, and day-care or close school contacts should receive prophylactic therapy with rifampin. A vaccine for the most common serogroups is available and is recommended for high-risk groups, such as college students and military recruits.

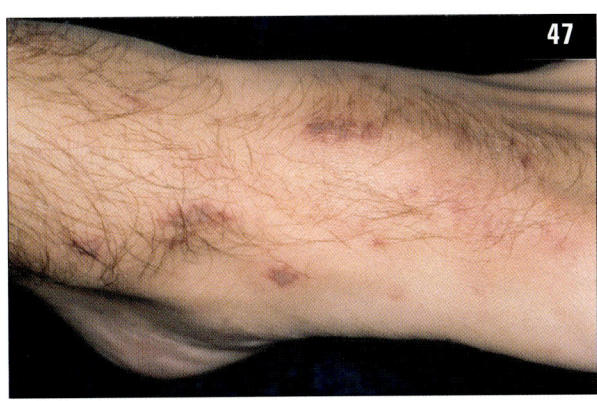

47 Meningococcemia. Note the characteristic stellate lesions with a gun metal gray interior.

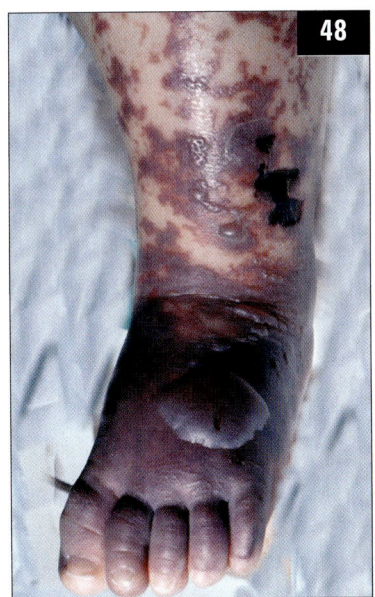

48 Meningococcemia. Acral purpura, bullae, and necrosis suggest ensuing purpura fulminans.

CAT-SCRATCH DISEASE

Cat-scratch disease (49), caused by the Gram-negative bacillus *Bartonella henselae*, is the most frequent cause of chronic lymphadenopathy in children and young adults. Tender lymphadenopathy develops 2–4 weeks after a cat scratch or bite and can last from 2 to 5 months. Adenopathy is regional and typically involves the axilla. Suppuration occurs in less than one-quarter of cases. A papule or pustule is present 3–5 days after a cat scratch or bite in two-thirds of patients. This usually heals within a few weeks without lymphangitis. Rarely, fever, malaise, fatigue, and headache occur. Culture confirmation of infection is difficult because organisms infrequently grow from pus or nodal tissue. Serological testing supports the diagnosis; however, there is cross-reactivity with *B. quintana* and testing may be negative early in the disease. Routine histology and special stains (Warthin–Starry) of the skin or node, in conjunction with the clinical history, support the diagnosis.

This is a spontaneously resolving disorder and use of antibiotics has had variable and less than dramatic results. Some advocate the use of trimethoprim-sulfamethoxazole, ciprofloxacin, or azithromycin (Windsor, 2001).

CHANCROID

Chancroid (50, 51) is a sexually transmitted disease caused by the Gram-negative bacillus *Haemophilus ducreyi*. It generally begins as an inflammatory macule or pustule on the genitalia, 1–5 days after sexual exposure. The pustule ruptures with formation of a punched-out, tender ulceration with a purulent base. Autoinoculation often results in kissing lesions. Painful, usually unilateral, inguinal lymphadenopathy or bubo formation is present in half of patients. These may rupture after becoming an abscess. Subsequent scarring can be a permanent complication. Definitive diagnosis requires identification by culture. However, culture is unreliable and insensitive. Specimens for culture should be taken from the ulcer base or active border and inoculated in the clinic on special media. If cultures are going to be positive, they usually grow organisms within 3 days. Interpretation of Gram stain of smears from the ulcer base can be complicated by polymicrobial contamination. The characteristic parallel rods have been described as 'schools of fish'. PCR is sensitive but is not, however, usually performed on site, causing a delay in diagnosis. A probable diagnosis is made if the patient has one or more painful ulcers with painful adenopathy and no evidence of syphilis (darkfield examination of ulcer exudate) or herpes simplex virus. Serologic testing for other coincident sexually transmitted diseases, such as syphilis and human immunodeficiency virus (HIV), should be performed. Chancroid is rare in the United States. It is more common in areas of low socioeconomic status such as Africa, Asia, and the Caribbean.

The treatment of choice is azithromycin, which can be given in a single oral dose. Erythromycin, ceftriaxone, and ciprofloxacin are also acceptable alternatives. Aspiration of fluctuant buboes may be required.

GRANULOMA INGUINALE (DONOVANOSIS)

Granuloma inguinale (GI) is a sexually transmitted disease caused by *Calymmatobacterium granulomatis*, a Gram-negative pleomorphic bacillus. It has an incubation period that ranges from 1 week to 3 months. Soft, red nodules arise at the site of inoculation and eventually ulcerate. These ulcers are painless with raised rolled margins and hypertrophic granulation tissue that is beefy red and friable (52–54). Autoinoculation is a common feature, resulting in lesions on adjacent skin. In men, the lesions are most common on the prepuce or glans, and in women, on the labia. Lymphadenopathy does not occur unless there is a secondary bacterial infection. Although culture of the organism has been reported, it is extremely fastidious and is beyond the capability of most laboratories. The most effective method of establishing a diagnosis is visualization of the organisms within the macrophages as bipolar staining, safety pin-shaped intracytoplasmic inclusions, known as Donovan bodies. Wright–Giemsa or Warthin–Starry stained tissue smears or biopsy specimens demonstrate the Donovan bodies. It should not be overlooked that other venereal disease often co-exist with GI. Testing for other sexually transmitted diseases, including HIV, is warranted. GI is endemic in Western New Guinea, the Caribbean, Southern India, South Africa, southeast Asia, Australia, and Brazil. In the United States, most cases are thought to be due to foreign travel.

Trimethoprim–sulfamethoxazole or doxycycline is the recommended treatment. Alternatives include ciprofloxacin, erythromycin, or azithromycin. If there is no response, gentamicin may be added. Untreated, the lesions may continue to expand for years. Systemic spread to internal organs occasionally occurs and may be fatal. Squamous cell carcinoma infrequently arises within the lesions. Once the lesions have healed, extensive scarring may lead to deformity, functional disability, and possible elephantiasis of the genitalia due to secondary lymphatic obstruction.

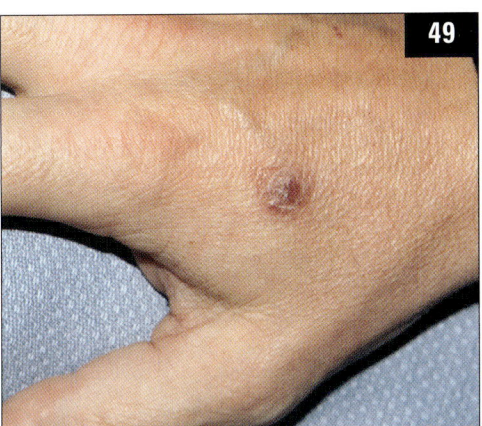

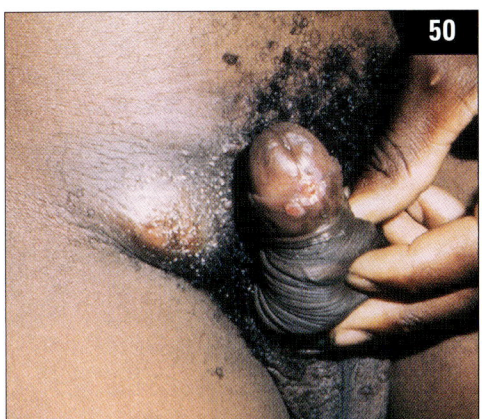

49 Papule at site of cat induced trauma, typically followed by tender lymphadenopathy in cat-scratch disease.

50 Painful ulcerations and lymphadenopathy of chancroid.

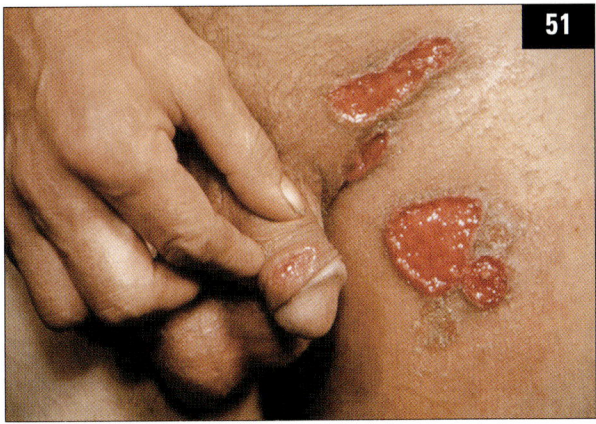

51 Autoinoculation resulting in tender punched-out 'kissing' ulcers in chancroid.

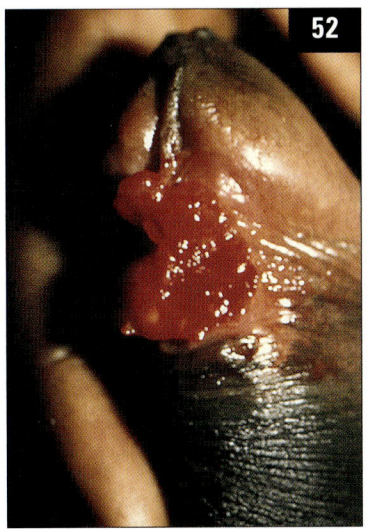

52 Beefy red and friable granulation tissue of granuloma inguinale.

53 Painless ulcer of granuloma inguinale.

54 Granuloma inguinale. Multiple ulcers are progressive and lead to tissue edema and deformity.

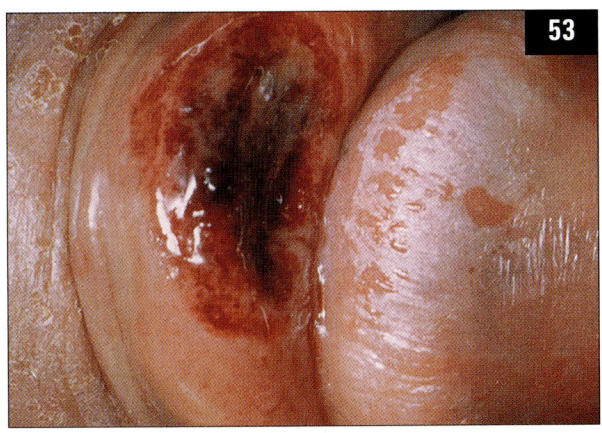

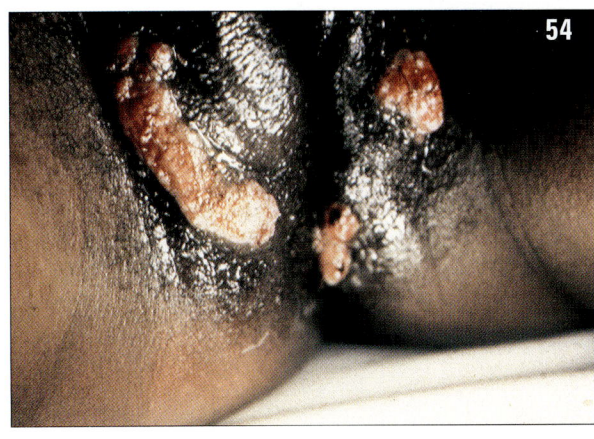

GONORRHEA

Gonorrhea (55–58) is caused by the Gram-negative, diplococcus, *Neisseria gonorrhoeae*. This sexually transmitted disease may present as an acute purulent urethritis or may produce asymptomatic infection. Disseminated infection is a complication of approximately 2% of mucosal infection (Anan & Culik, 1989). By the time disseminated disease is present, the primary site of mucosal infection may be normal in appearance. Women are predominantly affected with dissemination especially during pregnancy or menstruation. Disseminated gonococcemia is characterized by rash, fever, arthralgia, and arthritis. Infection may lead to meningitis or endocarditis. Skin lesions occur in crops, typically on acral sites, as small erythematous macules that evolve into vesiculopustules on a deeply erythematous or hemorrhagic base, or into purpuric macules. They heal in a few days and may leave small superficial scars. Skin lesions are usually in different stages of development at the time of clinical presentation. The skin lesions can be identical to those seen in meningococcemia, bacterial endocarditis, and rickettsial disease. Most patients have migratory polyarthralgia. Less often, purulent arthritis may affect a single joint, usually the knee. Tenosynovitis also is common, especially of the small joints of the hands.

By the time of dissemination, there may be no signs or symptoms at the primary site of mucosal infection. However, Gram stains and cultures of genital, rectal, conjunctival, and pharyngeal secretions should be obtained, even if the patient has no localized symptoms at any of those sites. Organisms are only rarely cultured from the skin lesions. Repeat Gram stain and culture of blood and aspirated fluid from affected joints is required. Cerebrospinal fluid should be stained and cultured if signs or symptoms of meningitis are present. Culture requires special growth conditions and enriched media. Other methods include immunologic and molecular biological techniques but these are not universally available. Testing for chlamydia, HIV, and syphilis should be considered.

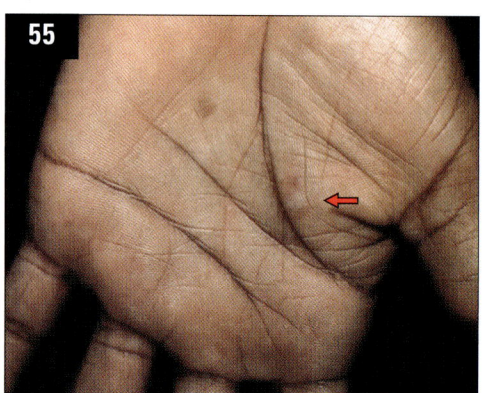

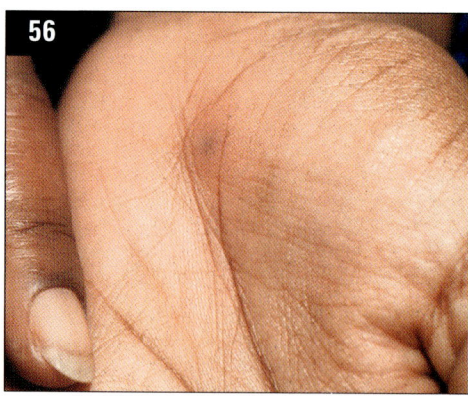

55 Acute pustule on a hemorrhagic base in disseminated gonococcemia.

56 Purpuric macules in disseminated gonococcemia.

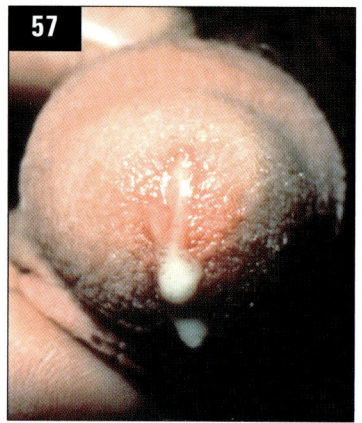

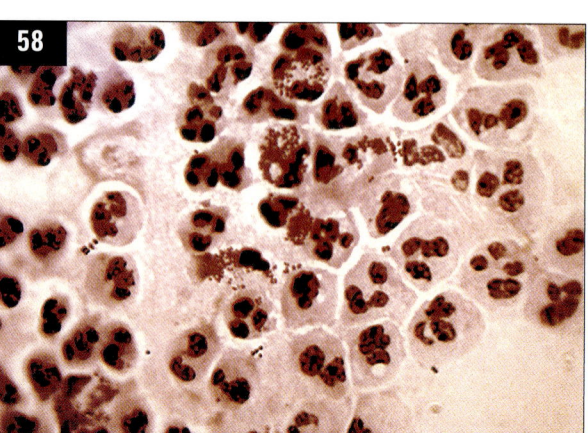

57 Acute purulent urethritis of gonorrhea.

58 Neutrophils and intracellular diplococci of gonorrhea.

Empiric treatment is often necessary because culture results are not available for 24–48 hours. The treatment of choice for disseminated gonococcal infection is ceftriaxone 1 g IM or IV every 24 hours with a switch to an oral equivalent, such as cefixime, ciprofloxacin, ofloxacin, or levofloxacin after improvement begins. Patients should be treated presumptively for concurrent chlamydial infection, unless appropriate testing excludes this infection (Low *et al.*, 2006).

TYPHUS

Typhus refers to a group of infectious diseases that occur when one of the *Rickettsia* bacteria is passed to a human through the bite of an arthropod vector. There are three main types of typhus: epidemic typhus, endemic or murine typhus, and scrub typhus (see below). These diseases are all somewhat similar, but with variable severity. The specific type of *Rickettsia* that causes the disease and the arthropod that transmits the bacteria vary. Typhus is a multisystem vasculitis and may cause a wide array of clinical manifestations but fever, headache, and rash are common symptoms.

Epidemic typhus is the prototypical infection of the typhus group. Epidemic typhus is caused by *R. prowazekii*. The vector is the body louse (*P. corporis*) that proliferates in the face of overcrowding with poor sanitary conditions, such as during war and natural disasters. Epidemic typhus is now found in the mountainous regions of Africa, South America, and Asia. While the louse feeds on the skin, it defecates and the organisms in the feces are scratched into the skin. Humans and flying squirrels are the animal reservoir. Fever, headache, weakness, and muscle aches abruptly occur followed in less than 1 week by a maculopapular rash. The rash starts on the trunk and axillary folds with peripheral spread. The face, palms, and soles are typically spared. The rash may become petechial and gangrene occasionally occurs. Multiorgan system involvement is possible. The central nervous and cardiovascular systems may be involved, as well as the lungs and kidneys.

Endemic (murine) typhus is caused by *R. typhi* that is transmitted to humans by the rat or cat flea (*Xenopsylla cheopis*, *Ctenocephalides felis*). Rats, mice, and cats are the natural reservoir. Murine typhus occurs in most parts of the world, particularly in subtropical and temperate coastal regions. In the United States, southern Texas and southern California have the largest number of cases. The peak incidence is in the summer and fall in urban areas. Endemic typhus (**59, 60**) causes about 12 days of high fever, with chills and headache. The skin manifestations, which occur in half of patients, are similar to those of epidemic typhus but less severe and gangrene does not occur.

Diagnosis of typhus may be confirmed using laboratory tests; however, more than 1 week may pass before patients mount a demonstrable immune response that can be measured serologically, so treatment is typically initiated on the basis of the patient's symptoms. Indirect immunofluorescence assay (IFA) or enzyme immunoassay (EIA) testing can be used to look for a rise in the antibody titers. PCR amplification of rickettsial DNA of serum or skin biopsy specimens can be used for diagnosing typhus (Rozmajzl *et al.*, 2006). The complement fixation (CF) test is a serological test that can be used to

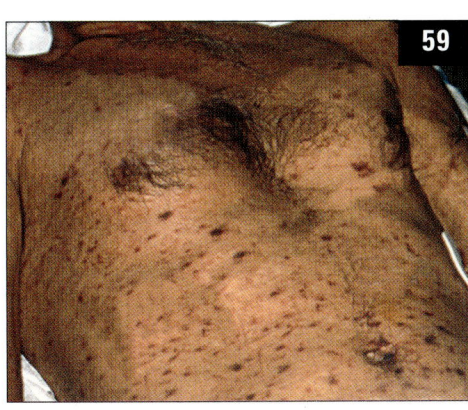

59 Endemic typhus. Multiple stellate necrotic lesions. (Courtesy of Richard DeVillez, MD.)

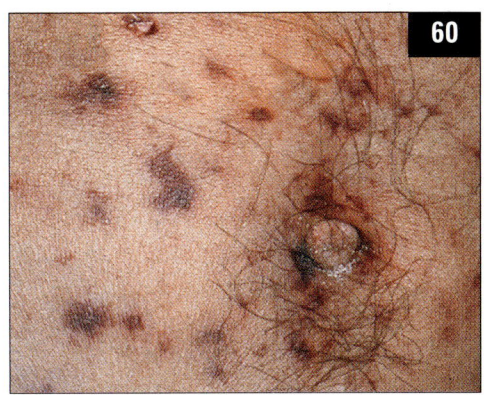

60 Endemic typhus. Stellate necrotic lesions. (Courtesy of Richard DeVillez, MD.)

demonstrate which specific rickettsial organism is causing disease by detection of specific antibodies.

Doxycycline and chloramphenicol are the antirickettsial agents of choice for treatment of typhus. Epidemic typhus has the most severe clinical presentation of the typhus group of rickettsial infections. The mortality rate is in excess of 10–15% (Raoult *et al.*, 2004). People usually recover uneventfully from endemic typhus, although the elderly and those with other medical problems may have a 1% death rate from the illness (Silpapojakul *et al.*, 1993).

SCRUB TYPHUS (TSUTSUGAMUSHI FEVER)

Scrub typhus is endemic in the Far East (Japan and southeast Asia). The trombiculid red mite larva (chigger) that infests wild rodents in low scrub vegetation transmits the causative organism, *Orientia tsutsugamushi*. An erythematous indurated papule occurs at the site of a mite bite (**61**). Vesiculation and ulceration with eschar and surrounding erythema subsequently develop. Approximately 1 week after the mite bite, fever, headache, and anorexia develop. This is followed in about one-third of patients with a self-limited erythematous macular eruption (**62**) on the trunk with peripheral extension that spares the palms and soles. Purpuric lesions are rare. Generalized adenopathy is frequent. The clinical picture varies with the virulence of the strain. Pneumonitis, myocarditis, deafness, conjunctivitis, and splenomegaly may occur. Laboratory studies of choice are serologic tests for antibodies because actual isolation and culture of rickettsiae is difficult, expensive, and dangerous. Diagnostic testing for this organism is in evolution (Blacksell *et al.*, 2007). The diagnosis may sometimes be made with indirect fluorescent antibody or indirect immunoperoxidase testing.

In patients who are not treated, the mortality rate is variable depending on the geographic area and the rickettsial strain. With proper antibiotic treatment, deaths are rare and the recovery period is short and is usually without complication. Treatment for scrub typhus is doxycycline, but chloramphenicol is also effective. Rifampin should be considered in areas with reduced susceptibilities to tetracyclines.

ROCKY MOUNTAIN SPOTTED FEVER

Rocky Mountain spotted fever (RMSF) is the most common fatal tick-borne disease in the United States. *Rickettsia rickettsii* are introduced into humans after an infected wood tick, dog tick, or Lone Star tick feeds for more than 6 hours. The tick bite is painless and frequently goes unnoticed. Small rodents are the primary reservoir. Disease onset is classically characterized by fever, myalgias, headache, and a petechial rash (**63**). North Carolina, Oklahoma, South Carolina, Tennessee, and Georgia account for the majority of cases (Chapman *et al.*, 2006a). Less than 2% of the total number of cases are found in the Rocky Mountain states. The peak incidence is between May and June.

Approximately 1 week after the tick bite, there is fever, myalgia, headache, and malaise. A few days after this prodrome, a maculopapular eruption appears on the ankles and wrists with centripetal

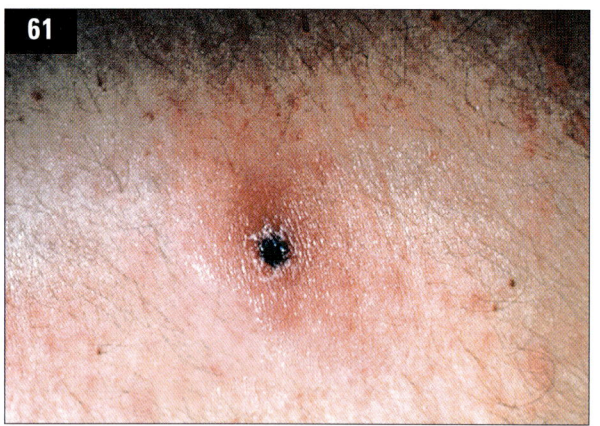

61 Eschar with surrounding erythema at the site of a mite bite in scrub typhus, caused by *Orientia tsutsugamushi*.

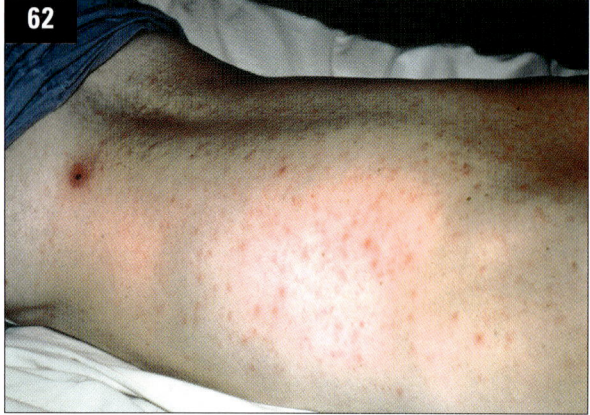

62 Erythematous macular eruption of scrub typhus. The eschar is visible on the buttock.

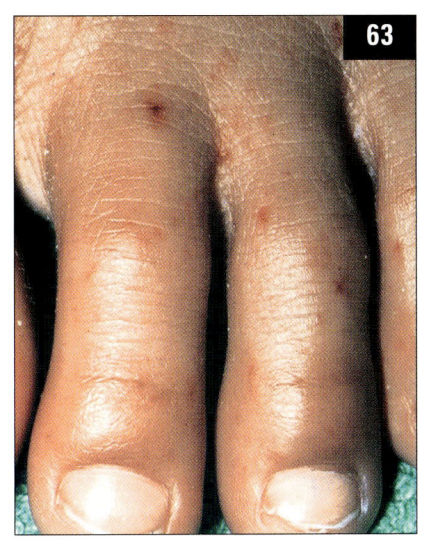

63 Petechial eruption with centripetal spread to the trunk in Rocky Mountain spotted fever caused by *Rickettsia rickettsii*.

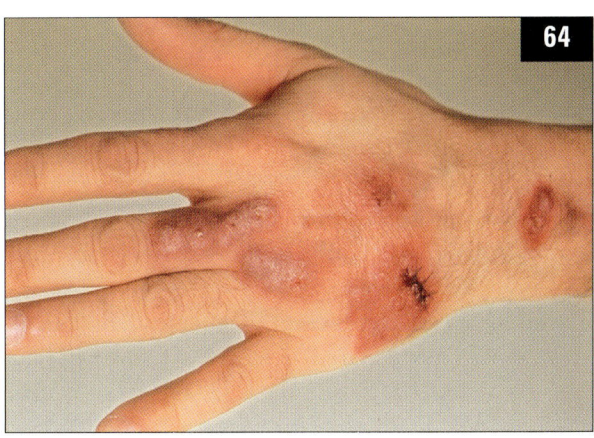

64 Verrucous papules and plaques of fish tank granuloma caused by *Mycobacterium marinum*, often with successive nodules along the lymphatics.

spread to the trunk. There is rapid progression to petechial and hemorrhagic lesions with rare gangrene. The palms and soles are typically involved. Widespread infectious vasculitis results in a multisystem disease with potential nausea, vomiting, diarrhea, gastrointestinal bleeding, pneumonitis, pulmonary edema, myocarditis, muscle necrosis, azotemia, interstitial nephritis, seizures, coma, ataxia, blindness, and deafness.

A high index of suspicion is the most important aspect of diagnosis. Indirect hemagglutination assay (IHA) and IFA tests are sensitive and specific. However, serology is only of interest retrospectively based on acute and convalescent studies. Treatment should be started on the basis of clinical grounds. Organisms may be identified in skin specimens by immunofluorescence or immunoperoxidase methods, where available.

The untreated case fatality rate is as high as 30% and up to 4% with treatment (CDC, 2004). Early intervention with appropriate antibiotics and supportive care reduces mortality (Chapman *et al.*, 2006b). Doxycycline or chloramphenicol is administered for 1 week or until the patient has been afebrile for 2 days.

FISH TANK GRANULOMA

Acid-fast mycobacteria that do not cause tuberculosis or leprosy are grouped under the term 'atypical' mycobacteria. *Mycobacterium marinum* is the most common cause of cutaneous atypical mycobacterial infection in the United States, including fish tank and oyster shucker's granulomas (Van Seymortier *et al.*, 2004). The usual source is an aquarium, salt water, or marine animals. Fishermen, oyster workers, swimmers, and aquarium workers are predisposed. An injury precedes or occurs simultaneously with exposure to contaminated water. A lesion (**64**) develops about 3 weeks after exposure as a verrucous papule or plaque, most commonly on the hand. Usually there is no necrosis or ulceration. In approximately 20% of patients, successive nodules occur along the lymphatic drainage in a sporotrichoid distribution (Iredell *et al.*, 1992). Fever, localized lymphadenopathy, and systemic infection rarely are observed, with the exception of immunosuppressed patients. Osteomyelitis, tenosynovitis, bursitis, septic arthritis, and disseminated infection rarely occur.

Culture from tissue requires special media and appropriate incubation time and temperature. Growth occurs after 7–14 days. Histology is helpful but does not always distinguish from sporotrichosis. Acid-fast organisms occasionally can be seen with special stains on histopathologic sections.

Spontaneous resolution rarely occurs. *M. marinum* is resistant to antituberculosis medications. This organism is sensitive to minocycline, doxycycline, trimethoprim–sulfamethoxazole, and clarithromycin. Response is slow and may take months. Treatment should continue 1–2 months after clinical resolution. If empiric therapy fails, multidrug treatment should be based on laboratory sensitivities.

LYME DISEASE

Lyme disease is caused by the bite of *Ixodes* ticks that harbor the spirochete, *Borrelia burgdorferi*. Subspecies of *B. burgdorferi* are geographically restricted and cause variable clinical presentations. Most parts of the world, especially the United States and Europe (particularly Scandinavia and central Europe), are affected. Lyme disease occurs year-round but most cases present in summer. These ticks are common in woodland areas and are so small that they go unnoticed in over one-third of cases (Melski *et al.*, 1993). Erythema chronicum migrans (ECM) (65, 66) is the characteristic eruption of Lyme disease and is identified in approximately 80% of cases about 1 week after the tick bite (McGinley-Smith & Tsao, 2003). It classically starts as an erythematous papule at the bite site and evolves into spreading annular erythema, sometimes with central clearing. It is usually asymptomatic and may go unnoticed but may have a burning sensation or rare pruritus or pain. With dissemination, secondary lesions of ECM are seen in 17–57% of patients but are typically smaller, less migratory, and less indurated (McGinley-Smith & Tsao, 2003). ECM clears spontaneously within approximately 1 month.

Other findings in Lyme disease include regional lymphadenopathy and mild flu-like symptoms. Sixty percent of untreated cases develop arthritis, especially of large joints such as the knee (Steere *et al.*, 1987). Cardiac manifestations occur in 8% with the most common finding being conduction defects (Nagi *et al.*, 1996). Neurologic disorders occur in 15%, mostly in European cases, and include meningitis, cranial nerve palsies, encephalitis, and radiculoneuritis (Sorensen, 1989).

Acrodermatitis chronica atrophicans (ACA) is almost exclusively seen in a minority of European cases associated with the subspecies *B. afzelii*. This cutaneous manifestation occurs 1 or more years after the initial infection. It is characterized by erythematous nodules or plaques with central clearing on acral sites that progress over months to years to atrophic, cigarette paper-like areas with prominent superficial blood vessels (poikiloderma).

Lymphadenosis benigna cutis (lymphocytoma cutis) is a cutaneous lymphoid hyperplasia that occurs almost exclusively in Europe where unique *Borrelia* subspecies are present. These reddish, violaceous nodules or plaques are identified predominantly on the earlobe of children or areola of adults.

Confirmation of the diagnosis of Lyme disease is mainly by serology, although this is often negative in the first few weeks after inoculation, and for this reason the diagnosis is made through recognition of ECM. The confirmatory serologic studies available include ELISA and Western blot. PCR is expensive and not widely available. Biopsy from the periphery of the lesions of ECM and lesions of ACA may reveal spirochetes with silver stains. Culture is of low yield.

If the tick is removed in less than 24 hours, transmission can generally be avoided. In uncomplicated cases, amoxicillin, cefuroxime, or doxycycline orally is advised. After dissemination, severe infections require IV treatment with ceftriaxone (Feder *et al.*, 2006).

SYPHILIS (LUES)

Syphilis is an infectious disease caused by the spirochete *Treponema pallidum*. It almost always is transmitted by sexual contact, but it also can be transmitted *in utero* and via blood transfusion. Classically, there are four phases of syphilis: primary, secondary, latent, and tertiary.

Primary

The chancre (67, 68) is the primary lesion of syphilis. This painless lesion occurs at the site of inoculation, usually on the genitalia, about 3 weeks after exposure. It begins as a papule that rapidly becomes ulcerated and indurated. The ulcer is punched out with scant, yellow, serous discharge. Spontaneous healing occurs in 1–4 months. The chancre usually is associated with painless regional non-suppurative, lymphadenopathy. About the time of the disappearance of the chancre, constitutional symptoms, including fever, generalized lymphadenopathy, and flu-like symptoms occur, in association with the signs of generalized secondary syphilis. Occasionally, primary syphilis occurs as a syphilic balanitis (69) without a chancre. This is more common in uncircumcised males.

Bacterial Infections

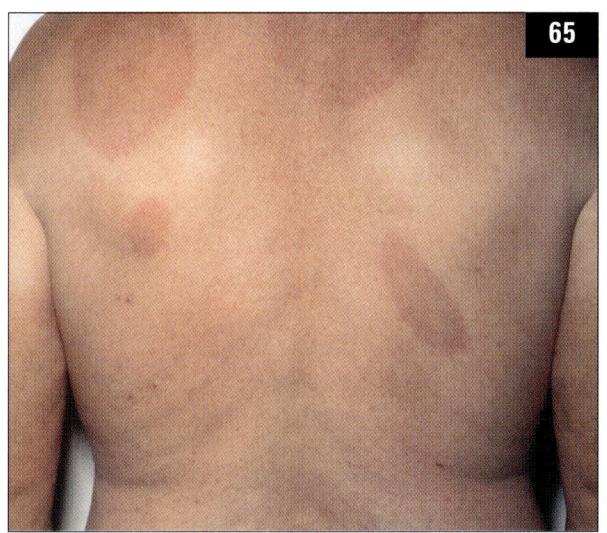

65 Erythema chronicum migrans in Lyme disease.

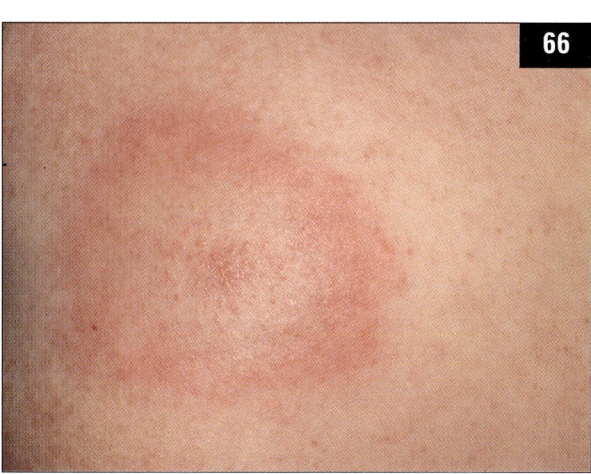

66 Erythematous papule at a tick bite site with spreading annular erythema and central clearing, characteristic of erythema chronicum migrans in Lyme disease.

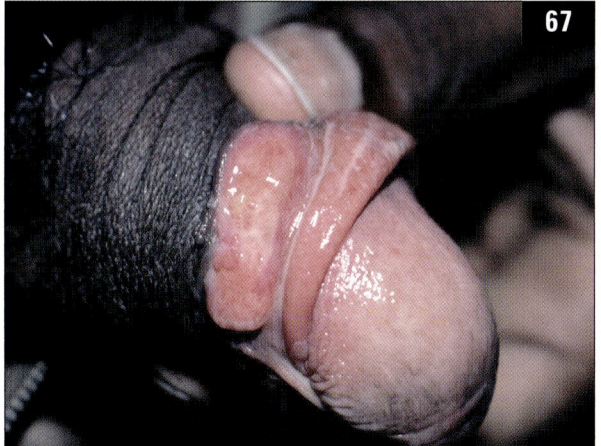

67 Characteristic hard chancre of syphilis.

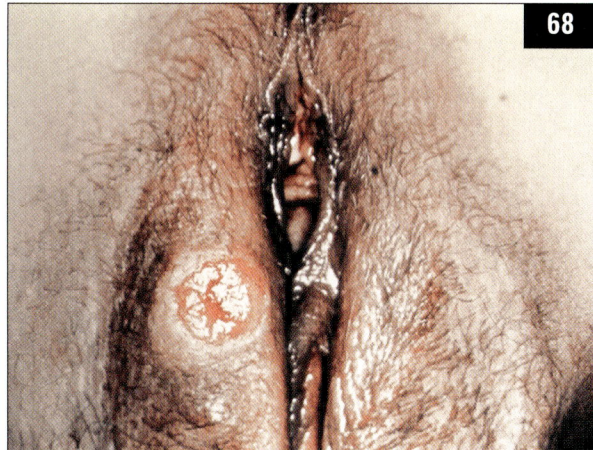

68 Chancre in syphilis. Note the underlying edema.

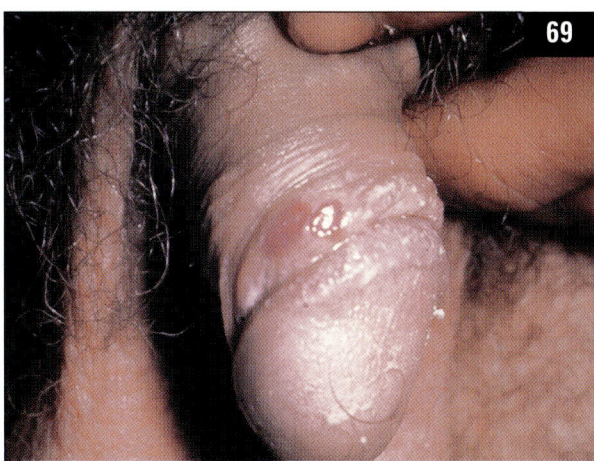

69 Syphilic balanitis.

Secondary

The exanthem of secondary syphilis (70, 71) is bilaterally symmetric and may be macular, papular, or mixed. These non-pruritic lesions are discrete and sharply demarcated and have a copper hue. There is a special predilection for the palms and soles. Lues maligna is a rare form of secondary syphilis with severe ulcerations and pustules, and is accompanied by severe constitutional symptoms. Syphylitic alopecia is irregularly distributed with a moth-eaten appearance and occurs in up to 7% of patients with secondary syphilis (Singh & Romanowski, 1999). Papular or plaque lesions on moist, intertriginous areas are called condylomata lata (72). They are elevated, reddish-brown or gray, flat-topped, moist, and teeming with spirochetes. Mucous patches are the most characteristic mucous membrane lesion of secondary syphilis. They are usually painless, superficial mucosal erosions with a grayish-white membranous base that may develop on the tongue, oral mucosa, lips, and female genitalia.

Other, less common, manifestations of secondary syphilis include acute glomerulonephritis, gastritis, or gastric ulceration, proctitis, hepatitis, acute meningitis, optic neuritis, and polyarthritis. Symptomatic secondary syphilis usually resolves without treatment in a few weeks or as long as 1 year. The disease then enters a latent stage.

Latency

During latency there are no signs or symptoms of infection but the serologic tests are reactive.

Tertiary

As many as 40% of untreated infections can develop into tertiary disease (Singh & Romanowski, 1999). The cutaneous lesions of tertiary syphilis may be nodular, nodulo-ulcerative, or gummatous, and are chronic, painless, asymmetrical, slow growing, and destructive. Patients may have symptoms related to the cardiovascular, musculoskeletal, or central nervous systems.

The spirochete cannot be cultivated *in vitro* and is too small to be seen under the light microscope. Therefore, direct visualization of the organism by darkfield microscopy (73), immunofluorescent staining, or serologic testing is necessary for diagnosis of syphilis. Serology is positive 5–6 weeks after infection, shortly before the chancre heals. Darkfield microscopic diagnosis of oral lesions should be avoided because of the difficulty in distinguishing *T. pallidum* from commensal oral treponemes. The nontreponemal serologic studies, VDRL and rapid plasma reagent (RPR), are nonspecific. A positive VDRL should be quantified and titers followed at regular intervals to follow response to treatment. Biologic false positives occur; therefore, patients with a reactive VDRL or RPR should have a confirmatory specific treponemal test, such as fluorescent treponemal antibody absorption (FTA-ABS) or the microhemagglutination assay for *T. pallidum* (MHA-TP). Biopsy may reveal spirochetes with appropriate silver stains, such as Warthin–Starry, or immunoperoxidase staining. All patients with syphilis should be tested for HIV. Syphilis enhances the risk of transmission of HIV. Cerebrospinal fluid (CSF) evaluation is recommended if neurologic or ophthalmologic findings are present, and in late tertiary syphilis.

The drug of choice is penicillin G. For primary, secondary, and early latent syphilis, IM benzathine penicillin G is recommended. Alternative regimens for penicillin-allergic patients include doxycycline, tetracycline, or desensitization and standard drug therapy. Macrolide resistance is emerging (Marra *et al.*, 2006).

A self-limited Jarisch–Herxheimer reaction may occur a few hours following the onset of treatment, with transient fever and flu-like symptoms. Existing lesions may intensify temporarily. The reaction is quite common and is believed to be due to the breakdown of the spirochetes.

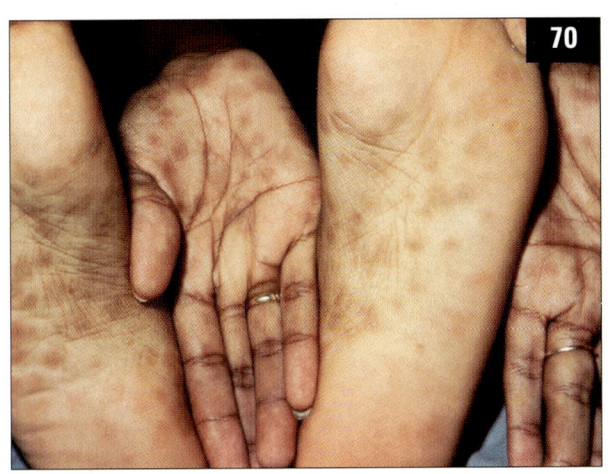

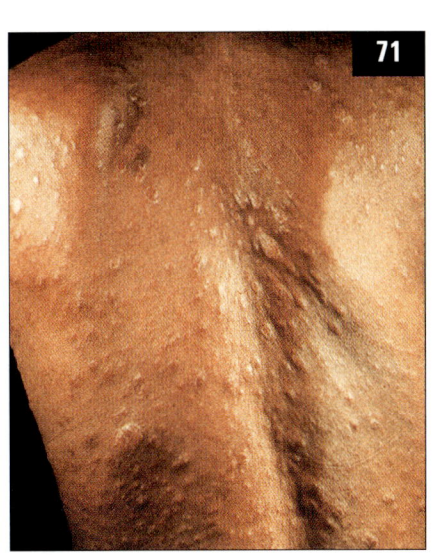

70 Discrete copper colored macules involving the palms and soles in secondary syphilis.

71 Diffuse 'pityriasis rosea-like' exanthem of secondary syphilis.

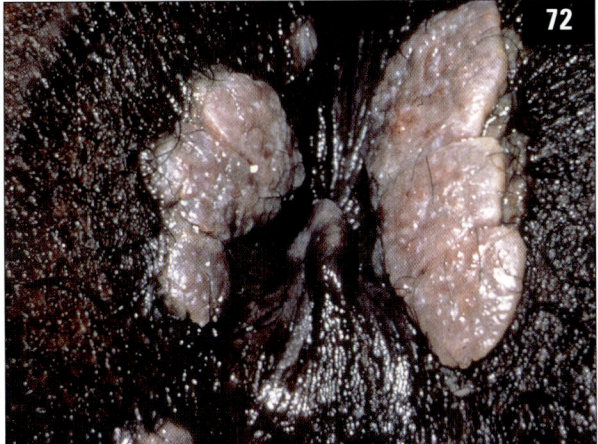

72 Gray flat-topped condylomata lata of secondary syphilis.

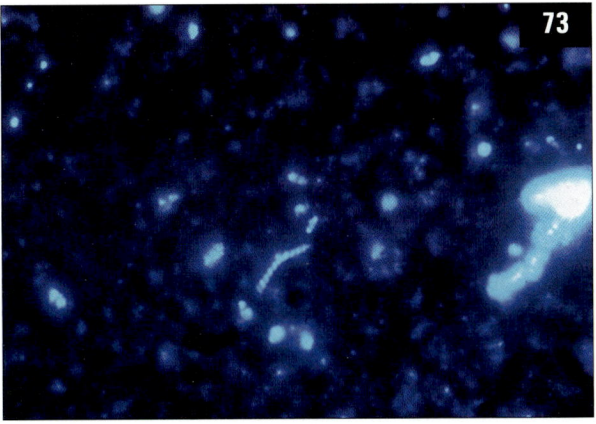

73 *Treponema pallidum* visualized by darkfield microscopy.

CHAPTER 2

FUNGAL INFECTIONS

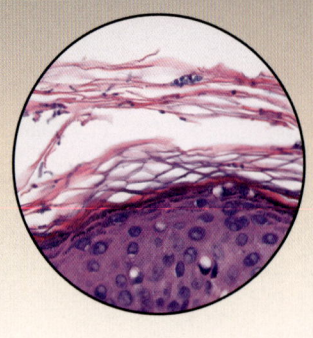

Whitney A High

INTRODUCTION

Fungal infections are common in the skin, an organ system exposed to a barrage of insults from the environment. Cutaneous fungal infections are often divided into 'superficial' and 'deep' forms. Superficial fungal infections include such commonplace conditions as tinea pedis ('athlete's foot'), tinea cruris ('jock itch'), tinea corporis ('ring worm'). Deep fungal infections are more unusual and range from sporotrichosis, a worldwide affliction, to those conditions associated chiefly with immunocompromised states, such as cryptococcosis or penicilliosis. Finally, because of overlapping clinical features, diagnostic modalities, and treatment modalities, rare cutaneous infections caused by algae-like organisms are traditionally discussed with fungal infections.

SUPERFICIAL FUNGAL INFECTIONS

Superficial fungal infections affect the epidermis, mucosa, nails, and hair. Most of these superficial infections are caused by dermatophytes. Non-dermatophytes, such as *Candida* and *Pityrosporum*, also produce skin infections.

DERMATOPHYTOSIS

Dermatophyte infections are referred to collectively as 'tinea'. Additional Latin names are attached to subclassify the infection based upon the site of involvement (*Table 1*). The degree of inflammation engendered by a dermatophyte infection is variable. It depends chiefly upon the virulence of the fungus and the intensity of the patient's immune response. In general, infections acquired from animals or soil (zoophilic or geophilic species) yield greater inflammation than those acquired from other humans (anthropophilic).

TINEA CAPITIS

Tinea capitis is a dermatophyte infection of the hair and scalp. Three-quarters of cases occur between 2 and 9 years of age. Over 95% of tinea capitis in the United States is caused by a single dermatophyte species, *Trichophyton tonsurans* (Foster *et al.*, 2004). Worldwide, *T. tonsurans* and *T. violaceum* account for the vast majority of tinea capitis (Borman *et al.*, 2007).

The clinical presentation of tinea capitis ranges from scaling with minimal inflammation ('gray patch tinea') (**74, 75**) to vigorous inflammation ('a kerion') (**76**). Occipital lymphadenopathy is

---

Table 1 Nosology of dermatophyte infections

Tinea is a Latin word meaning 'gnawing worm or moth'. Additional Latin descriptors are added to indicate the area of the skin involved:

- Tinea capitis – scalp infection
- Tinea facei – facial infection
- Tinea corporis – truncal infection
- Tinea cruris – groin infection
- Tinea manum – hand infection
- Tinea pedis – foot infection
- Tinea unguium – nail infection

common in tinea capitis, but its absence does not exclude the diagnosis (Williams *et al.*, 2005). *T. tonsurans* produces endothrix, meaning it grows inside the hair shaft. Structural compromise leads to breakage of the hairs at the scalp surface. Broken and dilated follicular ostia may yield the appearance of 'black-dot tinea'. Tinea may also resemble patches of seborrheic scale (77). In histologic sections it is possible to identify the hyphae and conidia of an endothrix within the hair shafts or ectothrix surrounding the hair shaft (78).

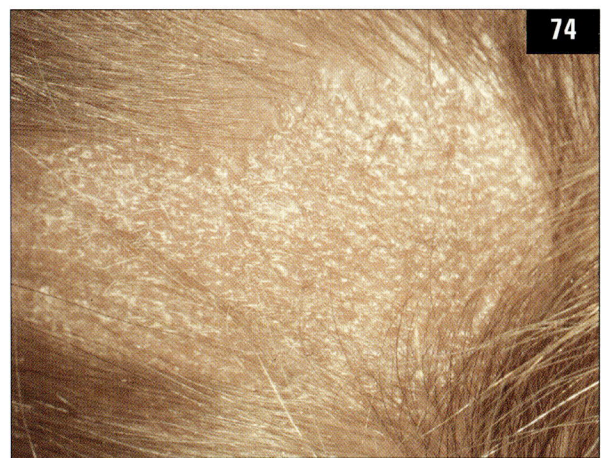

74 'Gray patch tinea' in tinea capitis.

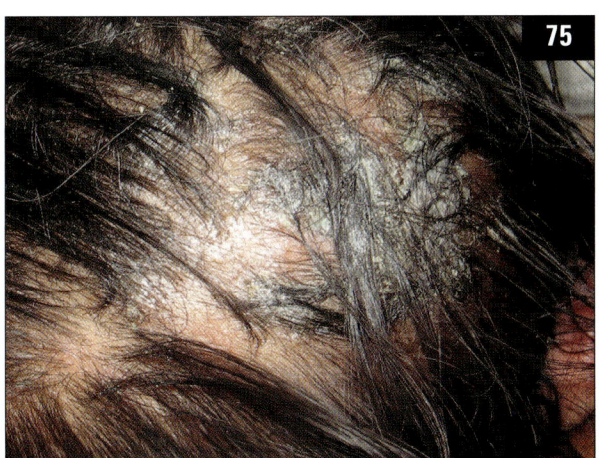

75 'Gray patch tinea' in tinea capitis.

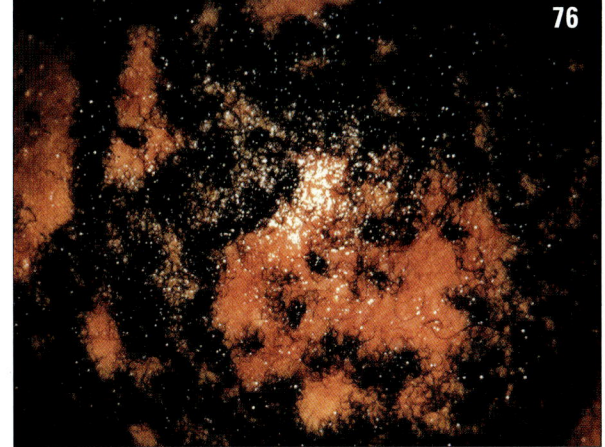

76 A kerion in tinea capitis.

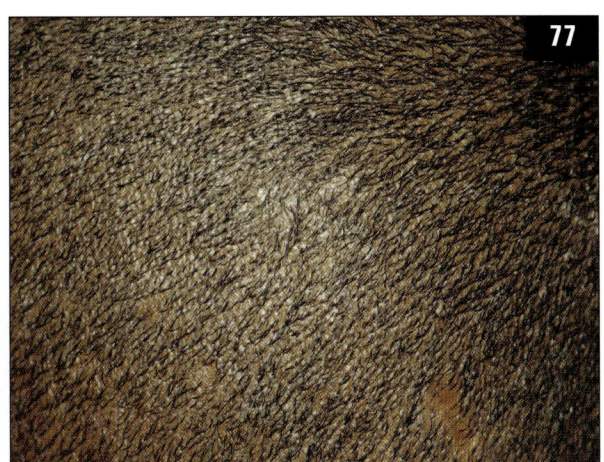

77 Tinea resembling patches of seborrheic scale.

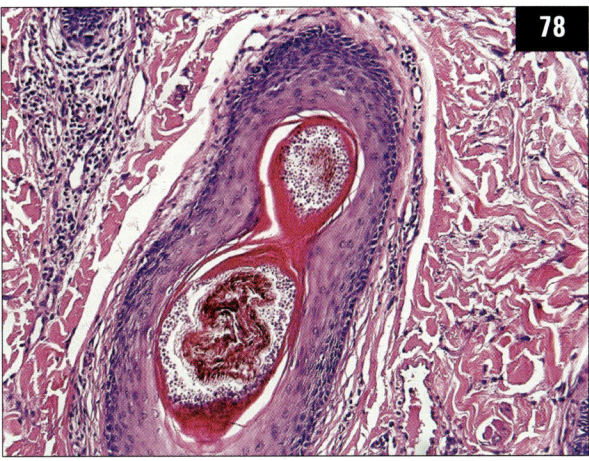

78 Hyphae and conidia of an ectothrix surrounding the hair shaft.

When tinea capitis is suspected, it is appropriate to perform a potassium hydroxide (KOH) examination of hairs plucked from the affected area (**79**), or upon material collected by rubbing the area with moistened gauze. A toothbrush may be used to collect material for culture. Kerions are often misdiagnosed as bacterial infections. (O'Donnell *et al.*, 1990; Brook, 2002). Superinfection with *Staphylococcus* may confound superficial swab-cultures. Because of the potential for scarring and permanent alopecia, a high degree of suspicion for fungal infection is recommended in all pediatric patients with alopecia and a scaling and/or purulent plaque on the scalp.

Oral antifungal agents must be used in the management of tinea capitis. Griseofulvin currently remains the treatment of choice because of its affordability and long safety record (Roberts & Friedlander, 2005). Shorter treatment courses with oral triazoles and oral allylamines may lead to modification of this recommendation in the future. Adjuvant use of antifungal shampoo decreases fungal shedding. Children may return to school with commencement of treatment. The sharing of brushes and hats should be strictly avoided.

TINEA CORPORIS AND TINEA FACEI

Tinea corporis is often referred to by laypersons as 'ring worm', due to its tendency to form annular lesions with peripheral active scaling and central clearing (**80–84**). This radial spread is due to the utilization of keratin within the stratum corneum. The plaques are usually intensely pruritic.

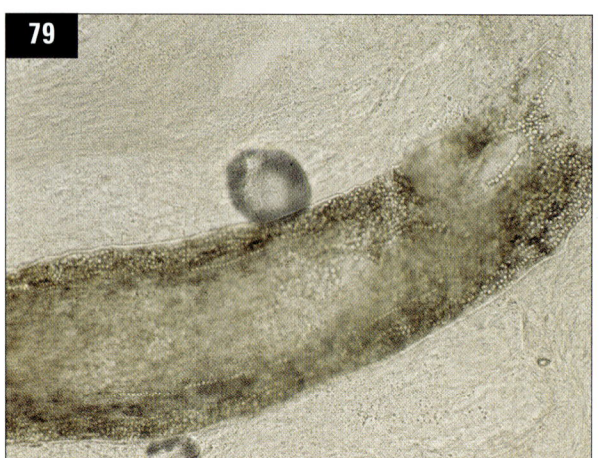

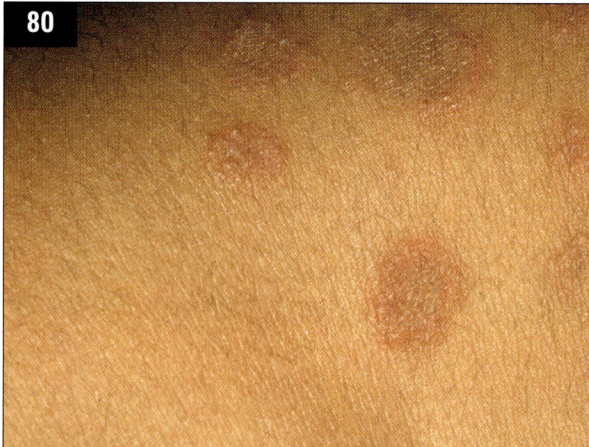

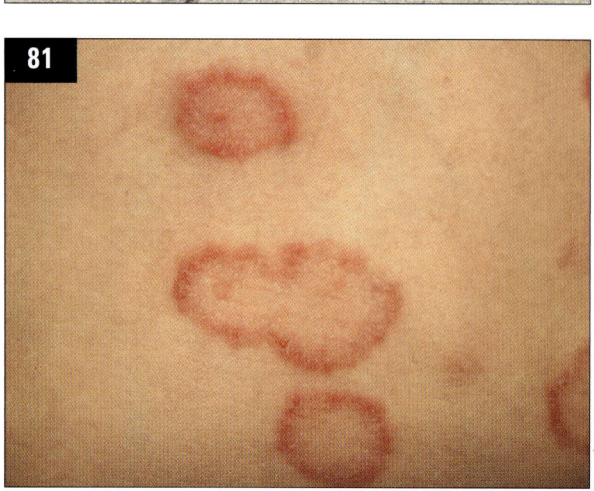

79 Potassium hydroxide examination of hair in suspected tinea capitis.

80 Tinea corporis demonstrating an active edge with erythema.

81 Tinea corporis demonstrating an active scaling edge and central clearing.

Fungal Infections

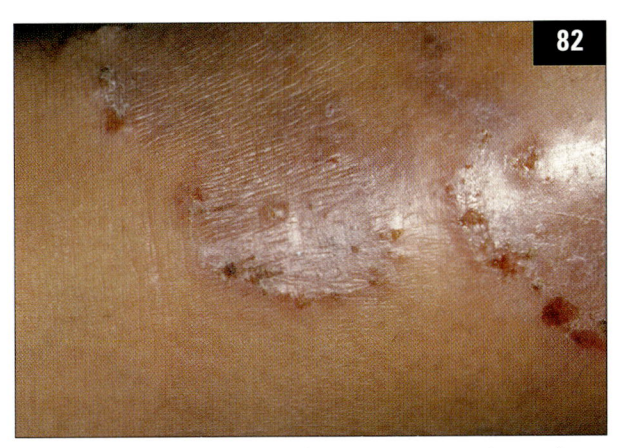

82 Tinea corporis with focal follicular accentuation at the margin.

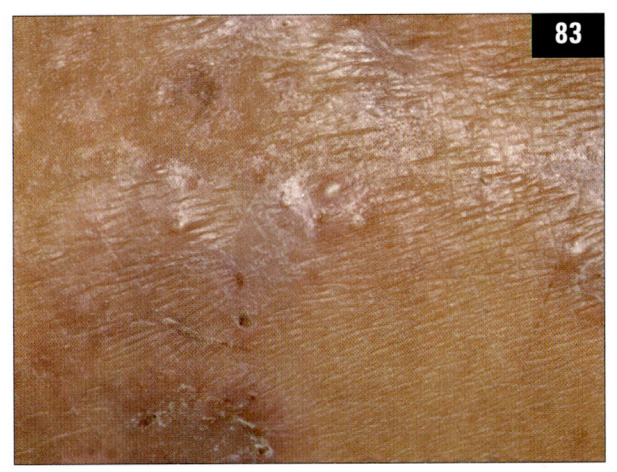

83 Tinea corporis with pustule formation at sites of follicular accentuation.

84 Tinea corporis with multiple scaling plaques with central clearing on the trunk and extremities.

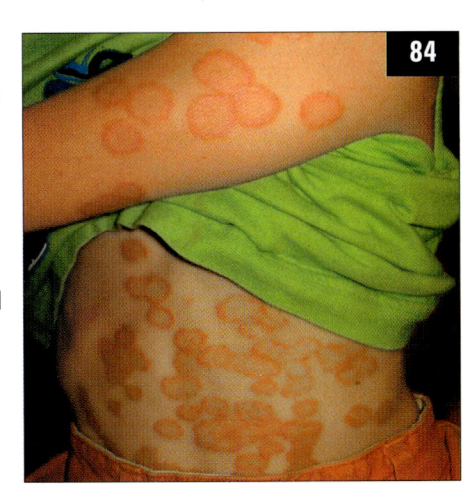

Fungal Infections

A significant number of cases of tinea corporis are associated with new pets or farm animals, and this information must always be sought in the clinical history. Fungi acquired from an animal tend to be more highly inflammatory. Tinea facei represents an essentially identical condition of the facial skin or upper neck (85–93).

It is not uncommon for tinea corporis to be misdiagnosed as eczema, with potent topical steroids mistakenly applied to the area. Associated symptoms initially improve due to the anti-inflammatory properties of the steroid, yet local immunosuppresion allows the fungus to extend

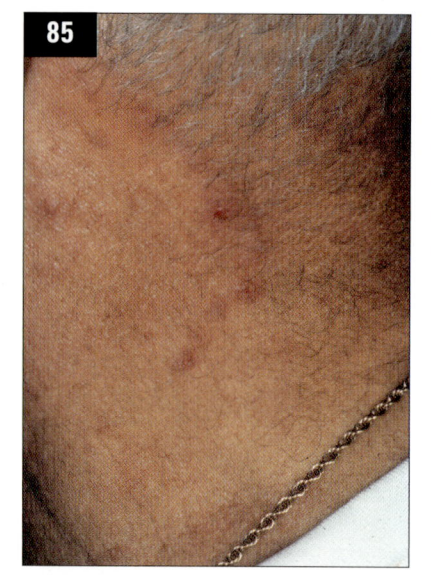

85 Tinea facei on the lateral neck with subtle erythematous follicular papules coalescing into an annular plaque.

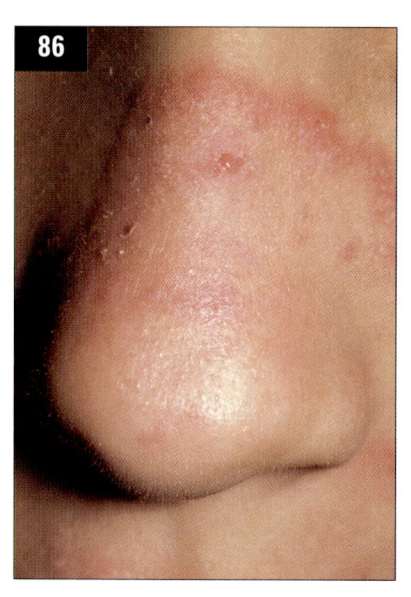

86 Tinea facei on the nose with an erythematous annular active edge of scale.

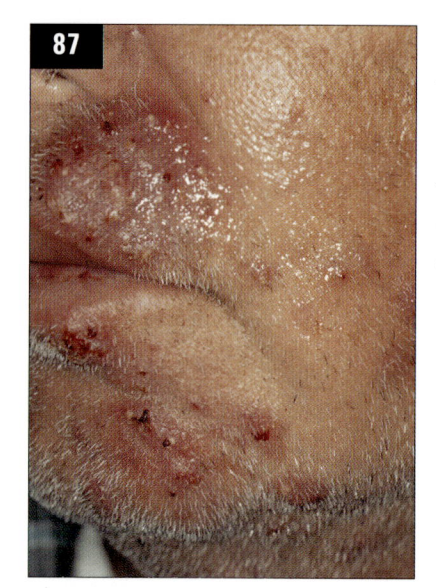

87 Tinea facei on the bearded face (tinea barbae) leading to follicular pustules occurring within an annular plaque.

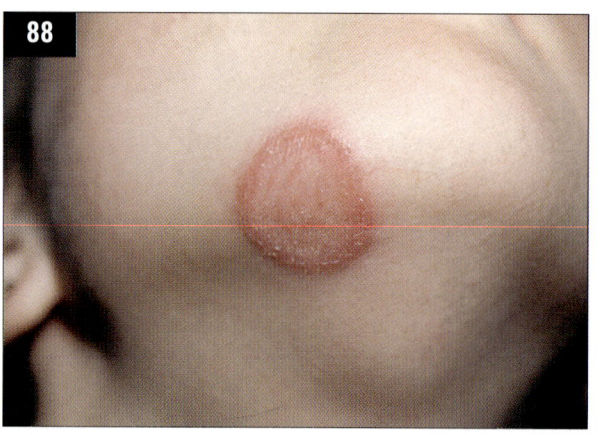

88 Tinea facei leading to an active erythematous and scaling edge with central clearing.

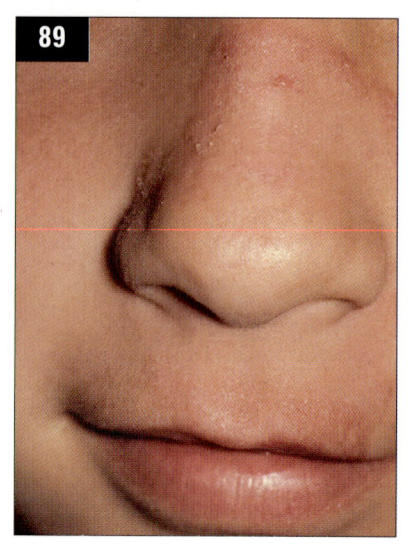

89 Tinea facei on the peri-nasal area with erythematous peripheral scaling and some central clearing.

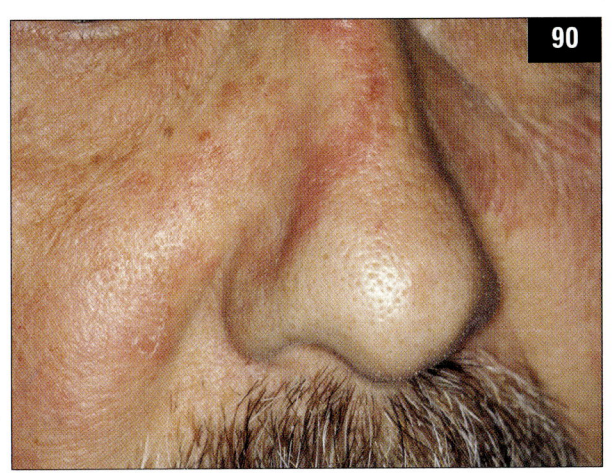

Fungal Infections

90 Tinea facei on the nose of a middle-aged man yielding a subtle annular erythema and scaling.

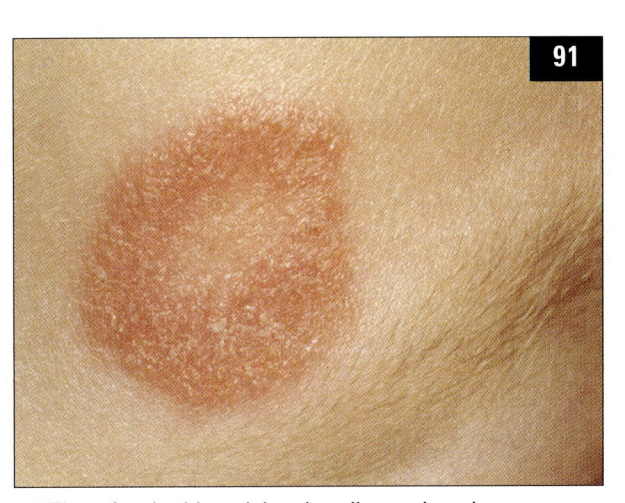

91 Tinea facei with peripheral scaling and erythema.

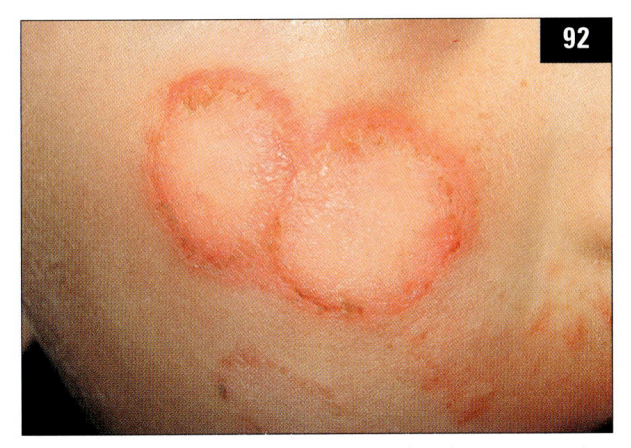

92 Tinea facei leading to multiple annular plaques upon the face with peripheral scaling and erythema and central clearing.

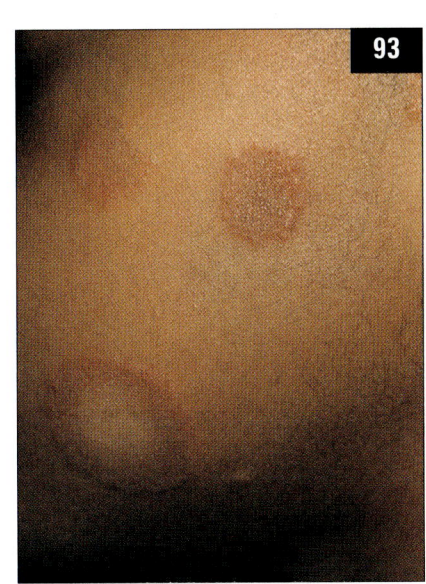

93 Tinea facei on more darkly pigmented skin showing the same peripheral activity with central clearing.

down follicular epithelium (Oklota & Brodell, 2004). The resultant fungal folliculitis is referred to as Majocchi's granuloma (**94–97**) (Janniger, 1992). Patients on oral or strong topical corticosteroids or topical calcineurin inhibitors are predisposed to extensive tinea corporis (**98–101**).

The diagnosis of tinea corporis is made readily by microscopic examination of a KOH scraping taken from the scaling margin. Fungal hyphae are identified as refractile, septate structures that disregard the boundaries of polygonal keratinocytes (**102, 103**). Various dyes such as chlorazole black E can be used to stain the hyphae during a KOH examination.

Treatment of tinea corporis typically involves use of topical antifungal agents, unless extensive surface area is involved or fungal folliculitis (Majocchi's granuloma) is present, in which case oral agents are recommended.

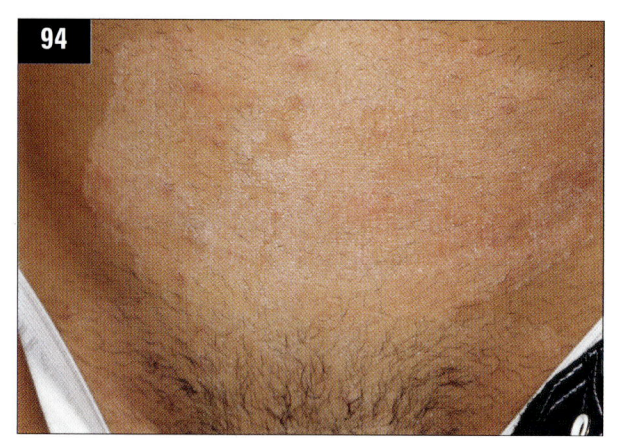

94 Majocchi's granuloma caused by follicular infiltration of terminal hairs in the suprapubic region. Often the local immunosuppressive effects of topical corticosteroids will foster such follicular involvement.

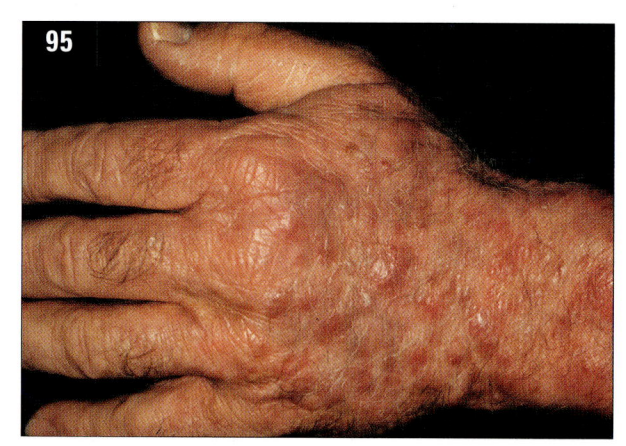

95 Majocchi's granuloma caused by follicular infiltration of the terminal hairs on the back of a man's hand.

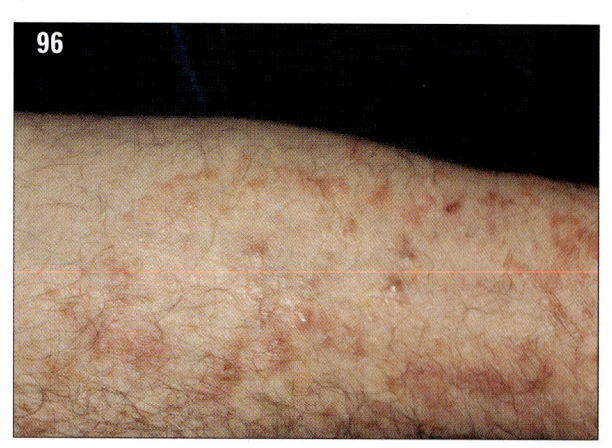

96 Majocchi's granuloma caused by follicular infiltration of the terminal hairs on the leg.

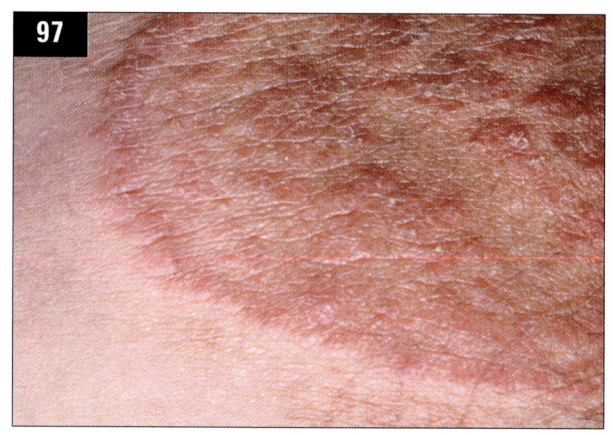

97 Close examination of a plaque of tinea showing follicular papules diagnostic of Majocchi's granuloma.

Fungal Infections

98 Topical calcineurin inhibitors, acting as local immuno-modulators, can lead to extensive tinea infections.

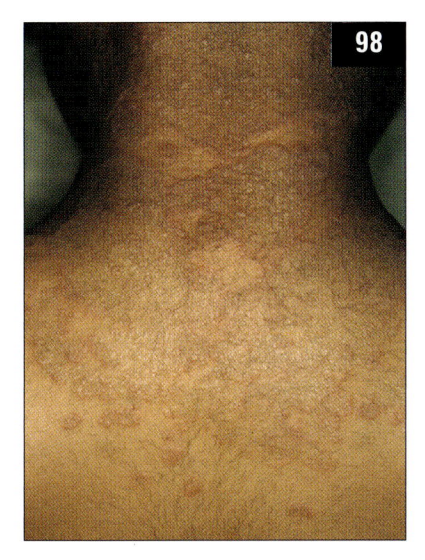

99 Tinea incognito is the name often given to widespread tinea mimicking unresponsive dermatitis.

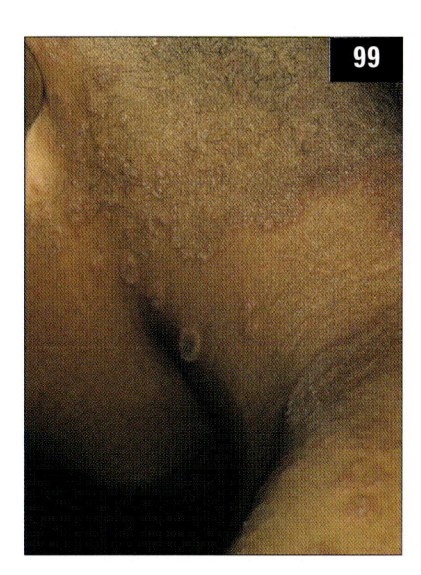

100 The combination of clotrimazole and betamethasone can lead to extensive tinea infections with Majocchi's fungal folliculitis.

101 Extensive tinea secondary to a topical calcineurin inhibitor.

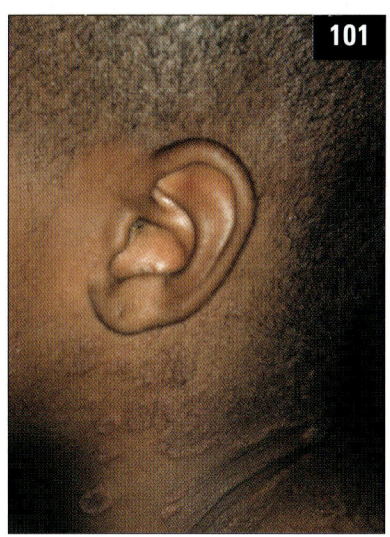

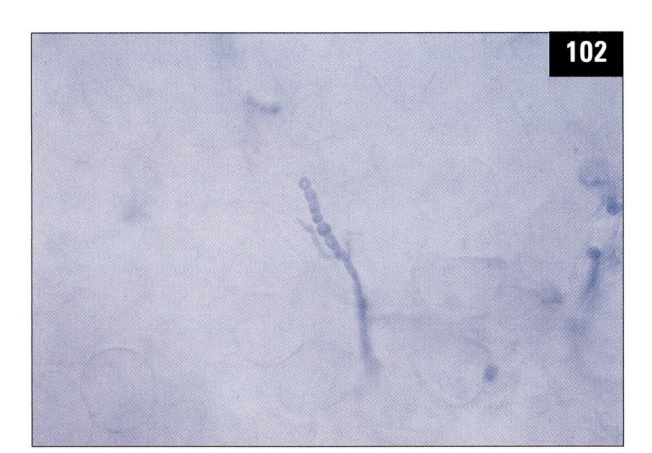

102 Fungal hyphae in the center of the field highlighted with chlorazole black E stain. The light appearing mosaic lines in the background are the cell boundaries of keratinocytes.

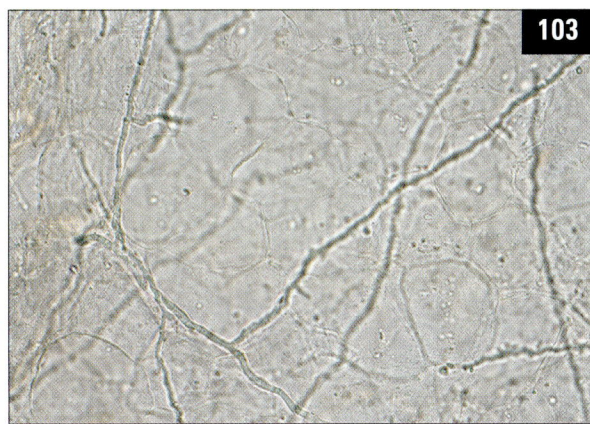

103 Fungal hyphae intersecting and branching. The light appearing mosaic lines in the background are the cell boundaries of keratinocytes.

Tinea cruris

Tinea cruris, or 'jock itch' is a common condition afflicting men. It is a rare infection in women. A multitude of dermatophyte species may yield tinea cruris, and it is not uncommon to see 'jock itch' and other forms of tinea (tinea pedis) in the same person. Clinically, tinea cruris most often yields an annular scaling eruption on the inner thighs and inguinal folds. Tinea cruris rarely affects the scrotum, but may extend to the buttocks (**104**) (La Touché, 1967).

Tinea cruris must be distinguished clinically from erythrasma, a superficial bacterial infection caused by corynebacterium. Erythrasma does not tend to have such a scaly active margin, nor does it typically manifest central sparing. A Wood's lamp may be used to solidify the distinction, as erythrasma yields a 'coral-red' fluorescence, while tinea cruris does not (Miller & David-Bajar, 2004).

The diagnosis of tinea cruris may be substantiated using a KOH preparation in a manner similar to that described for tinea corporis. It is not unusual to see small epidemics among men housed in close quarters (athletic teams, prisons, military barracks). Treatment is similar to that of tinea corporis.

Tinea pedis/Tinea manuum

Tinea pedis is the single most common fungal infection in mankind, and it is a caused primarily by one benefit of civilization – shoes. Shoes maintain a warm and moist environment that fosters the growth of fungus. Generally, two forms of tinea pedis are distinguished. Interdigital tinea pedis is characterized by maceration and scaling between the digits (**105**). Plantar or dorsal foot tinea pedis (**106–111**) is characterized by hyperkeratosis, scaling and erythema which extends 'like a moccasin' across the entire plantar surface or presents with multilocular bullae. The most common cause of tinea pedis is *Trichophyton rubrum*, not coincidentally the most common cause of onychomycosis (Foster *et al.*, 2004).

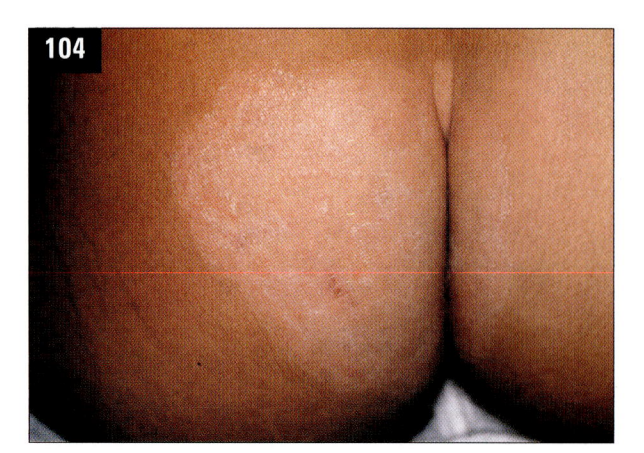

104 Tinea on the buttocks, arms and legs is often misdiagnosed as psoriasis.

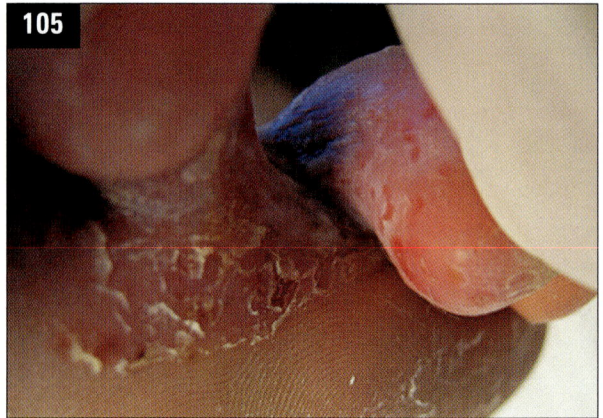

105 Interdigital tinea pedis often yields a macerated appearance.

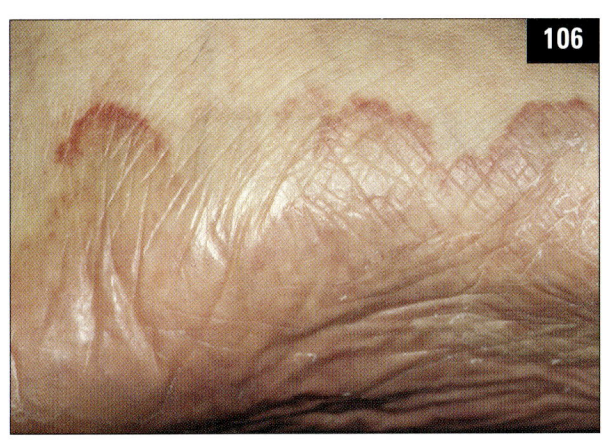

Fungal Infections

106 Tinea pedis affecting the plantar surface with a well demarcated scaling border on the lateral foot.

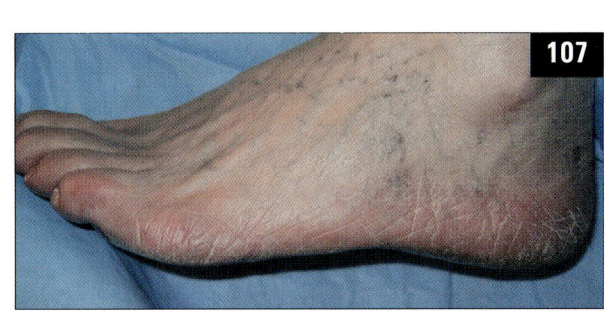

107 Tinea pedis upon the bulk of the plantar surface creating a dry, hyperkeratotic appearance is often referred to as 'moccasin-like' tinea pedis.

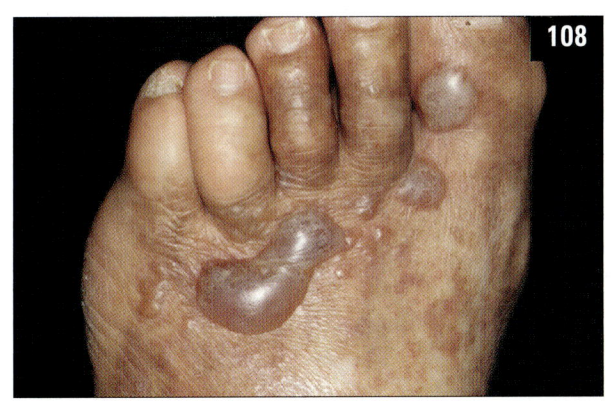

108 Bullous tinea pedis is caused by an exuberant inflammatory response leading to separation in the epidermis. It is more common on soft surfaces, such as the instep and along the dorsal surfaces of the foot rather than the plantar surface itself.

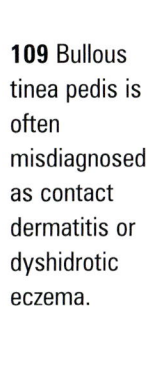

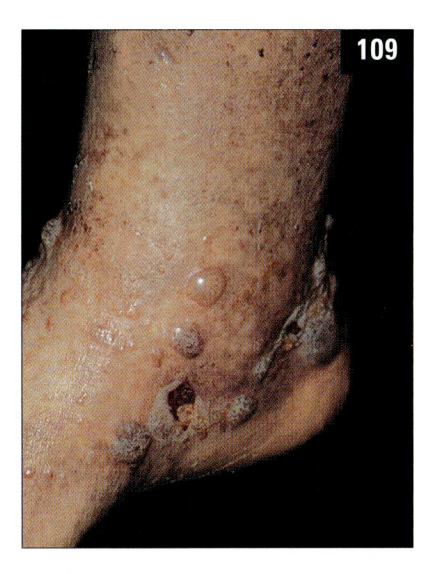

109 Bullous tinea pedis is often misdiagnosed as contact dermatitis or dyshidrotic eczema.

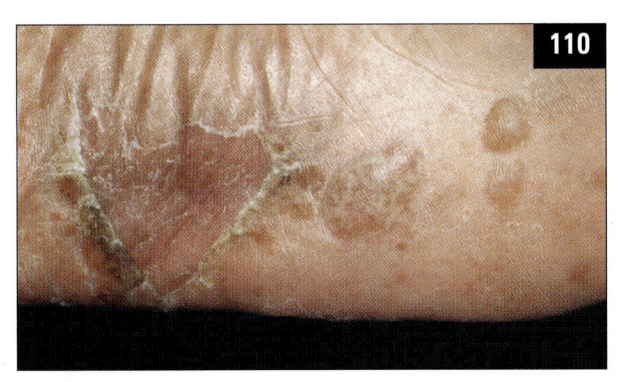

110 Extensive bullous tinea pedis can affect the plantar surface.

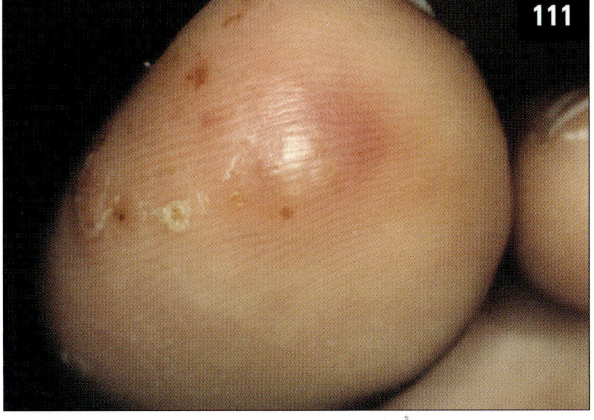

111 The lateral surfaces, in addition to the interdigital areas, may be involved with tinea pedis.

In comparison to tinea pedis, tinea manuum, fungal infection of the palmar skin, is much less common. tinea manuum (**112–118**) usually presents as hyperkeratosis, peeling and mild erythema of the palmar skin. Often, one hand and both feet are involved with tinea manuum and tinea pedis, respectively. Bullae may be present. The reasons for this 'one hand, two feet syndrome' are not entirely clear; it does not appear to pertain to strict handedness (Daniel *et al.*, 1997).

The diagnosis of tinea pedis or tinea manuum may be substantiated using a KOH preparation in a manner similar to that described for tinea corporis. Treatment usually involves topical antifungal agents. Moccasin-like tinea pedis is often recalcitrant to treatment, and oral antifungal agents may be required.

ONYCHOMYCOSIS

Onychomycosis is a broad term that refers to any fungal infection affecting the fingernails or toenails. Tinea unguium refers to the largest subclass of onychomycosis: specifically those cases of fungal infection of the nail caused by dermatophytes (Foster *et al.*, 2004). Onychomycosis commonly causes nail dystrophy (onychodystrophy), separation of the nailplate from the nailbed (onycholysis), hyperkeratosis with increased subungual debris, and discoloration of the nail plate material (**119–121**).

Four subtypes of onychomycosis are distinguished: distal subungual (the most common), lateral subungual (a variant of distal), proximal subungual (associated with immunocompromised states), and superficial onychomycosis (on the surface of the nailplate).

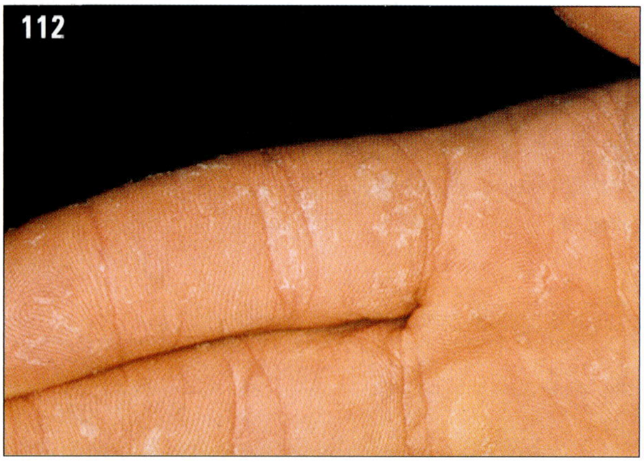

112 Tinea manuum causes scaling and peeling of the hands and is often misdiagnosed as eczema. It tends to involve a single hand.

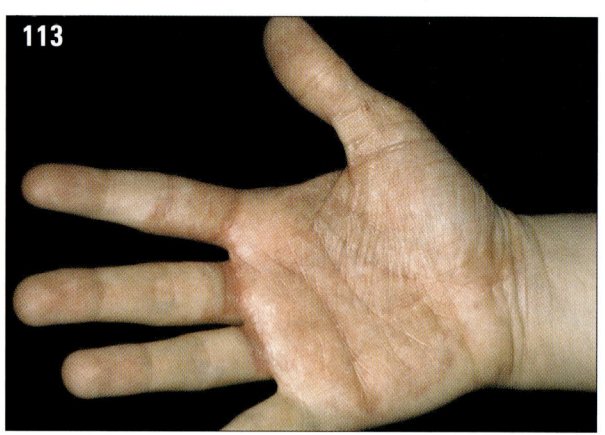

113 Tinea manuum may yield an erythematous and fissured appearance on the palmar surface.

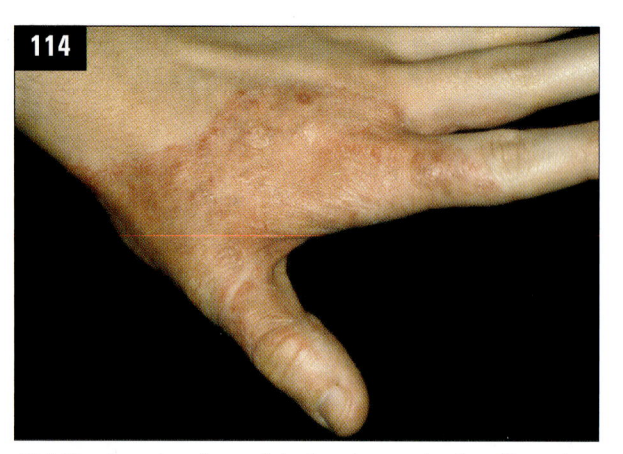

114 The dorsal surface of the hand may also be affected by tinea manuum.

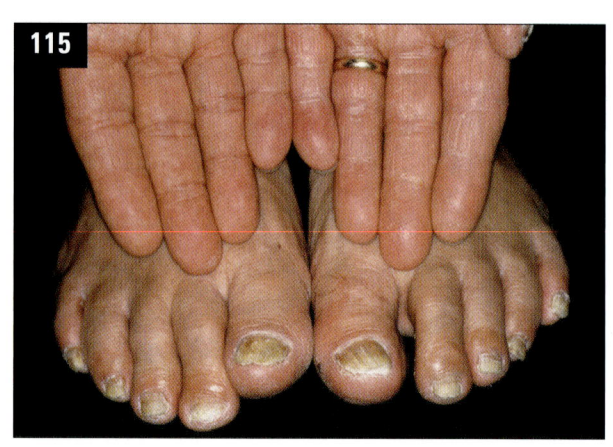

115 It is not uncommon for patients to have two feet and one hand affected by tinea.

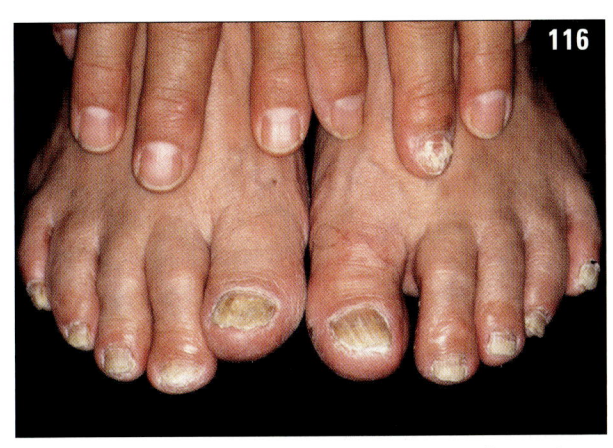

Fungal Infections

116 Nails may be affected in patients with persistent tinea pedis and tinea manuum, as in this patient with both the skin and nails of two feet and one hand involved.

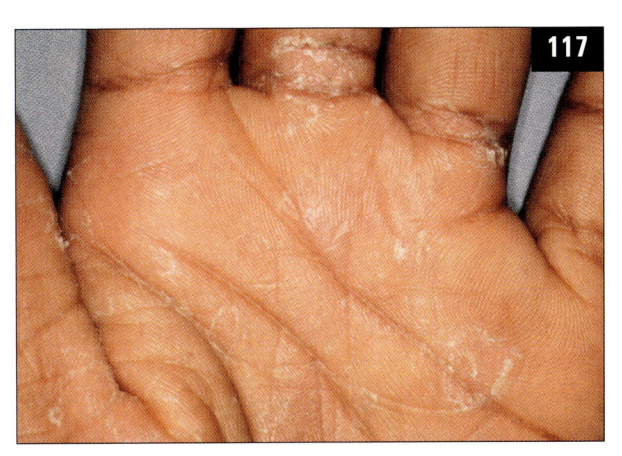

117 Tinea manuum may involve moist areas of the hand including the base of the digits.

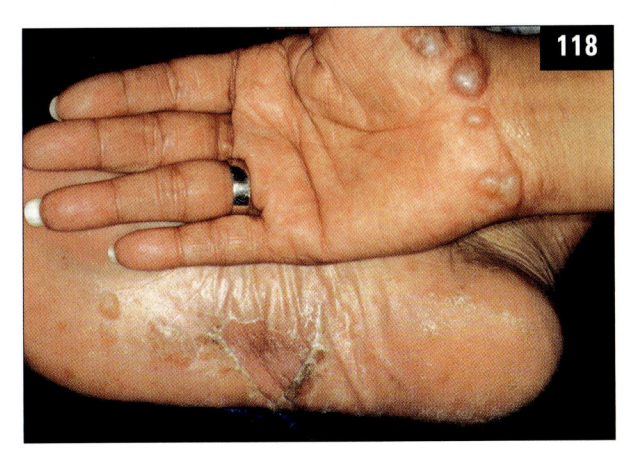

118 Bullous tinea pedis may produce a bullous 'id' reaction on the hands. KOH of the hand will not show hyphae.

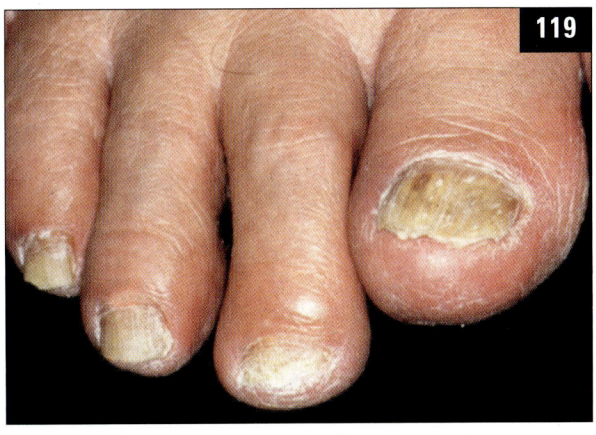

119 Onychomycosis often presents as thickening, crumbling, and discoloration of the toenails.

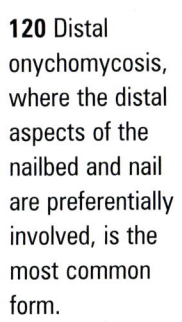

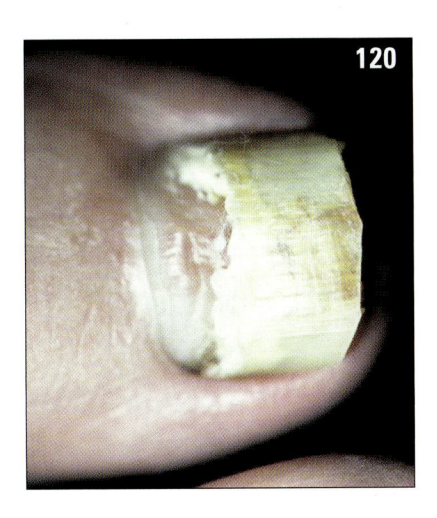

120 Distal onychomycosis, where the distal aspects of the nailbed and nail are preferentially involved, is the most common form.

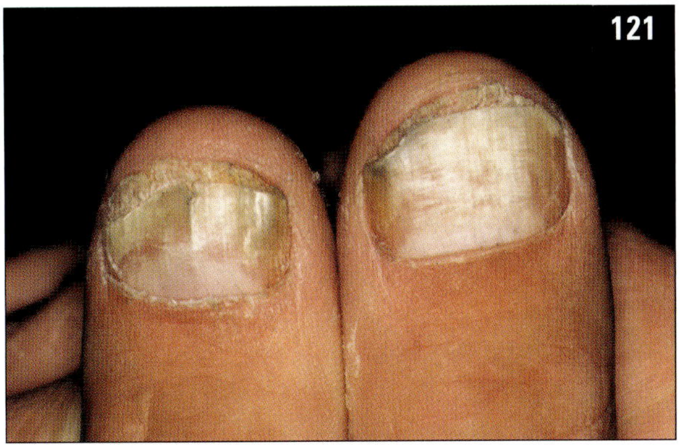

121 In white superficial onychomycosis, the fungal infection occurs on the superficial aspects of the nail plate.

Proximal subungual onychomycosis may be the initial cutaneous sign of human immunodeficiency virus/acquired immunodeficiency syndrome (HIV/AIDS) infection (**122**) (Daniel *et al.*, 1992).

It is important to stress that onychodystrophy is not equivalent to onychomycosis. Psoriasis, lichen planus, lichen striatus, pressure deformities, or even the aging process may result in a dystrophic nail (Weinberg *et al.*, 2005; High & Fitzpatrick, *in press*). The diagnosis of onychomycosis may be substantiated through microscopic examination of a KOH preparation derived from subungual debris, via fungal culture, or by formal histological examination of nail clipping using periodic acid-Schiff (PAS) staining or toluidine blue staining (**123, 124**). Recent studies have suggested that histological examination enjoys the highest sensitivity as long as a representative sample is obtained (Reisberger *et al.*, 2003; Weinberg *et al.*, 2003).

If patients are asymptomatic, deferral of treatment may be acceptable. Diabetics, those with peripheral vascular disease, a history of recurrent cellulitis, pain upon ambulation, or a major impact on social functioning likely benefit from treatment. Topical nail lacquers are of limited efficacy, and treatment of onychomycosis generally requires oral antifungal agents. Even with use of oral terbinafine, the 5-year recurrence rate may be as high as 50% (Gupta & Lynch, 2004). Treatment failure is more likely when the infecting organism is not a dermatophyte.

CANDIDIASIS

Candidiasis is a generic term used to refer to all mucocutaneous infections with *Candida*, a yeast normally found upon the skin and mucosa. *C. albicans* is the most common pathogen, but other species may yield candidiasis. Maceration, diabetes mellitus, recent antibiotic therapy, or immunosuppression may predispose to overgrowth of *Candida* with resultant disease. *Candida* does not utilize keratin for energy, but instead prefers glucose.

CANDIDAL INTERTRIGO

The most common form of candidiasis in adults is candidal intertrigo (**125, 126**). The groin, axilla, and inframammary crease may be involved. *Candida* prefers the high humidity of these areas for

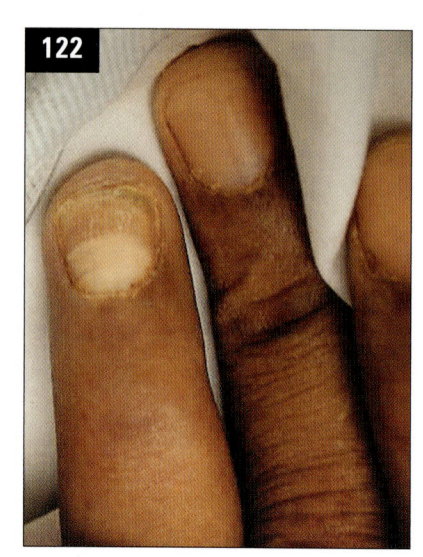

122 Proximal onychomycosis, where the proximal aspects of nail bed and nail are involved is associated with immunocompromised disease states, chiefly HIV/AIDS.

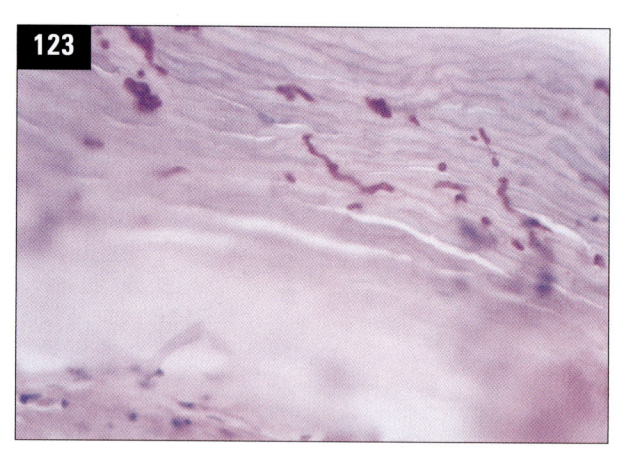

123 Periodic acid-Schiff (PAS) staining of nail clippings often highlights PAS-positive (purple-red) hyphal elements in the nail plate.

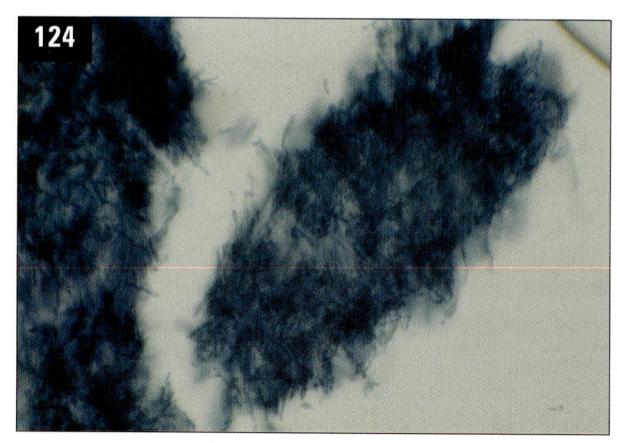

124 Microscopic examination in onychomycosis (Toluidine blue stain).

optimum growth. Maceration in these areas affords easier vertical penetration into the tissue. Brightly erythematous skin with 'satellite lesions' studding the periphery is a common presentation. Denuded areas may demonstrate a fire-red color. Of course, simple intertrigo may occur without *Candida* overgrowth, in which case skin reactions are caused simply by maceration and irritation alone. Candidal diaper dermatitis, at its essence, is merely a variant of candidal intertrigo.

One form of candidal intertrigo, unusual both in name and frequency, is erosio interdigitalis blastomycetica (Adams, 2002). In this disorder, chronic moisture of the hands leads to overgrowth of *Candida* in the finger webbing. The skin between the third and fourth fingers is most often involved, as in most people this is the longest webspace with the greatest occlusion.

Candida infections of the genitalia may be moist or dry and psoriasiform. They may involve the glans, shaft, or scrotum.

Candidiasis is typically diagnosed based upon the clinical presentation. Microscopic examination of scrapings using KOH preparation will demonstrate yeast and pseudohyphae. Scrapings may also be cultured on Sabouraud's fungal medium, *Candida*-specific media such as Nickerson's agar, or even on standard agar.

Candidiasis responds to most antifungal medications used for dermatophyte infections, except for tolnaftate and griseofulvin (High, 2007). Based on efficacy and affordability, topical imidazoles are often recommended as first-line therapy. Nystatin, a topical polyene, has efficacy against most *Candida* species encountered in dermatology. Topical ciclopirox olamine may also be used. Simple 'airing out' of the lesions, with prevention of retained moisture, will often improve the condition substantially.

ORAL CANDIDIASIS

Oral candidiasis may yield thrush or perleche. Oropharyngeal candidiasis, thrush, most often affects newborns, the elderly, diabetics, or immunocompromised patients. It presents as white-yellow, stuck-on papules and confluent plaques in the oropharynx. Perleche consists of cracks or fissures at the corners of the mouth with adherent white exudates and surrounding erythema. It is often associated with thrush but it may also occur independently (Driezen, 1984).

The diagnosis of oral candidiasis and/or perleche is typically established based upon the clinical appearance. If desired, a scraping with microscopic examination using KOH preparation techniques would demonstrate findings similar to cutaneous candidiasis. Standard treatment for thrush includes clotrimazole troches or nystatin oral suspension. Perleche responds rapidly to twice daily application of a topical antifungal agent.

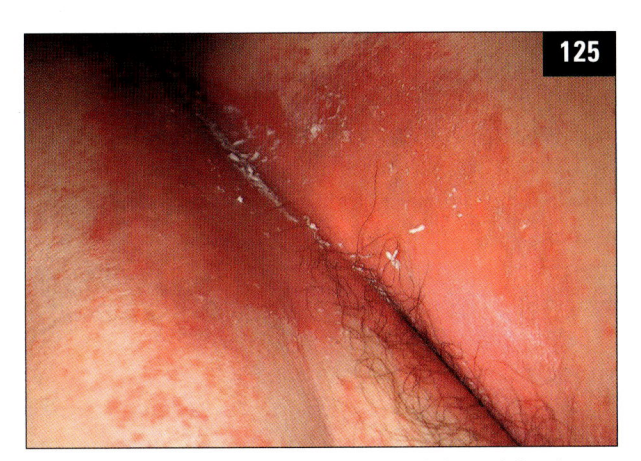

125 Candida intertrigo often causes a bright and 'beefy-red' erythema with surrounding satellite pustules in the body folds.

126 Candidiasis may also affect the genitalia proper, leading to eroded and brightly erythematous plaques.

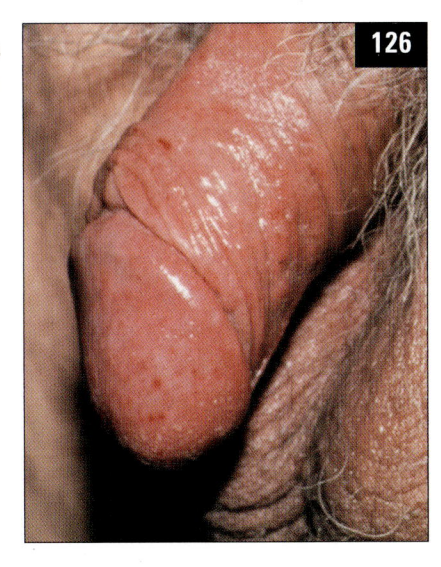

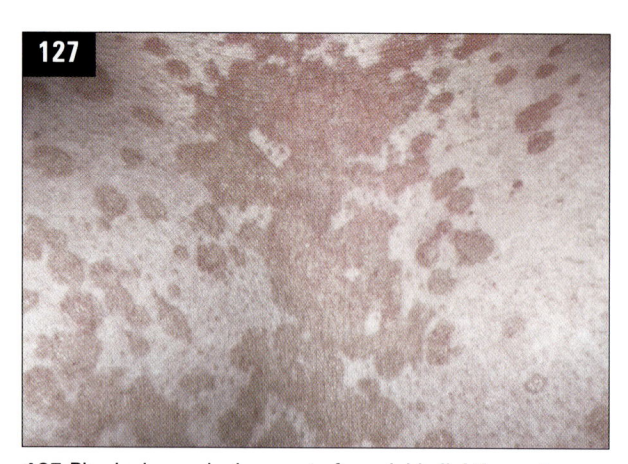

127 Pityriasis versicolor most often yields lightly scaling 'fawn-colored' plaques upon the skin in areas of high sebaceous activity, such as the upper chest.

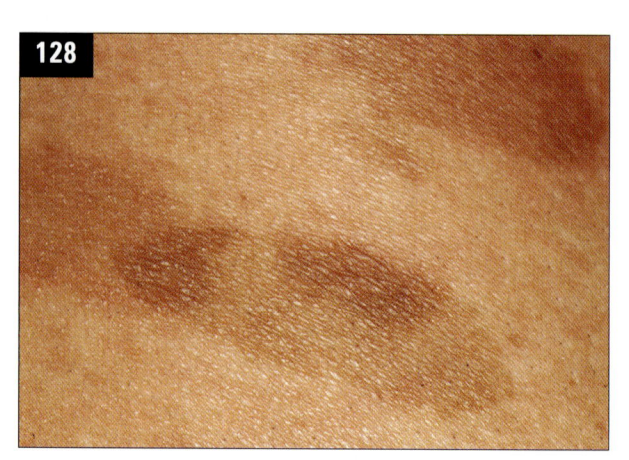

128 In darker skin types, the plaques of pityriasis versicolor may be hyperpigmented.

PITYRIASIS VERSICOLOR

Pityriasis versicolor refers to a superficial infection of the epidermis caused by the commensal yeast *Pityrosporum*. Older references may use the term 'tinea versicolor', but 'tinea' implies infection with a dermatophyte, and use of this terminology is discouraged. The pathogenic hyphal phase of this yeast may also be referred to as *Malassezia* (Crespo-Erchiga & Florencio, 2006).

Pityriasis versicolor presents as tan, hypopigmented, hyperpigmented, pink or fawn-colored plaques (**127, 128**). As *Pityrosporum* utilizes sebum for energy, involvement of the upper trunk is common. Close inspection often reveals a fine, bran-like scale. Occasional patients may complain of mild pruritus. Substances elaborated by the yeast (azelaic acid derivatives) interfere with melanin synthesis and distribution, and hypopigmentation may be noticed in affected skin.

The diagnosis of pityriasis versicolor is most often based upon the clinical presentation. Microscopic examination with KOH preparation may be performed using a skin scraping, or alternatively, by touching the lesions with clear cellophane tape ('tape stripping') (**129**). Visualization of short hyphae and round yeast ('spaghetti and meatballs') confirms the diagnosis (**130**). *Pityrosporum* yeast are normal follicular flora. In early disease, organisms are often identified in larger numbers adjacent to the follicular ostia (**131**).

TINEA NIGRA

Tinea nigra (**132**) represents a superficial fungal infection common to tropical regions of the world. The infection is most often caused by *Hortaea werneckii* (formerly *Phaeoannellomyces werneckii* or *Exophiala werneckii*) (Perez et al., 2005). It is believed that tinea nigra occurs due to traumatic inoculation with contaminated soil, sewage, wood, or compost.

This pigment-producing fungus remains confined to the stratum corneum, and clinically it creates a visibly hyperpigmented macule. The lesion is often on the palmar surface of the hand, and it may be confused with a melanocytic process such as acral lentiginous melanoma (Hall & Perry, 1998).

The diagnosis may be made using microscopic examination of skin scrapings treated with KOH preparation (**133**). Thick, septate, branching hyphae with dark pigment are visualized. Culture of skin scrapings on Sabouraud's fungal agar yields growth in about 1 week. Initially, shiny, black, and mucoid colonies are present, although pigment production wanes with time. Because of confusion with a melanocytic process, a lesion may be occasionally biopsied. Hyperkeratosis, mild acanthosis, and septate, pigmented hyphae are identified in the stratum corneum (**134**).

Topical antifungal agents have variable efficacy in treating tinea nigra. Because the infection is confined to the stratum corneum, potent keratolytics, like salicylic acid, are also effective in treatment (Sayegh-Carreno et al., 1989).

Fungal Infections

129 'Tape stripping' with cellophane tape placed directly onto slides with a drop of appropriate stain is a valuable diagnostic technique for pityriasis versicolor.

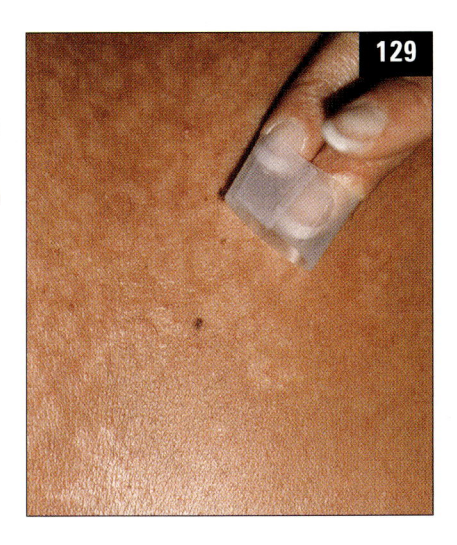

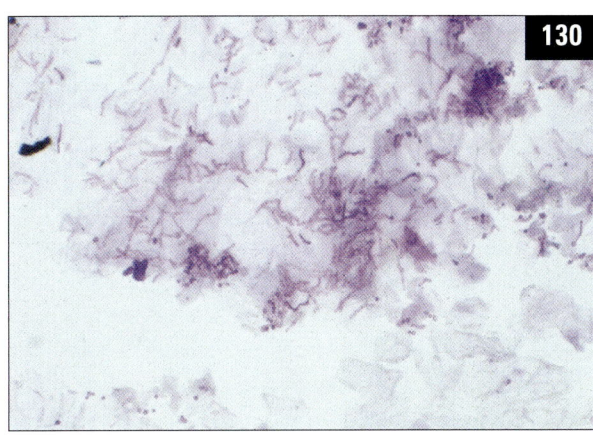

130 Short hyphae and round yeast ('spaghetti and meatballs') in pityriasis versicolor (Swartz–Lamkin stain).

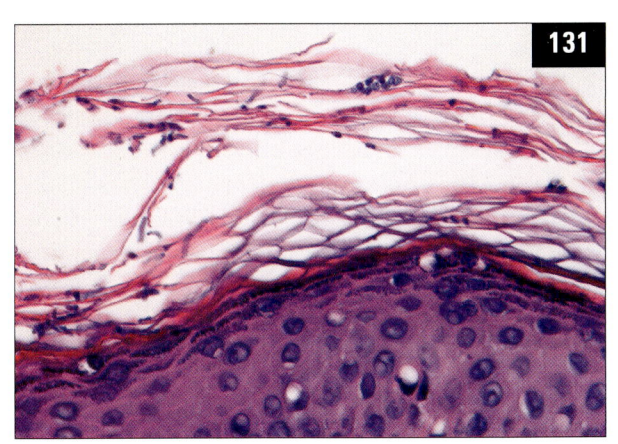

131 Pityriasis organisms are often basophilic and interspersed with normal basket-weave keratosis within the stratum corneum in pityriasis versicolor.

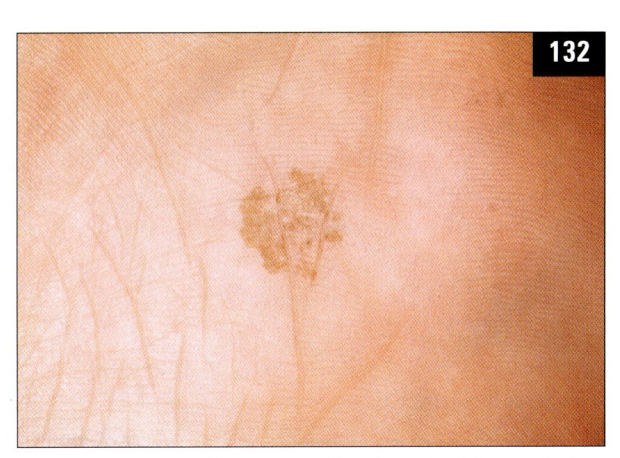

132 Tinea nigra, a fungus capable of synthesizing melanin, often creates hyperpigmented plaques on the acral surfaces that are confused with pigmented lesions.

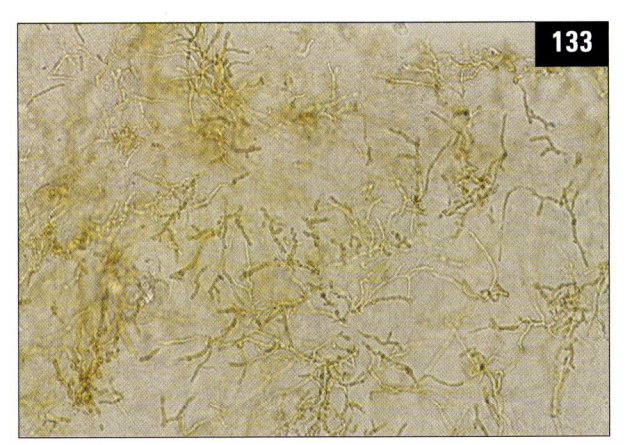

133 The hyphae caused by species of fungi causing tinea nigra produce pigment which is visible on KOH preparations without any additional staining.

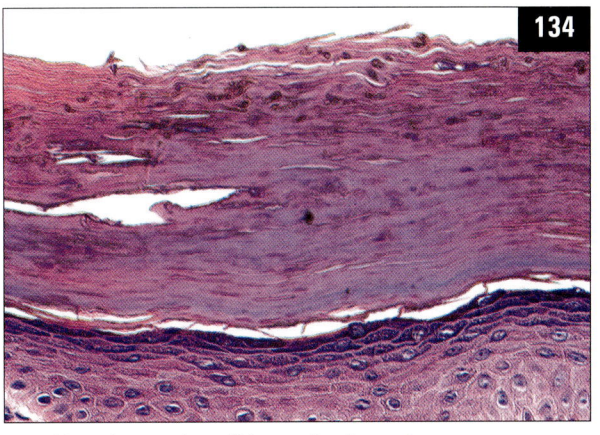

134 Hyperkeratosis, mild acanthosis, and septate, pigmented hyphae in the stratum corneum.

DEEP FUNGAL INFECTIONS

Some fungal infections may invade into the deeper layers of soft tissue. Alternatively, others may involve the skin secondarily, or they may eventuate in systemic disease from initial skin infections. In dermatology, these infections are collectively referred to as deep fungal infections. Some deep fungal infections, such as sporotrichosis, may occur in otherwise healthy persons. Others, such as cryptococcosis and penicillosis, are associated with immunocompromised states, in particular HIV/AIDS.

CHROMOBLASTOMYCOSIS

Chromoblastomycosis is an infection that may be caused by any of several pigment-producing fungi, including species of the genus *Cladosporium*, *Phialophora*, *Rhinocladiella*, or *Fonsecaea* (Lupi et al., 2005). Chromoblastomycosis is most often an infection of agricultural workers, particularly men, living in tropical and subtropical climes (see Chapter 4, Tropical Diseases).

SPOROTRICHOSIS

Sporotrichosis (**135–138**) is a deep tissue infection caused by the dimorphic fungus *Sporothrix schenckii*. It is a disease described throughout the world. Sporotrichosis is most often an infection of farmers, gardeners, and horticulturists (Morris-Jones, 2002). It is often referred to as 'rose gardener's disease', due to its association with traumatic implantation via rose bush thorns.

Following traumatic implantation into the skin, an erythematous papule develops within 1–10 weeks. Classically, lymphangitic spread leads to the formation of secondary lesions extending proximally or radially following lymphatic drainage. Satellite lesions are common. However, this characteristic pattern of extension ('sporotrichoid spread') is not unique to sporotrichosis, but may also be seen with atypical mycobacterial infections, cat-scratch disease, tularemia, nocardiosis, and leishmaniasis (Kostman & DiNubile, 1993). Widespread dissemination may be seen in immunosuppressed patients, particularly those with HIV/AIDS (Hardman et al., 2005).

The diagnosis is usually made via tissue culture. Sporotrichosis develops rapidly, with most cultures showing positivity within 1–2 weeks. Sporotrichosis may be difficult to identify upon histopathologic examination, even when fungal stains are used. The absence of organisms in tissue does not exclude the diagnosis and culture is recommended. Occasionally, cigar-shaped yeast may be identified in tissue specimens stained with PAS, Gomori methenamine-silver (GMS), or immunohistochemical stains (Bullpitt & Weedon, 1978). Extracellular asteroid bodies comprised of eosinophilic spicules surrounding a central yeast form are thought to be distinguished from asteroid bodies of other granulomatous reactions that are typically intracellular (Rodriguez & Barrera, 1997).

Sporotrichosis is often best treated with oral itraconazole (Koga et al., 2003). Supersaturated potassium iodide (SSKI) represents an alternative, but it often produces gastrointestinal distress. Disseminated cases are treated with IV forms of amphotericin B.

HISTOPLASMOSIS

Histoplasmosis (Darling's disease) refers to a broad category of fungal infection caused by the dimorphic fungus *Histoplasma capsulatum*. This fungus may be found throughout the world, but it is particularly prevalent in the Ohio, Missouri, and Mississippi River valleys of the United States (Conces, 1996). Highly infectious soil occurs in areas inhabited by birds and bats.

Exposure to histoplasmosis typically occurs through inhalation of aerosolized conidia. Most infected individuals are entirely asymptomatic, but

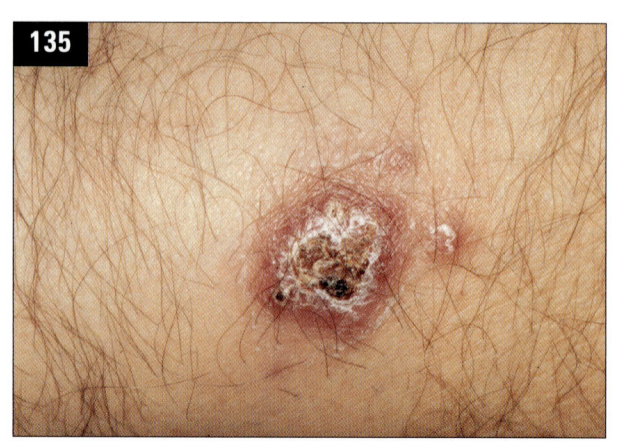

135 Lesions of sporotrichosis are typically nodules or indurated plaques with a keratotic surface.

Fungal Infections

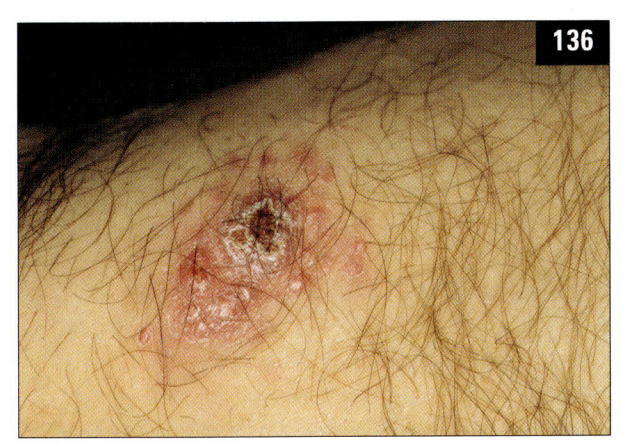

136 Sporotrichosis often produces keratotic lesions with surrounding satellites.

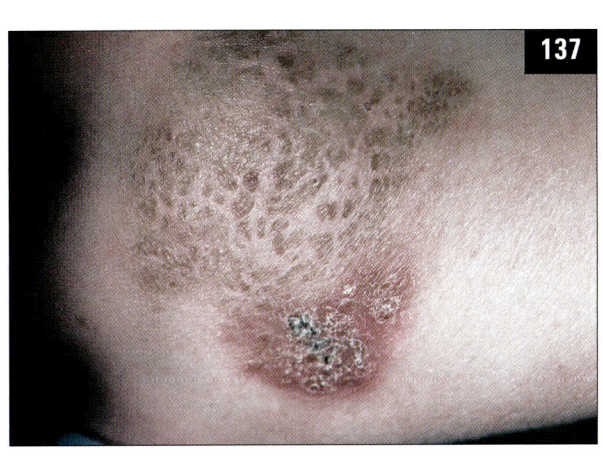

137 Fixed cutaneous sporotrichosis demonstrates radial spread via lymphatic channels.

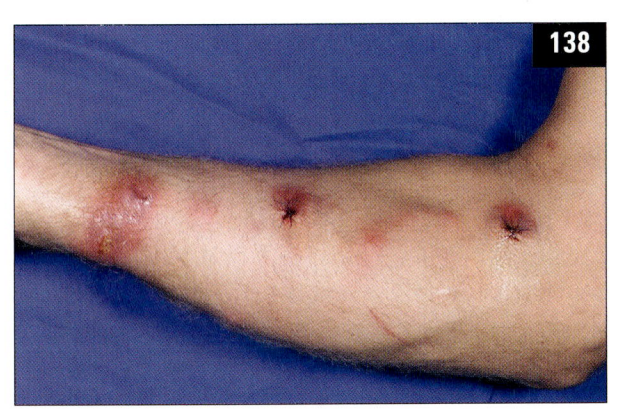

138 Sporotrichosis is a deep-tissue fungal infection that often yields scaling and/or weeping nodules that migrate up the lymphatic drainage patterns of an extremity.

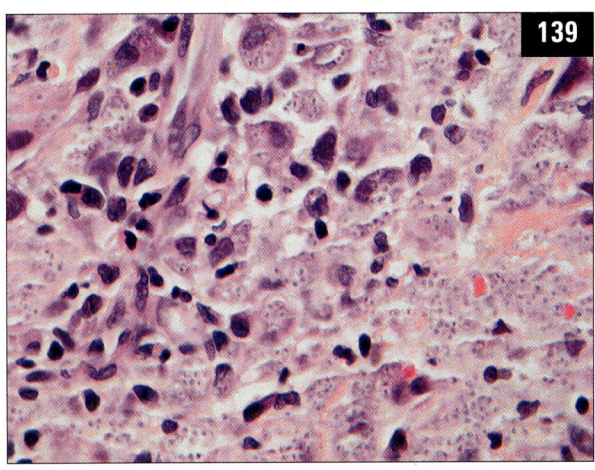

139 In tissue, *Histoplasma capsulatum*, the causative organism of histoplasmosis, exists as an intracellular organisms (2–5 microns) within histiocytes.

later may develop a small granuloma within the lungs. The minority of patients who develop clinically appreciable disease are usually immunocompromised (HIV/AIDS) or are exposed to very large inoculums (spelunkers in caves with bat guano) (Lottenberg *et al.*, 1979). Disseminated forms of histoplasmosis may involve the reticuloendothelial system, the bone marrow, the nervous system, or the skin. Cutaneous lesions are present in only about 10% of patients with disseminated disease (Cohen *et al.*, 1990). Maculopapular eruptions, skin ulcerations, or oropharyngeal lesions may be observed.

Tissue biopsy from skin lesions of histoplasmosis may reveal yeast within macrophages (**139**). The sensitivity in some series, however, has been less than 50% and often multiple diagnostic modalities are employed (Wheat, 2006). The histopathologic appearance is roughly similar to leishmaniasis; however, yeast forms of histoplasmosis are evenly spaced, demonstrate a pseudocapsule, and lack the kinetoplast common to amastigotes of leishmaniasis (Olofinlade & Cacciarelli, 2000).

Isolated and asymptomatic pulmonary histoplasmosis requires no treatment. Patients with disseminated histoplasmosis are often treated with IV amphotericin B, possibly with oral itraconazole used as a maintenance medication (Kauffman, 2002).

NORTH AMERICAN BLASTOMYCOSIS

North American blastomycosis (Gilchrist's disease) refers to an unusual fungal infection caused by the dimorphic fungus *Blastomyces dermatitidis*. This fungus is particularly prevalent in the central and southeastern United States (the Mississippi and Ohio river valleys and the Great Lakes region), with hyperendemic areas noted in Wisconsin (Davies & Sarosi, 1997). North American blastomycosis has been associated with exposure to shallow lakes and waterways, and it is a common fungal infection in dogs (Bromel & Sykes, 2005; Baumgardner *et al.*, 2006). Despite the name, North American blastomycosis has been described throughout the world.

Exposure to blastomycosis occurs through inhalation of aerosolized conidia. Unlike histoplasmosis, blastomycosis leads to disseminated infection in about 50% of cases. Those with immunocompromised states or chronic health issues may be predisposed to systemic infection. The skin is the most common extra-pulmonary site of infection, with involvement in approximately 20% of disseminated cases; other sites of involvement may include the bones (15%), and the central nervous system (5%) (Lemos *et al.*, 2000).

In cutaneous blastomycosis, lesions usually occur upon the face, neck, and extremities. The skin lesions are non-specific. Early in the course, papules or pustules may exist, and ulceration and scarring may eventuate. Often the lesions may be verrucous in appearance (Bradley *et al.*, 2006).

Tissue biopsy of blastomycosis may reveal yeast 8–20 μm in diameter, with broad-based buds and doubly refractile walls (**140**) (Adams *et al.*, 2002). In this regard, blastomycosis may be cautiously distinguished from other fungal infections that exhibit narrow-based budding, such as cryptococcosis. Tissue culture may be used to solidify this morphologic distinction.

Patients with severe blastomycosis, including central nervous system involvement, should be treated with high-dose IV amphotericin B, while oral itraconazole is the drug of choice for mild-to-moderate disease (Bradsher *et al.*, 2003). Prolonged treatment may be necessary in patients with fungal osteomyelitis (bone involvement).

PARACOCCIDIOIDOMYCOSIS (SOUTH AMERICAN BLASTOMYCOSIS)

Paracoccidioidomycosis (South American blastomycosis) refers to fungal infection caused by the dimorphic fungus *Paracoccidioides brasiliensis* (see Chapter 4, Tropical Diseases).

COCCIDIOIDOMYCOSIS

Coccidioidomycosis (**141**) is a fungal infection caused by the dimorphic fungus *Coccidioides immitis*. While sporadic cases occur throughout the world, coccidioidomycosis is particularly associated with the Sonoran Desert of the United States and Mexico, often being referred to as 'San Joaquin Valley Fever' (Crum-Cianflone *et al.*, 2006).

Coccidioidomycosis is caused by the inhalation of arthrospores. Sixty percent of cases are asymptomatic and resolve spontaneously (Chiller *et al.*, 2003). Low-grade fever, chest pain, or chills may be present in some limited pulmonary infections.

In immunocompromised patients (HIV/AIDS), certain ethnic subgroups (blacks and Filipinos), or occasionally in pregnant women or those with chronic health issues, disseminated disease may occur (Rosenstein *et al.*, 2001). In the disseminated form (<5% of symptomatic cases), the infection may spread to the bones, lungs, liver, meninges, visceral organs, or skin. Skin lesions are often non-specific (Crum, 2005).

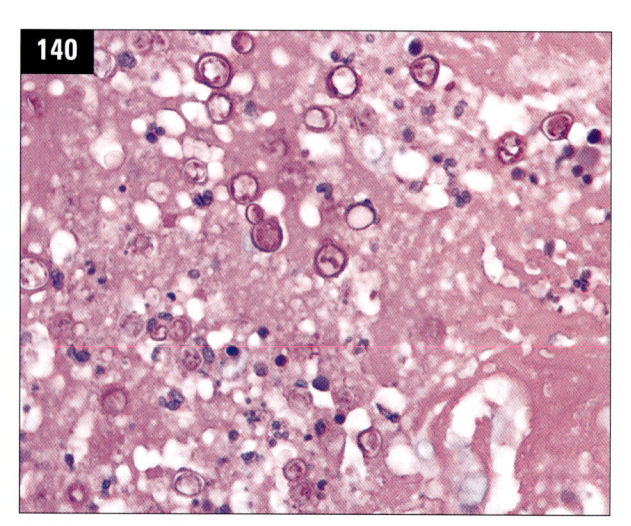

140 In tissue, *Blastomyces dermatitidis*, the causative organism of blastomycosis, exists as yeast that produces daughter cells via broad-based budding.

Fungal Infections

Also, cutaneous reactions to the infection, including erythema nodosum and erythema multiforme may occur in patients with coccidioidomycosis (**142**) (DiCaudo *et al.*, 2006). The development of erythema nodosum has often been associated with a favorable prognosis, particularly during pregnancy (Arsura *et al.*, 1998).

Tissue biopsy of coccidioidomycosis often reveals characteristic 30–60 µm spherules that contain numerous endospores (**143**). These spherules of coccidioidomycosis are much smaller than those of rhinosporidiosis. The diagnosis is easily confirmed with culture or serologic studies. If culture is performed, it is imperative to notify the laboratory of the suspected diagnosis beforehand, due to the high infectivity of the arthrospores that will develop within cultured material (CDC, 1993). Rarely, an interstitial granulomatous dermatitis without organisms, assumed to be reactive in nature, may be the presenting feature of pulmonary coccidioidomycosis (Dicaudo & Connolly, 2001).

Patients with asymptomatic or mild pulmonary coccidioidomycosis require no treatment. Those with disseminated disease may require oral fluconazole, oral intraconazole, or IV amphotericin B. Successful use of combination treatment with capsofungin and fulconazole has also been described (Park *et al.*, 2006).

141 The skin lesions of coccidioidomycosis are not specific, but disseminated disease is more common in immunocompromised persons and in certain ethnic groups, including blacks and Filipinos. (Courtesy of Larry Anderson, MD.)

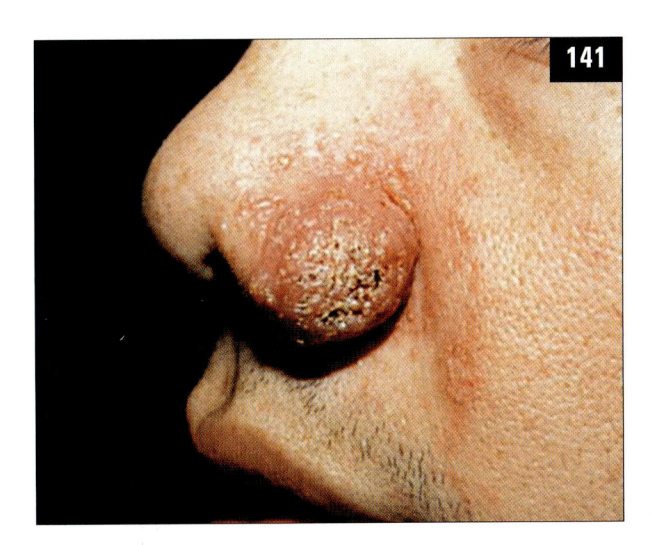

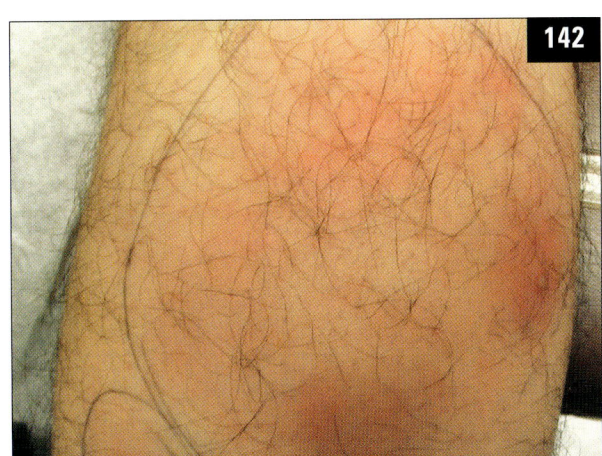

142 The skin lesions of coccidioidomycosis may be verrucous, nodular, or cellulitic.

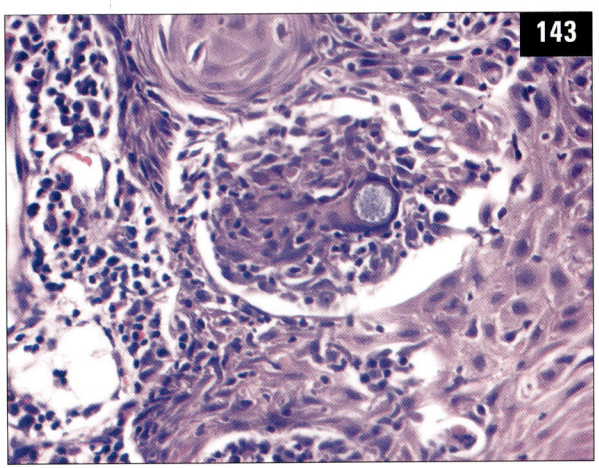

143 Skin biopsy of coccidioidomycosis demonstrates spherules (60–100 microns) in tissue with central endospores.

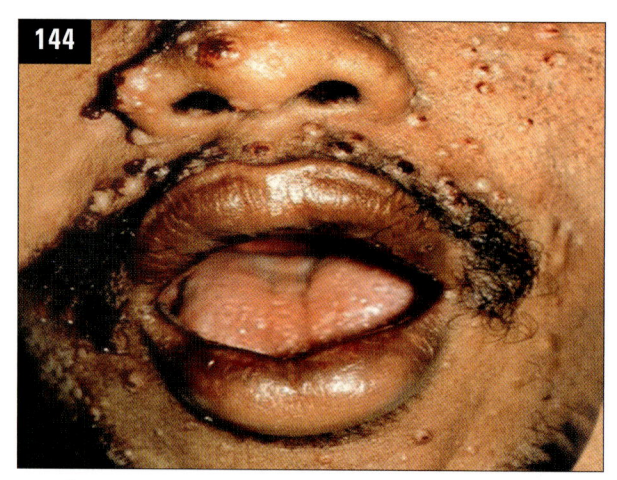

144 Cryptococcosis in immunocompromised patients often mimics the lesions of diffuse molluscum contagiosum.

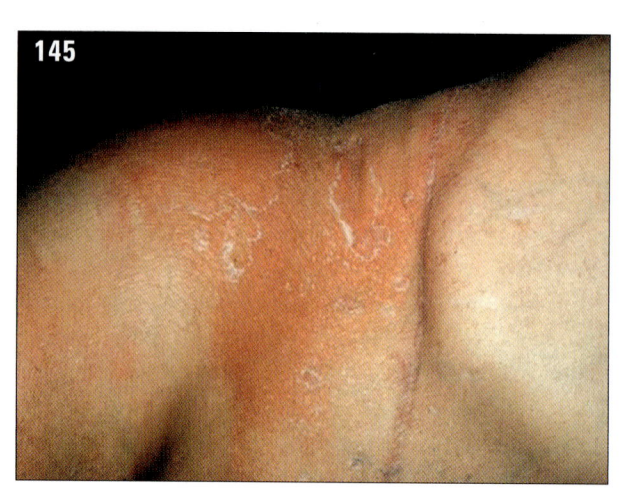

145 Cellulitis-like variant of cryptococcosis.

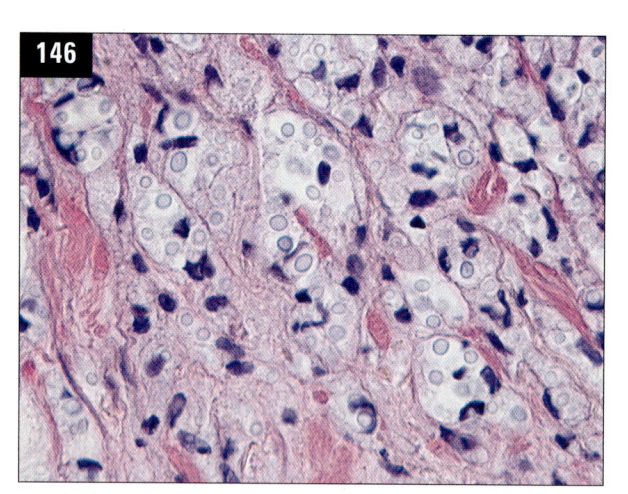

146 In tissue processed for histologic sections, the thick gelatinous capsule of *Cryptococcus neoformans* is lost leading to empty spaces surrounding pleomorphic organisms.

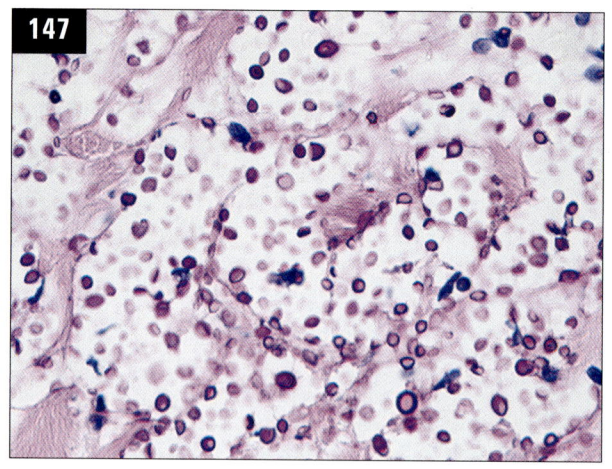

147 PAS staining of *Cryptococcus neoformans* highlights the cell wall and not the capsule.

CRYPTOCOCCOSIS

Cryptococcosis is a fungal infection caused by the encapsulated yeast *Cryptococcus neoformans*. Four serotypes exist: serotypes A and D (*C. neoformans var. neoformans*), and serotypes B and C (*C. neoformans var. gattii*). Serotypes A and D are most common in the United States, and are often found in association with pigeon excrement (Litvintseva et al., 2005). Worldwide, serotype A causes most cryptococcal infections in patients who are immunocompromised, particularly in those patients infected with HIV (Imwidthaya & Poungvarin, 2000).

Cryptococcosis is typically a systemic infection that begins in the lungs but disseminates widely. Often the disease is not diagnosed until meningeal symptoms are detected. The skin is affected in only about 10–15% of cases (Murakawa et al., 1996). Cutaneous lesions of cryptococcosis often resemble molluscum, another disease common to HIV/AIDS (**144**). A cellulitis-like variant of cryptococcosis is also well described in immunocompromised patients (**145**) (Anderson et al., 1992).

Tissue biopsy of cryptococcosis (**146, 147**) often reveals two general histological patterns: (1) a mucoid pauci-inflammatory form, and (2) a granulomatous inflammatory form. The yeast organisms are pleomorphic, and narrow-based budding may be identified. A thick mucoid capsule that surrounds them is lost to processing, leaving an empty halo. This mucoid capsule highlights with mucicarmine, while the fungal wall itself highlights with PAS staining. The diagnosis is easily further established with serologic studies (serum cryptococcal antigen). Performance of lumbar puncture after computed tomography (CT), is essentially requisite in all immunocompromised patients with evidence of extrapulmonary cryptococcosis, due to the high likelihood of meningeal involvement, even if it is subclinical (Saag et al., 2000).

Patients with disseminated cryptococcosis will require consultation with an infectious disease expert. Intravenous amphotericin B and chronic therapy with fluconazole are commonly utilized in treating disseminated disease.

LOBOMYCOSIS

Lobomycosis represents another largely regional fungal infection. The disease is caused by *Lacazia loboi* (formerly *Loboa loboi*), and most cases arise in the Amazon region (see Chapter 4, Tropical Diseases).

HYALOHYPHOMYCOSIS (ASPERGILLOSIS AND FUSARIOSIS)

Hyalohyphomycosis is an invasive fungal infection caused by various species of the genera *Aspergillus* and *Fusarium*. Typically, the infection begins first in the pulmonary system, via inhalation of spores, with subsequent dissemination to other organ systems, including the skin. In immunosuppressed patients, particularly those with neutropenia, aspergillosis is a major cause of morbidity and mortality. Severe disseminated aspergillosis has been associated with a mortality rate of 60–90% (Lin et al., 2001).

Clinically, cutaneous hyalohyphomycosis most often begins as erythematous or violaceous papules or plaques. Involvement of the extremities is more common than truncal lesions. The lesions are often tender. Because of the vasculotropic nature of the fungus, these papules and plaques often evolve rapidly into hemorrhagic vesicles and, ultimately, into black eschars (**148**). Primary cutaneous infections may also develop at sites of venous access, often due to contaminated dressing materials or abrasion of the skin by adhesive tape.

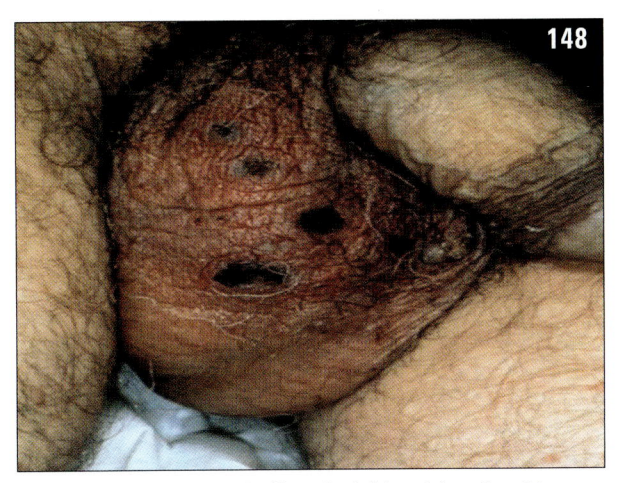

148 Hyalohyphomycosis (fusariosis) involving the skin often yields crusted and eschar-like lesions.

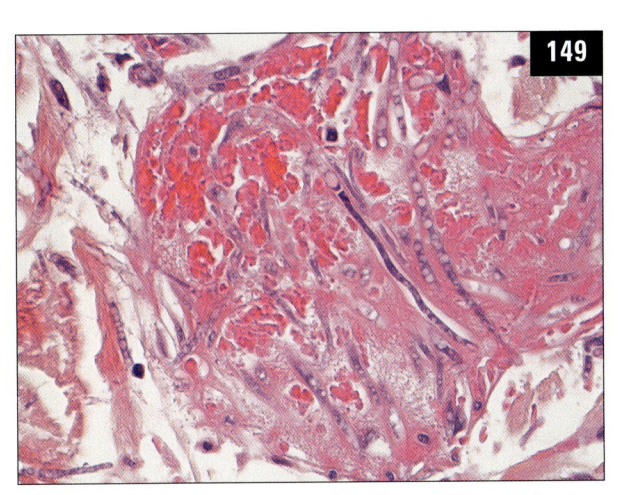

149 Hyalohyphomycosis caused by *Aspergillus* species in tissue often demonstrates vasculotropic hyphae with prominent cytoplasm with regular septae.

Histopathologic examination of cutaneous aspergillosis often demonstrates vasculotropic hyphae of less than 5 μm in diameter, with prominent cytoplasm, a thin delicate wall, and associated inflammation and vessel destruction (**149**). It is widely taught that aspergillus demonstrates dichotomous branching (45°), but in truth this quality is difficult to appreciate in histologic sections. Subtle but regular septae may be identified within the hyphae of aspergillus, and this is a point of discrimination from *Mucor* and *Rhizopus* species. *Fusarium* may look identical in tissue or may demonstrate characteristic vesicular swellings (**150**). The diagnosis may be confirmed with culture, as apergillus forms characteristic fruiting heads which readily facilitate identification.

The new antifungal voriconazole has emerged as the drug of choice for disseminated aspergillosis (Mays *et al.*, 2006). Still, systemic aspergillosis, particularly when associated with a persistent or uncorrectable neutropenia, often heralds a disappointing outcome (van Burik *et al.*, 1998).

Risk factors for disseminated fusariosis include severe immunosuppression, neutropenia, lymphopenia, and corticosteroids use (Dignani & Anaissie, 2004). It should be emphasized that it may be impossible to discriminate between aspergillus and fusarium species based on histopathology alone and culture is almost always necessary (Sampathkumar & Paya, 2001). On culture, fusarium forms characteristic canoe-shaped or banana-shaped macroconidia. Mortality from disseminated fusarium infections in immunocompromised patients is high (>80%), particularly when an accompanying neutropenia cannot be corrected. Limited success has been reported with high-dose amphotericin B, voriconazole, and posaconazole.

PHAEOHYPHOMYCOSIS

Phaeohyphomycosis (**151**) occurs in immunocompetent patients as indolent cystic lesions after traumatic implantation of a splinter. In immunocompromised patients, disseminated phaeohyphomycosis presents with leathery eschars with erythematous edematous rims (**152**) similar to those of hyalohyphomycosis. Itraconazole has been used most frequently, but antifungal therapy is unreliable and surgical debridement is an essential aspect of therapy.

MUCORMYCOSIS

Mucormycosis (**153–155**) is a term that refers to several different diseases due to fungi in the order Mucorales. Mucorales includes ubiquitous fungi commonly found in soil or decaying matter. *Rhizopus* is the most common causative genus, but various species of *Rhizomucor*, *Absidia*, and *Mucor*, among others, have been implicated (Chayakulkeeree *et al.*, 2006). Despite prevalence in the environment, mucormycosis is an unusual infection because of low virulence of the organisms, which affect mainly those with immunocompromising conditions. Hosts with

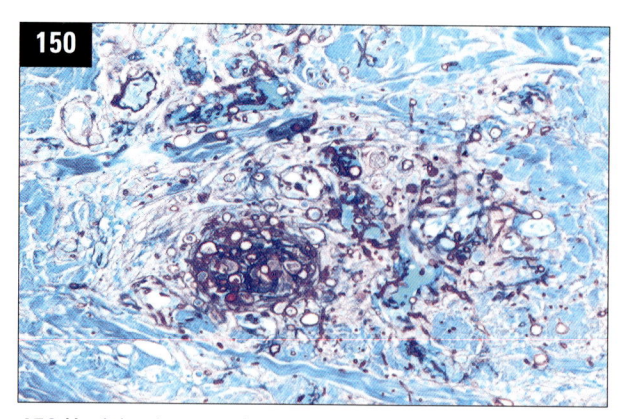

150 Hyalohyphomycosis caused by *Fusarium* species in tissue may appear identical to that of *Aspergillus* species, or it may demonstrate characteristic vesicular swellings.

Fungal Infections

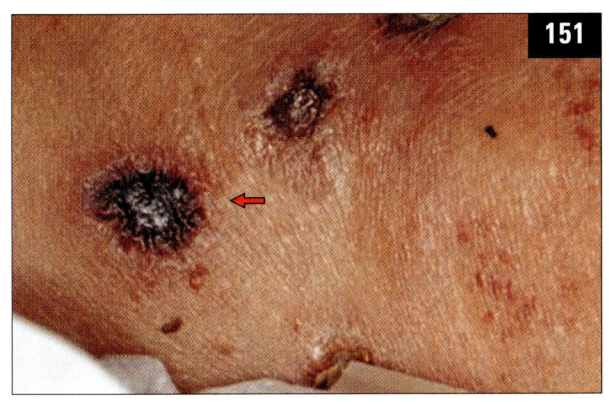

151 Disseminated phaeohyphomycosis in the skin often yields eschar-like lesions with surrounding erythema similar to those of hyalohyphomycosis.

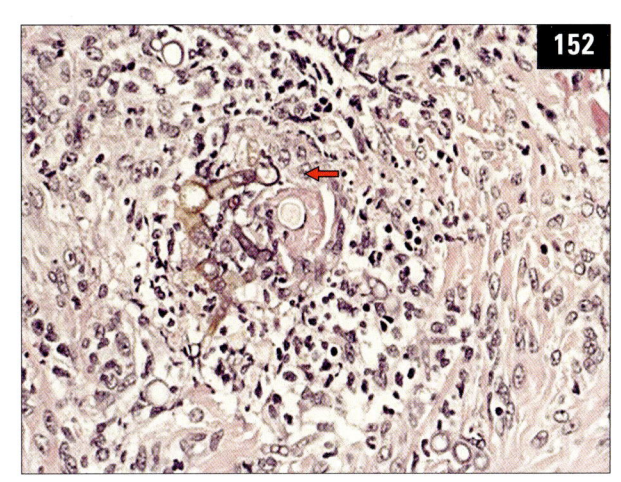

152 In tissue, phaeohyphomycosis produces pigmented hyphae with thick refractile walls, vesicular swellings, and visible cytoplasm.

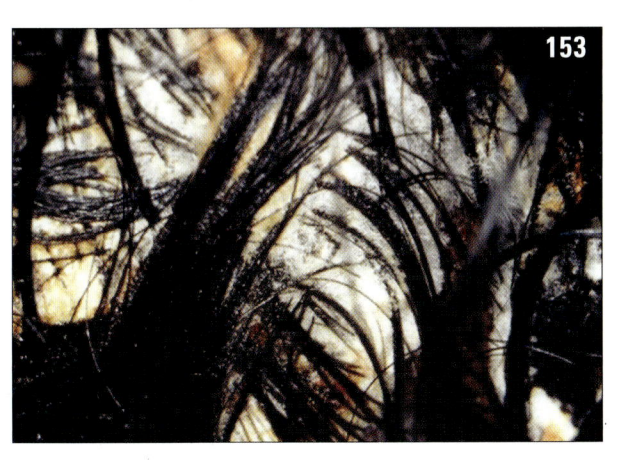

153 Mucormycosis is caused by rapidly proliferating pathogens that can create white, cotton-like growths on the surface of the affected skin, in this case, the scalp.

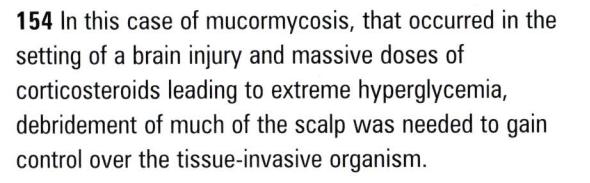

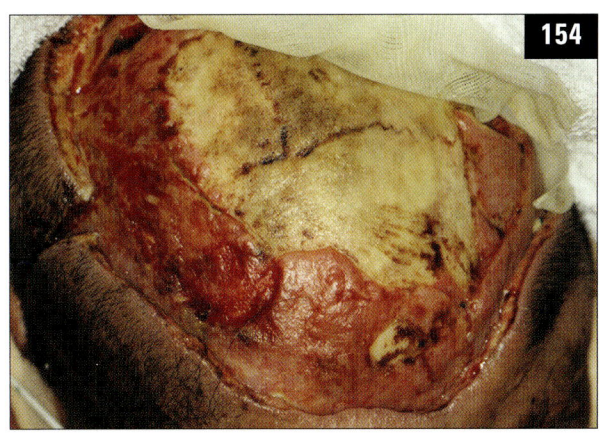

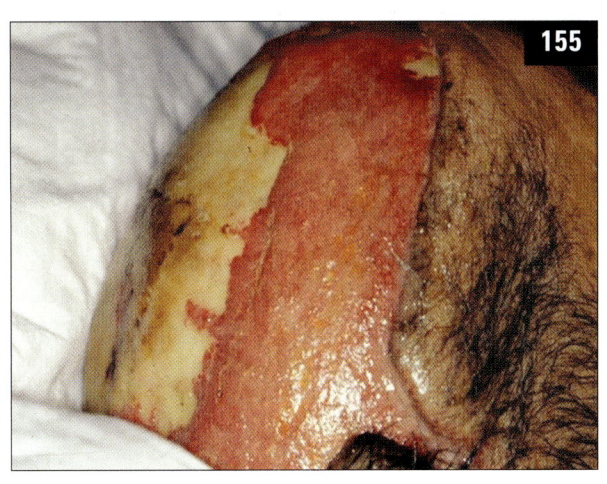

154 In this case of mucormycosis, that occurred in the setting of a brain injury and massive doses of corticosteroids leading to extreme hyperglycemia, debridement of much of the scalp was needed to gain control over the tissue-invasive organism.

155 The presence of granulation tissue over the exposed calvarium after cure of the infection by surgical excision.

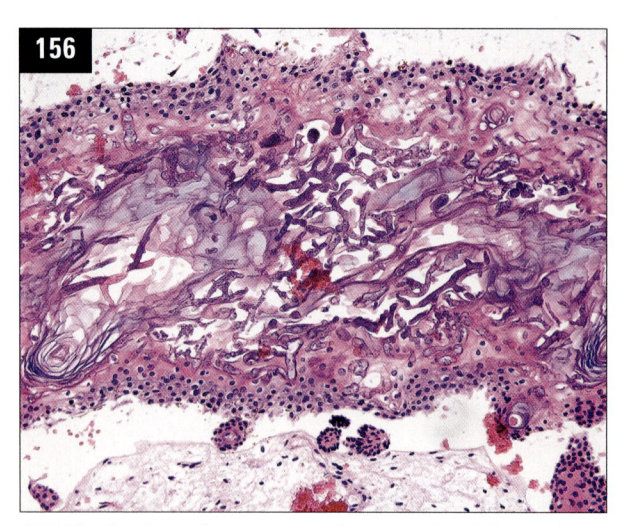

156 The hyphae of mucormycosis are eosinophilic, hollow, broad, aseptate, and often demonstrated obtuse branching.

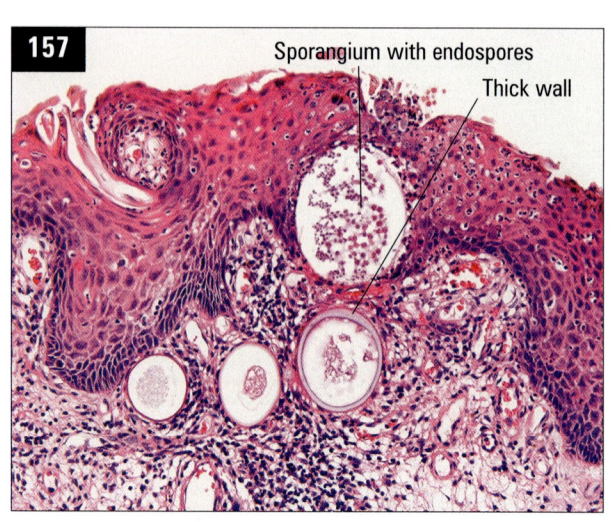

157 Rhinosporidiosis in tissue is characterized by large sporangium (100–450 microns in diameter) with central endospores.

poorly controlled diabetes mellitus (especially with ketoacidosis), those placed on high-dose glucocorticoids, and those with profound neutropenia are at particular risk for mucormycosis. Rare cutaneous-limited disease has been associated with patch testing using ground plant matter (Lesueur *et al.*, 2002).

Cutaneous findings of disseminated mucormycosis, like aspergillosis, include progressive black necrotic lesions caused by vascular invasion and destruction. The central face is a common area of involvement, and is of particular concern as invasion into the central nervous system yields disastrous results. Histopathology of mucormycosis demonstrates broad (5–20 µm), essentially non-septate to sparsely septate, ribbon-like hyphae (**156**) (Frater *et al.*, 2001). In contrast to aspergillosis, the hyphae of mucormycosis are associated with right-angle branching, although this may be difficult to appreciate on thin histologic sections. Neutrophilic abscesses, vessel invasion, and tissue infarction are often well-demonstrated. Tissue culture yields rapid confirmation of the suspected diagnosis.

Successful treatment of mucormycosis depends upon rapid diagnosis and aggressive coordinated medical and surgical therapy. High-dose amphotericin B and generous debridement of necrotic tissue are commonly employed. Even with such measures, the mortality in mucormycosis is often 50–85% (Mendoza *et al.*, 2005).

RELATED INFECTIONS

RHINOSPORIDIOSIS

Rhinosporidiosis was originally thought to be a fungal infection, but recent molecular techniques have shown the infecting organism, *Rhinosporidium seeberi*, to be an aquatic protistan parasite of fish and mammals (Hussein & Rashad, 2005). Although most cases of rhinosporidiosis occur in persons from the Indian subcontinent or Sri Lanka, the organism is also endemic to South America and Africa. The infection is acquired by traumatic implantation.

Clinically, rhinosporidiosis presents as a chronic granulomatous infection of mucosal epithelium. Infection of the nose and/or nasopharynx is observed in 70% of cases, while infection of the palpebral conjunctivae or lacrimal structures comprises around 15% of cases (Kumari *et al.*, 2005). Soft polyps result from infections and these sessile, friable, and hemorrhagic polyps are often described as 'strawberry-like' in appearance.

Tissue from rhinosporidiosis demonstrates large, thick-walled spherules 100–450 µm in diameter, that may contain up to several thousand endospores (**157**). These structures are similar in structure to the much smaller spherules of *Coccidioides immitis* (30–60 µm in diameter). An acute and chronic inflammatory infiltrate, papillomatous hyperplasia, and hypervascularity are also often observed.

There are limited anecdotal reports of medical treatment of rhinosporidiosis with dapsone, yet the treatment of choice remains surgical extirpation of involved skin (Vijaikumar et al., 2002). Wide local excision with electrocoagulation of the wound base is thought to decrease the incidence of recurrence.

PROTOTHECOSIS

Protothecosis, caused by *Prototheca wickerhamii*, represents another rare infection caused by an organism originally suspected to be a fungus, but then later reclassified as a type of achloric alga (Kantrow & Boyd, 2003). The organism is ubiquitous in aqueous locales, and infection occurs as a result of traumatic inoculation in contaminated water. Most cases in the United States occur in the southeast, although cases from virtually every region of the world have been reported.

Patients typically present with an isolated plaque or nodule of the skin, with or without ulceration. Erythema and pain may be reported. Patients with olecranon bursitis from protothecosis may present with painful swelling and mild erythema of the elbow. In severely immunocompromised individuals, cutaneous lesions can be widespread or the alga may be present in the blood.

Tissue from cutaneous protothecosis demonstrates characteristic sporangia consisting of a central rounded endospore (2–4 µm) surrounded by a corona of molded endospores forming a morula-like, frambesiform structure (158). The histologic diagnosis can be confirmed with tissue culture on Sabouraud's agar, which yields white-beige colonies within 48 hours when grown at room temperature.

Protothecosis is a difficult infection to treat. For cases amenable to surgical excision, this represents the preferred treatment. Patients with disseminated disease have been treated with IV amphotericin B. Ketoconazole, itraconazole, and fluconazole have also been wed according to anecdotal reports. Protothecosis has also been successfully treated with voriconazole, a triazole antifungal (Dalmau et al., 2006).

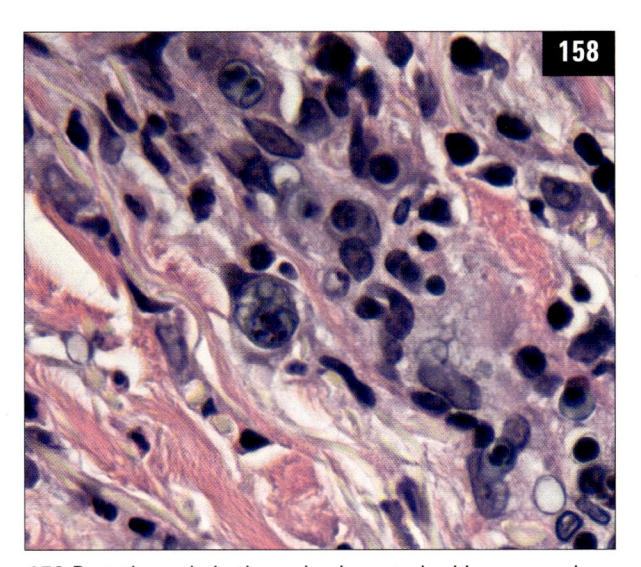

158 Protothecosis in tissue is characterized by sporangia consisting of a central rounded endospore surrounded by a corona of molded endospores yielding a morula-like ('soccer-ball' or 'berry-like') structure.

CHAPTER 3

VIRAL DISEASES

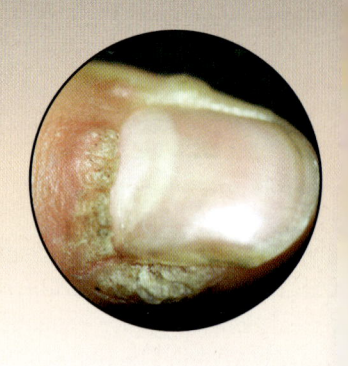

Anita Arora   Natalia Mendoza   Adriana Motta   Vandana Madkan   Stephen K Tyring

INTRODUCTION

Herpes and pox viruses are the most important viral skin pathogens. Herpes infection affects most of the human population at some time in their lives. Given the prevalence and morbidity associated with these diseases, physicians should be skilled in diagnosis and treatment.

HERPES SIMPLEX INFECTION

Herpes simplex virus type I (HSV-1) has been more frequently associated with orolabial herpes and herpes simplex virus type II (HSV-2) with genital infection (Wildly, 1973). However, recent studies have shown an increasing incidence of genital infection attributed to HSV-1 (Nahmias *et al.*, 1990). Transmission of HSV can occur during both asymptomatic and symptomatic episodes of viral shedding. HSV-1 is largely spread through direct contact with contaminated saliva or other infected secretions. HSV-2 is primarily spread through sexual contact.

HSV infections (**159–169**) are characterized by primary and recurrent vesicular eruptions.

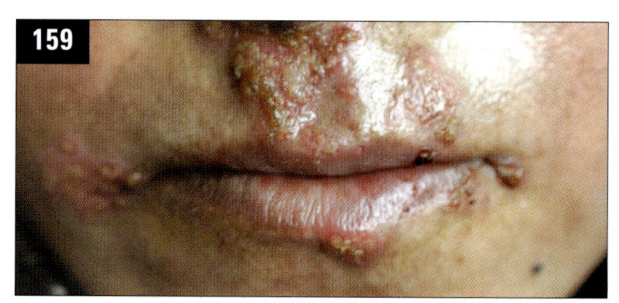

159 Herpes simplex infection in a typical distribution on the upper lip.

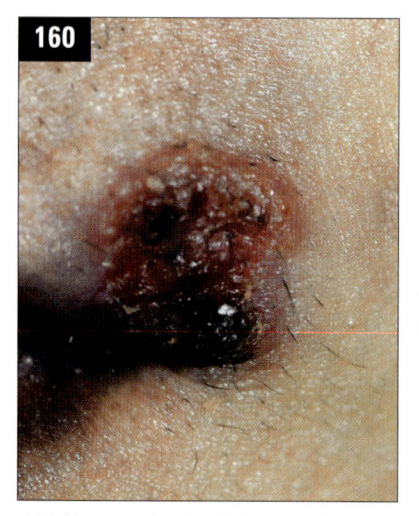

160 Herpes simplex infection. Crusted and hemorrhagic lesions are common.

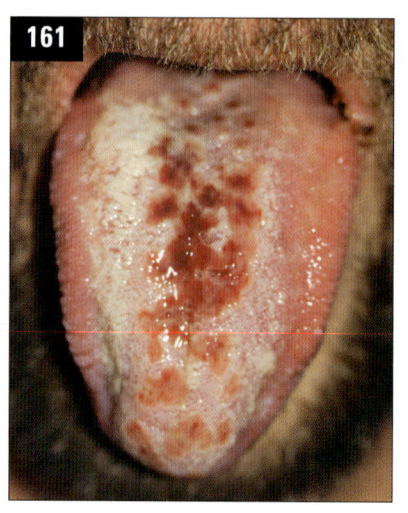

161 Herpes simplex infection. The herpetiform grouping of tongue lesions is characteristic.

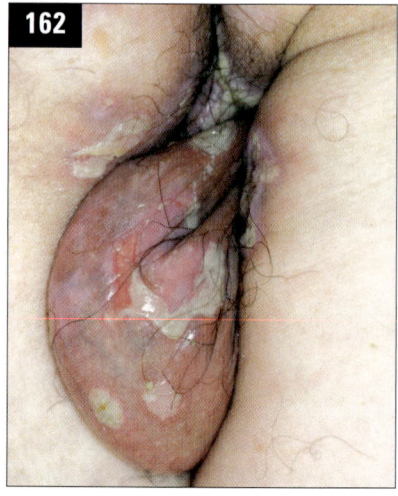

162 Herpes simplex infection. Lesions can be quite painful and spread locally via autoinoculation.

Viral Diseases

163 Chronic ulcerative herpes simplex infection is seen in immunosuppressed patients. The thread-like rolled border is characteristic.

164 Disseminated herpes simplex infection in an immunocompromized host.

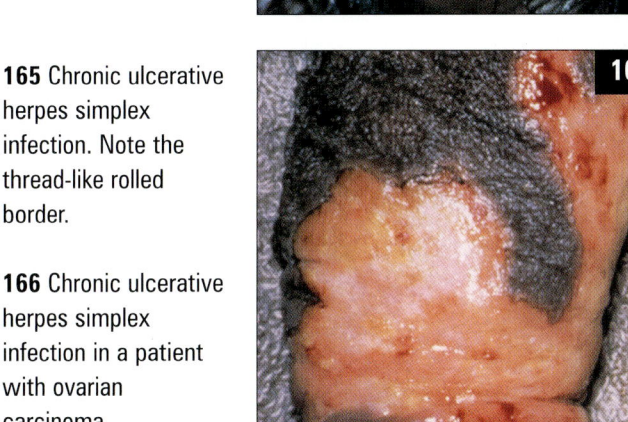

165 Chronic ulcerative herpes simplex infection. Note the thread-like rolled border.

166 Chronic ulcerative herpes simplex infection in a patient with ovarian carcinoma.

167 Herpes simplex infection with characteristic herpetiform grouping.

168 Herpes simplex infection with characteristic herpetiform grouping.

169 Herpes simplex infection reactivation after sun exposure.

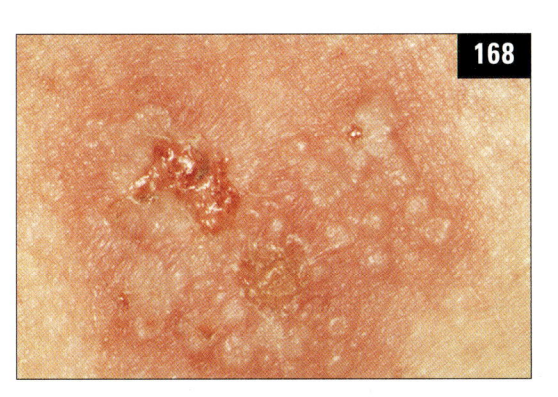

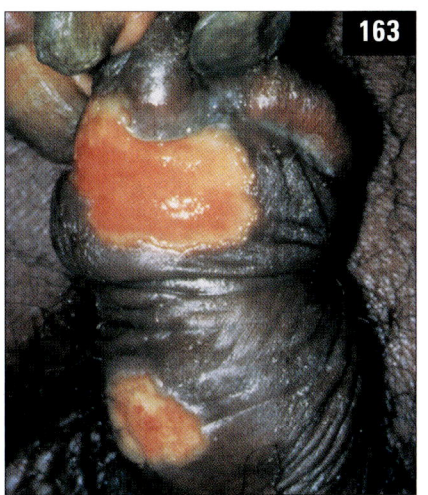

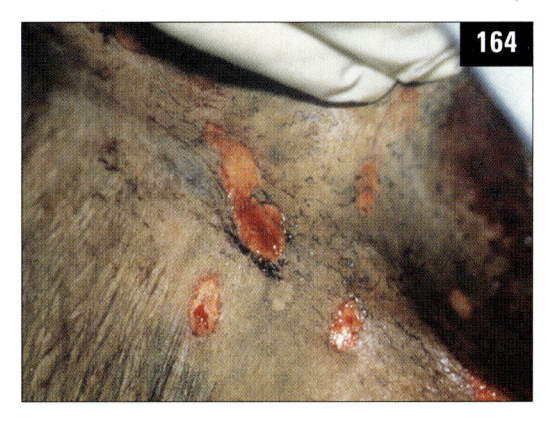

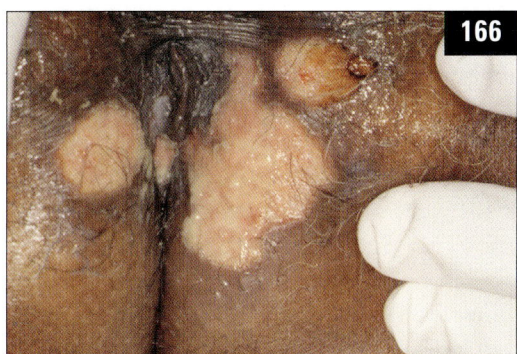

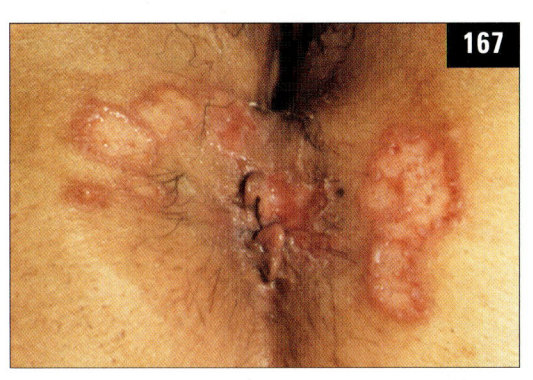

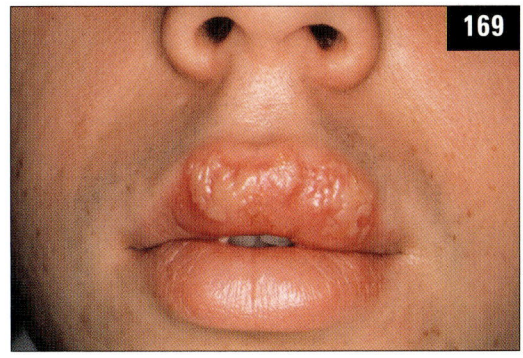

Viral Diseases

Initial infections of HSV usually present with multiple lesions that are often described as vesicles on an erythematous base, with progression to pustules and/or ulcerations. Healing often takes from 2–6 weeks for full crusting of the lesions and resolution of symptoms. Outbreaks following the initial infection are generally accompanied with fewer lesions as well as less associated prodrome such as burning, pain, or tenderness over the affected area. Initial infection with orolabial herpes presents as a gingivostomatitis in children. Subsequent lesions appear most often on the vermillion border of the lip. In immunocompromised individuals, recurrent herpes infections can affect the oral soft mucosa or result in chronic ulcers with a rolled border (Yeung-Yue et al., 2002b).

Genital herpes infections are generally linked to a more severe clinical picture, with resulting painful, erosive balanitis, vulvitis, or vaginitis. In women, in severe cases, the cervix, the buttocks, and perineum can be involved. In men, lesions tend to occur on the glans penis or penile shaft.

Severe HSV infections can occur in immunocompromised individuals. The most common clinical feature is an enlarging ulceration, although lesions can appear at multiple sites in addition to cutaneous dissemination. Lesions are often atypical, with verrucous, exophytic, pustular, or ulcerative appearance.

Herpetic whitlow is a HSV infection of the digits and often affects children, dental, and medical personnel who do not routinely use gloves (170).

Acquisition through digital/genital contact can also occur. Herpes gladiatorum results from those in contact sports such as wrestling, and generates a disseminated cutaneous infection subsequent to the athlete coming into direct contact with infected lesions. Further, females who are infected during childbirth with an ongoing infection and deliver vaginally, are at risk of infecting newborns. Infection often presents at the site of the fetal scalp monitor (171, 172). In newborns, cutaneous manifestations can progress to disseminated infections (Corey et al., 1983). In individuals with atopic dermatitis, widespread eczema herpeticum may occur (173–180). Finally, erythema multiforme and

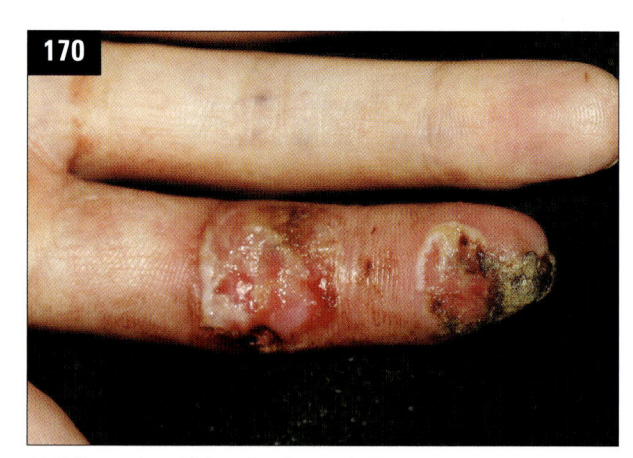

170 Herpetic whitlow is often misdiagnosed as bacterial infection.

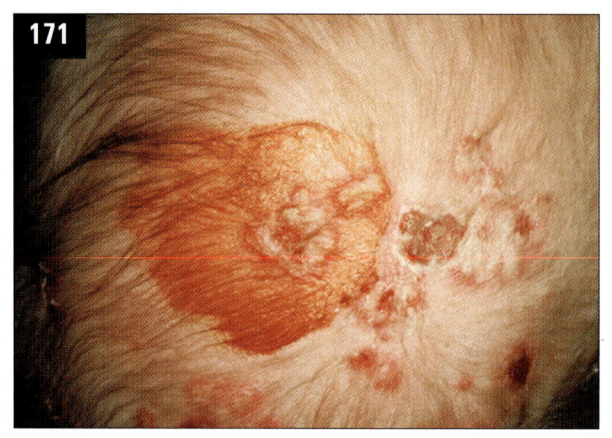

171 Infection with herpes simplex at the site of the fetal scalp monitor.

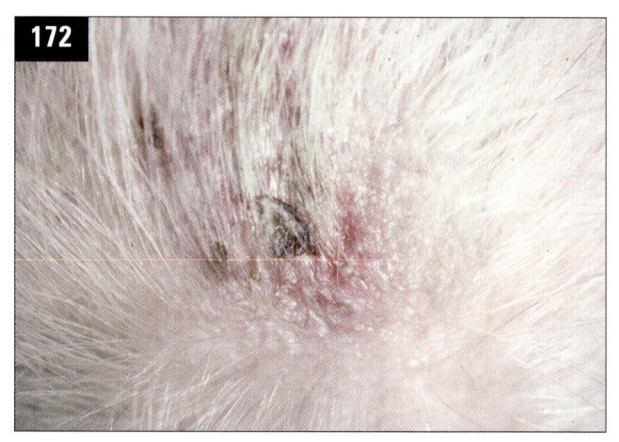

172 Infection with herpes simplex at the site of the fetal scalp monitor. The lesions present within hours to days after birth.

Viral Diseases

173 Eczema herpeticum is often misdiagnosed as impetiginized eczema.

174 Eczema herpeticum. The distinct umbilication of the lesions is characteristic.

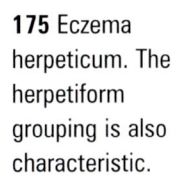

175 Eczema herpeticum. The herpetiform grouping is also characteristic.

176 Eczema herpeticum, heavily crusted lesions.

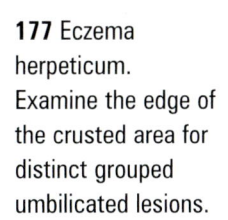

177 Eczema herpeticum. Examine the edge of the crusted area for distinct grouped umbilicated lesions.

178 Eczema herpeticum can involve most of the body surface in patients with atopic dermatitis.

179 Eczema herpeticum. Lesions often spread during shaving.

180 Eczema herpeticum. Distinct umbilication of the lesions.

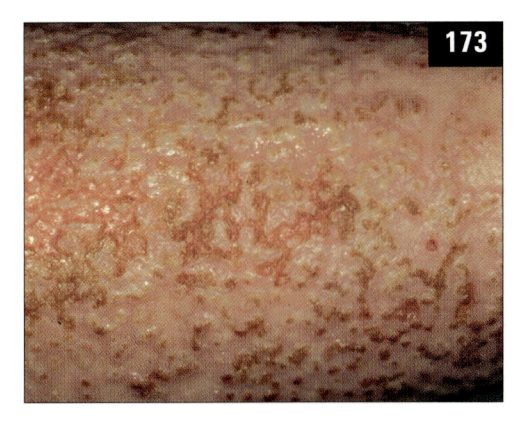

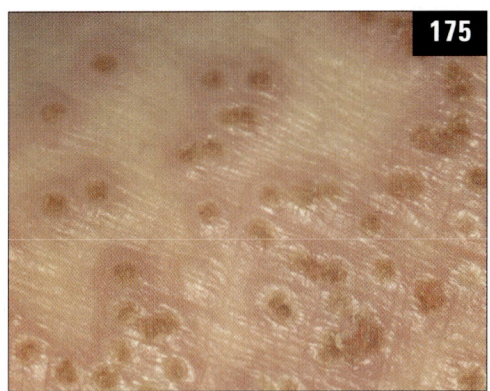

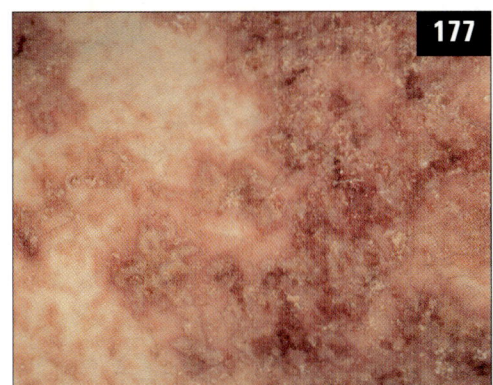

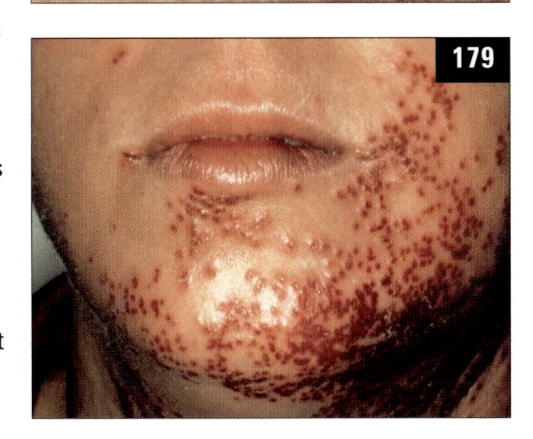

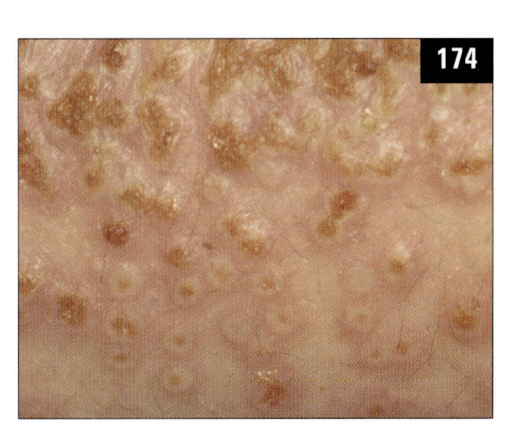

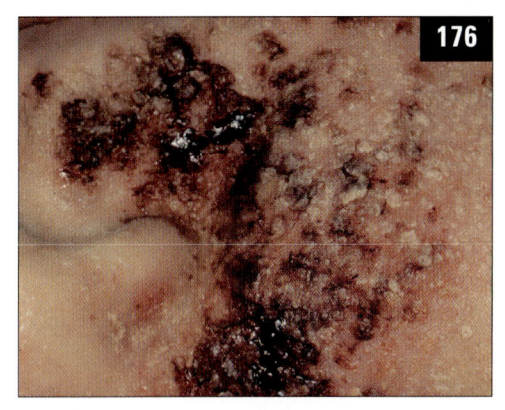

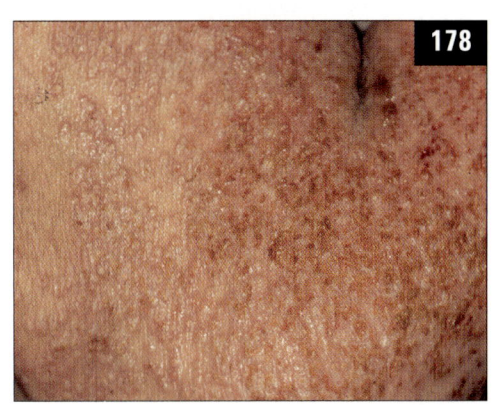

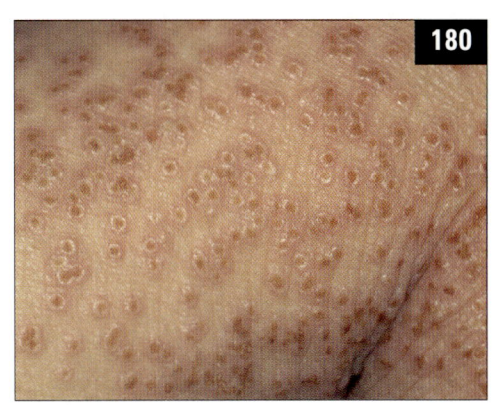

folliculitis are additional cutaneous manifestations of recurrent HSV infection.

HSV infection can be diagnosed by a variety of laboratory tests, including viral culture, direct immunofluorescence, molecular techniques, and serology. Western blot is 99% sensitive and specific for HSV antibodies, and is currently the gold standard of serological diagnosis (Ashley *et al.*, 1988). Four type-specific serologic assays based on type-specific glycoproteins gG-1 from HSV-1 and gG-2 from HSV-2 are currently approved by the United States' Food and Drug Administration (FDA) to distinguish between both HSVs (Corey *et al.*, 1983; Morrow *et al.*, 2005).

Tzanck smears taken from early lesions usually depict multinucleated, epithelial giant cells from the majority of herpetic lesions (Solomon *et al.*,1984) (**181, 182**). Biopsy demonstrates a blister with acantholysis and multinucleated giant cells with peripheral accentuation of nucleoplasm (**183, 184**).

Oral antiviral agents can be initiated at the first sign of symptom or infection and are most effective when taken within 48 hours. For the treatment of recurrent orolabial herpes, oral and topical antiviral creams are available, including oral acyclovir, valacyclovir, famciclovir, and penciclovir cream. In the treatment of primary and recurrent genital herpes, oral antivirals, including acyclovir, famciclovir, and valacyclovir, are available to

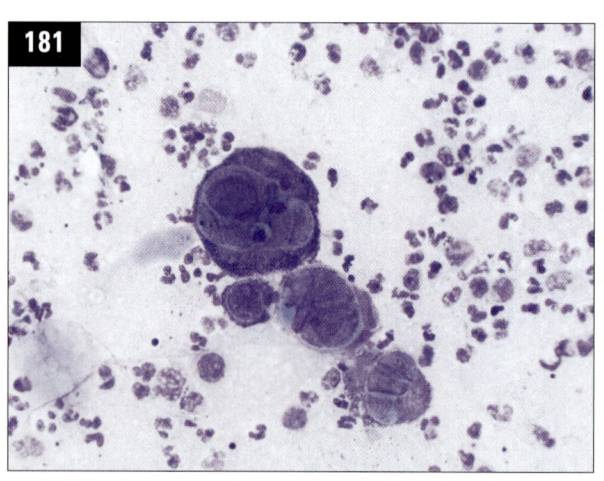

181 Tzanck smear of herpetic lesion. Ballooning degeneration of keratinocytes.

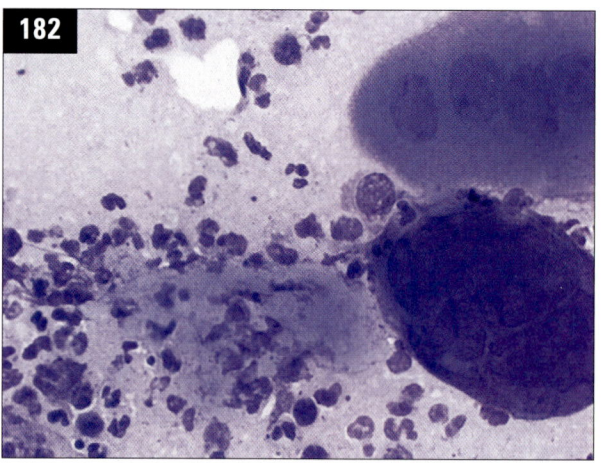

182 Tzanck smear of herpetic lesion. Nuclear molding within ballooned keratinocytes.

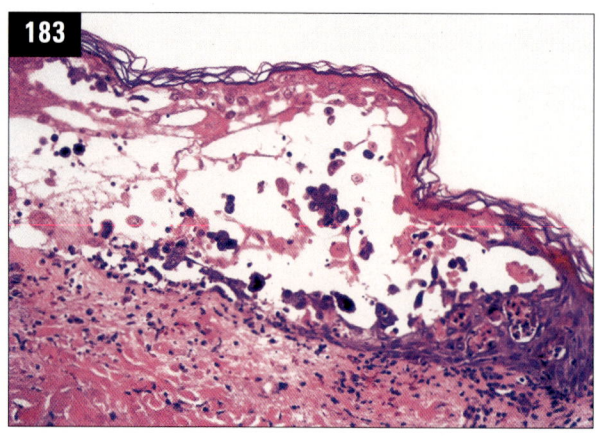

183 Biopsy histopathology. Acantholysis and ballooning degeneration.

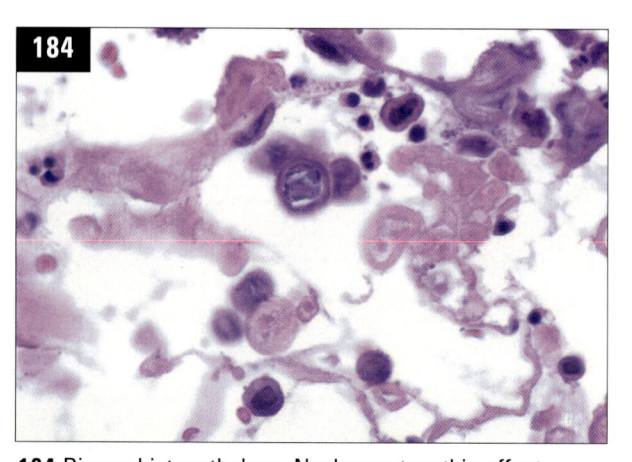

184 Biopsy histopathology. Nuclear cytopathic effect.

reduce the duration of viral shedding, pain, and time of healing (Whitley, 2006). Intravenous acyclovir is indicated for neonatal HSV infection (Kimberlin *et al.*, 2001), severe infections in immunocompromised individuals, and patients with systemic complications. Chronic suppressive therapy for those with recurrent genital herpes is generally reserved for those with six outbreaks per year (Yeung-Yue *et al.*, 2002a).

VARICELLA ZOSTER VIRUS INFECTION

Primary varicella (chickenpox) typically begins as a prodrome of mild fever, malaise, and myalgia followed by an eruption of pruritic, erythematous macules and papules starting on the scalp and face then spreading to the trunk and extremities (**185–188**). Varicella zoster virus (VZV) eventually travels from cutaneous and mucosal lesions to invade dorsal root ganglion cells where it remains until reactivation.

VZV, human herpesvirus 3 (HHV-3) is the etiologic agent of both varicella and herpes zoster. Airborne droplets are the usual route of transmission of primary varicella, although direct contact with vesicular fluid can spread the infection. The incubation period ranges from 10 to 20 days. The affected person can spread the virus until all of the vesicles have crusted (McCrary *et al.*, 1999).

During primary varicella infection, viremia occurs subsequent to an initial 2–4 days of

185 Varicella. Widespread vesicles and crusts in various stages.

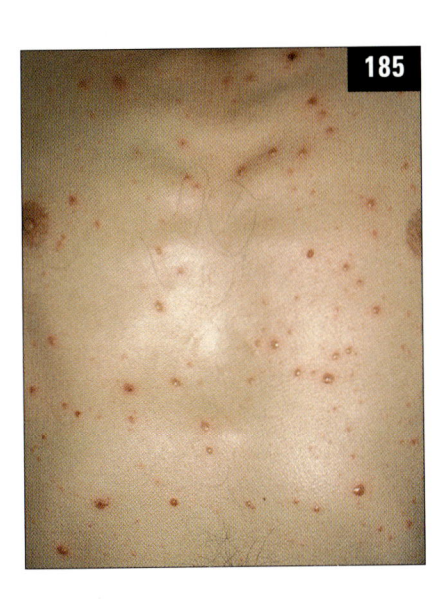

186 Varicella. When all lesions are crusted, the patient is no longer contagious.

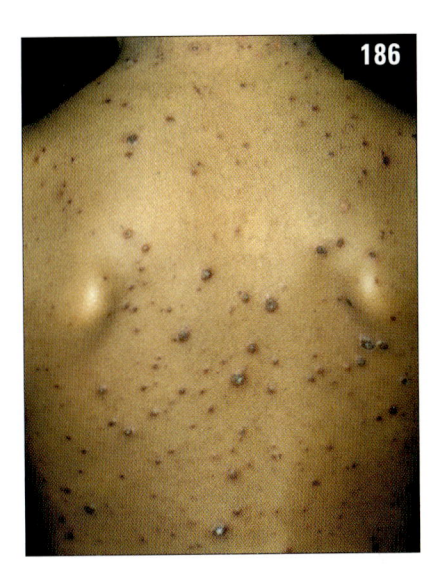

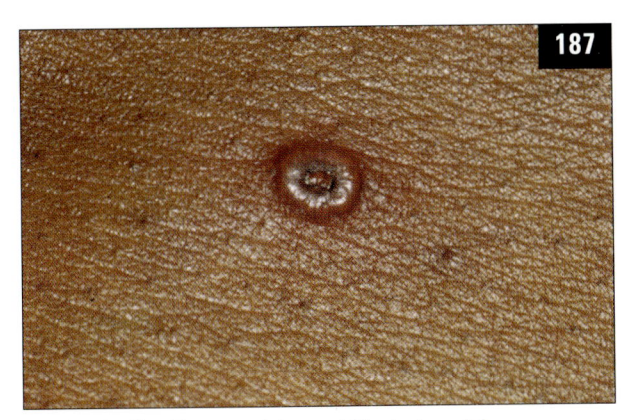

187 Varicella. Characterisitc umbilicated vesicle on an erythematous base.

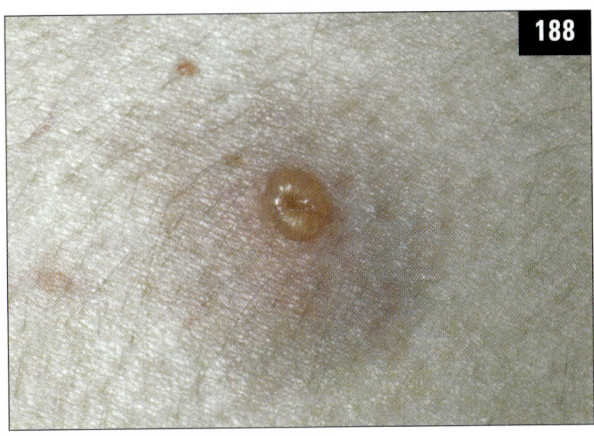

188 Varicella. Umbilicated vesicle. The erythematous base is more apparent in lighter skin.

replication in regional lymph nodes. A secondary viremia arises after a second cycle of viral replication in the liver, spleen, and other organs and seeds the entire body. Approximately 14–16 days post-exposure, the virus then travels to the epidermis by invasion of capillary endothelial cells.

Herpes zoster (shingles) appears upon reactivation of VZV, which can take place suddenly or may be triggered by stress, fever, radiation therapy, tissue damage, or immunosuppression. It often begins as a prodrome of intense pain associated with pruritus, tingling, tenderness, or hyperesthesia in more than 90% of patients. In the majority of cases, a painful eruption of grouped vesicles on an erythematous base develops within a sensory dermatome. The trunk is usually involved, but the face, neck, scalp, or extremity can be involved as well; further, the cutaneous eruption usually involves a single dermatome and rarely crosses the midline (**189–199**).

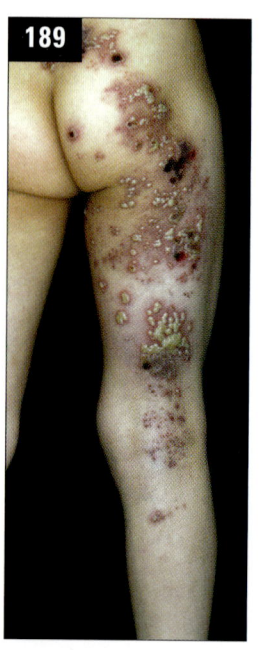

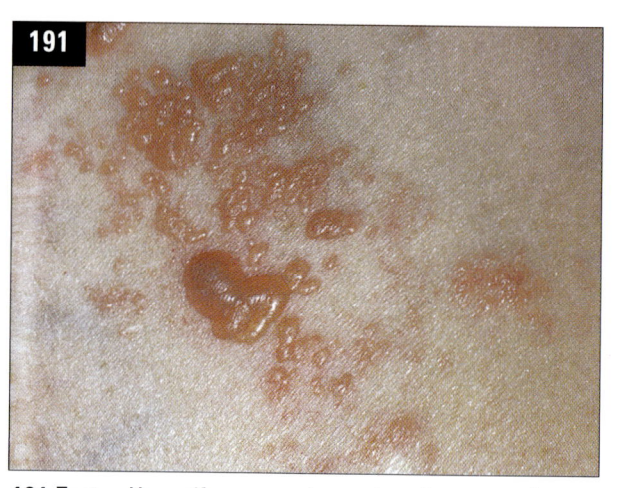

191 Zoster. Herpetiform grouping and coalescence of vesicles.

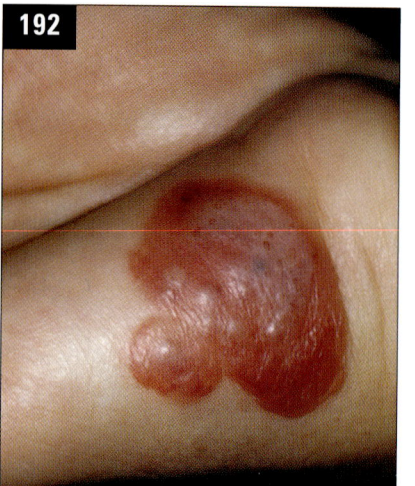

189 Zoster. Typical dermatomal involvement.

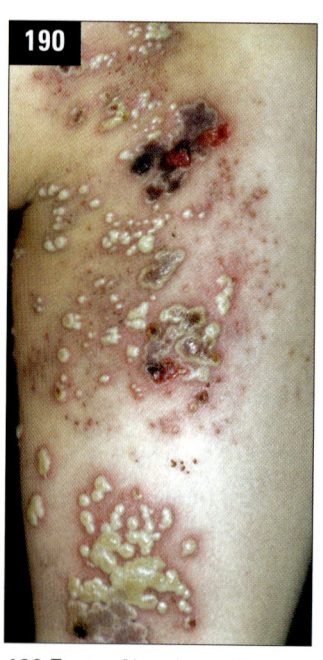

190 Zoster. Note herpetiform grouping of vesicles.

192 Zoster. Circinate grouping of lesions.

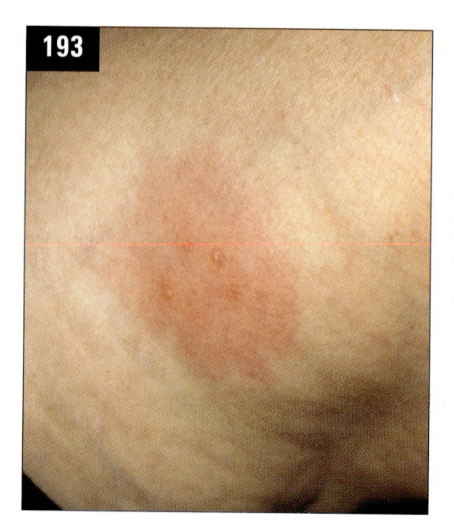

193 Zoster. Circinate zoster lesions are edematous and erythematous but may have few or no vesicles.

Viral Diseases

194 Zoster. Note unilateral distribution.

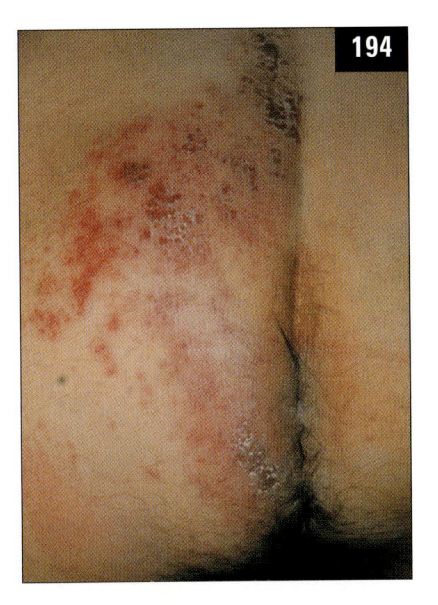

195 Zoster. Typical unilateral distribution.

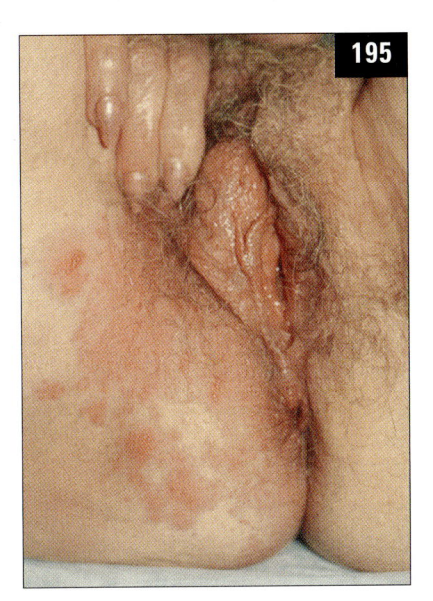

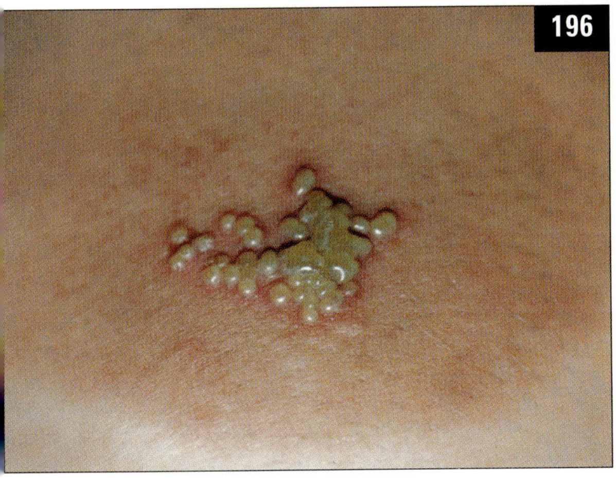

196 Zoster with pronounced herpetiform grouping of vesicles.

197 Zoster with sharp cut-off at midline.

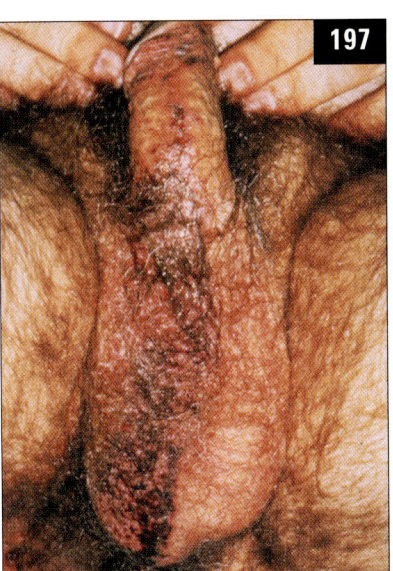

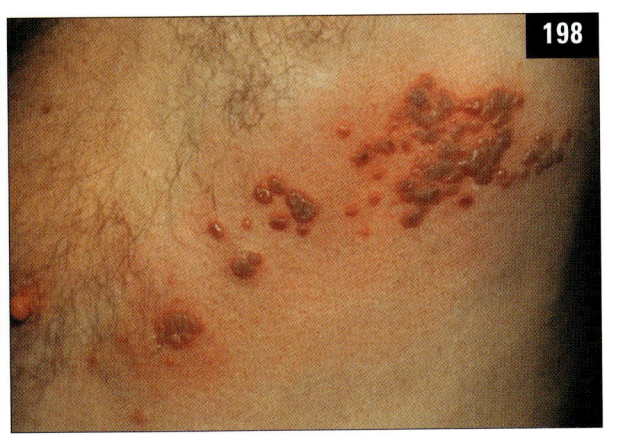

198 Zoster involving a thoracic dermatome.

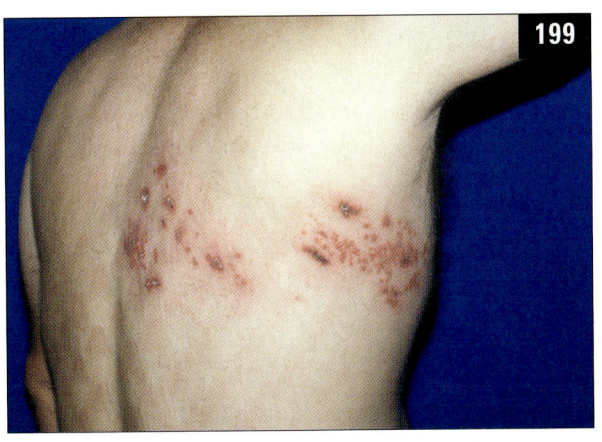

199 Zoster. Discrete groupings of blisters are often present within the dermatome.

A person with zoster can transmit varicella if a susceptible person comes in contact with vesicular fluid. Individuals with varicella or zoster cannot directly give another person zoster, since herpes zoster is caused by reactivation of latent VZV. Zoster usually resolves without complications in persons with intact immune systems. The elderly population and those with immune compromise typically endure more severe pain and resulting sequelae from zoster. Complications of zoster include post-herpetic neuralgia (PHN), secondary bacterial infection, scarring ophthalmic zoster, Ramsay–Hunt syndrome, meningoencephalitis, motor paralysis, pneumonitis, and hepatitis.

Most cases of varicella and herpes zoster are diagnosed based on history and clinical findings (Jemsek et al., 1983; McCrary et al., 1999). If further tests are required, a viral culture can be obtained from the base of a vesicle. A Tzanck smear demonstrating multinucleated giant cells can also confirm a diagnosis; however, this method cannot differentiate between HSV and VZV. Direct immunofluorescence of skin lesions is also available, but the highly sensitive molecular technique of polymerase chain reaction (PCR) is becoming the diagnostic test of choice (Schmidt et al., 1980; Nahass et al., 1992).

In uncomplicated cases of varicella, therapy consists of symptomatic relief with antipruritic lotions and antihistamines. If started within 24–72 hours after the onset of cutaneous eruption, oral acyclovir has been shown to decrease the duration of severity of varicella infection. Oral acyclovir is FDA-approved for treatment in adults and children over 2 years of age, and the intravenous form is indicated for varicella infection in the immunocompromised population (Lin et al., 2003). Varicella zoster immune globulin (VZIG) should be given to seronegative neonates, adolescents, adults, pregnant women, and immunocompromised hosts within 96 hours of exposure to reduce complications and decrease mortality (Ross, 1962). The varicella vaccine, approved by the FDA in 1995, should be administered to all healthy children starting at 1 year of age, as well as to seronegative adolescents and adults.

For the treatment of herpes zoster, analgesics, EMLA cream, lidocaine patches, capsaicin, narcotics, nerve blocks, biofeedback, gapapentin, and tricyclic antidepressants (TCAs) may provide pain relief (Bowsher, 1997). Acyclovir, valacyclovir, and famciclovir are FDA-approved for the treatment of zoster and result in decreased disease duration and pain. Intravenous acyclovir is indicated for immunocompromised individuals and those with serious complications (Lin et al., 2003). A live attenuated VZV vaccine has been recently approved by the FDA to prevent shingles in patients 60 years of age and older. In a randomized, double-blind, placebo-controlled study, the vaccine decreased incidence and morbidity from disease as well as reducing incidence of PHN (Mitka, 2006).

EPSTEIN–BARR VIRUS INFECTION

Epstein–Barr virus (EBV) is a human herpesvirus, HHV-4, and is associated with a variety of diseases including infectious mononucleosis syndrome, lymphoproliferative disorders, and oral hairy leukoplakia. The transmission is primarily through infectious saliva but it also has been demonstrated in genital secretions and breast milk (Andersson, 1991). The primary infection originates at the oropharyngeal epithelium within the epithelial cells and B-lymphocytes.

The most common disease caused by EBV is infectious mononucleosis, which usually affects young individuals (17–25 years old) (Ebell, 2004). The classical presentation begins after 30–50 days with the triad of pharyngitis, fever, and lymphadenopathy. Other symptoms include hepatomegaly, anorexia, nausea, cough, arthralgias, and tonsillitis (Bailey, 1994). The skin manifestations vary; the most common is an erythematous exanthem that lasts approximately 1 week. The exanthem can be morbilliform, urticarial, scarlatiniform, vesicular, or petechial. The exanthem starts at the trunk and upper extremities and subsequently spreads to the face and the forearms.

Diagnosis of infectious mononucleosis by currently available testing is somewhat problematic, especially early in the course of the illness. Testing initially with a complete blood count to detect atypical lymphocytes and further with a heterophile antibody titer is a good strategy. Tests for antibodies to Epstein–Barr viral capsid antigen (EBVCA) or Epstein–Barr nuclear antigen (EBNA) are the most sensitive and are highly specific (but also the most

Viral Diseases

expensive) for diagnosing infectious mononucleosis. The diagnosis is usually made by a positive monospot test and increased titers of heterophile antibodies (Bell *et al.*, 2006).

Usually the disease is self-limiting, and the therapy used is supportive. In severe cases, where hemolytic anemia or severe thrombocytopenia occurs, corticosteroids can be used (Andersson, 1991).

GIANOTTI–CROSTI SYNDROME (PAPULAR ACRODERMATITIS OF CHILDHOOD)

Gianotti–Crosti syndrome (200) has a worldwide distribution, and affects mostly young children 2–6 years of age (Brandt *et al.*, 2006). It is a self-limited cutaneous response to various infections including hepatitis B virus and EBV. This syndrome is usually preceded by an upper respiratory tract congestion and mild constitutional symptoms. The exanthem is symmetrical on the face, buttocks, and extensor surface of the extremities. The exanthem appears abruptly, it is monomorphous, and is characterized by pink and red edematous papules. Inguinal and axillary lymphadenopathy can be observed as well as splenomegaly and hepatomegaly (Hofmann *et al.*, 1997). The diagnosis is usually clinical. Skin biopsy can be done but the findings are not specific.

There are many potential etiologic agents associated with Gianotti–Crosti syndrome. The most common viruses are hepatitis B and EBV. Other viruses implicated include hepatitis A and C viruses, Coxsackie virus, respiratory syncytial virus, parvovirus B19, mumps virus, adenovirus, and human herpesvirus-6 among others (Ricci *et al.*, 2003; Brandt *et al.*, 2006). There is no specific treatment (Brandt *et al.*, 2006).

UNILATERAL LATEROTHORACIC EXANTHEM

This disease entity usually affects children around 3 years of age and it has a female predominance (ratio male: female 1:2). EBV is the most common etiologic agent associated with it. The majority of reports are from North America and Europe, especially during the spring season. The exanthem begins in a unilateral distribution at the axillary region followed by the trunk, arm, and thigh. The lesions are morbilliform or eczematous and tend to spread to the contralateral areas. An upper respiratory or gastrointestinal prodrome precedes the lesions. The patient can present with fever, diarrhea, rhinitis, or lymphadenopathy. The exanthem resolves spontaneously after 3–6 weeks (Resnick, 1997). The diagnosis is typically made by the clinical presentation. Skin biopsy is non-specific. There is no specific treatment.

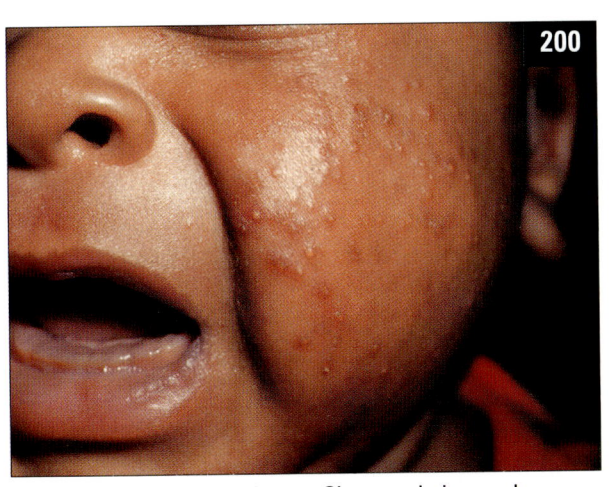

200 Gianotti–Crosti syndrome. Characteristic papular lesions on the cheeks.

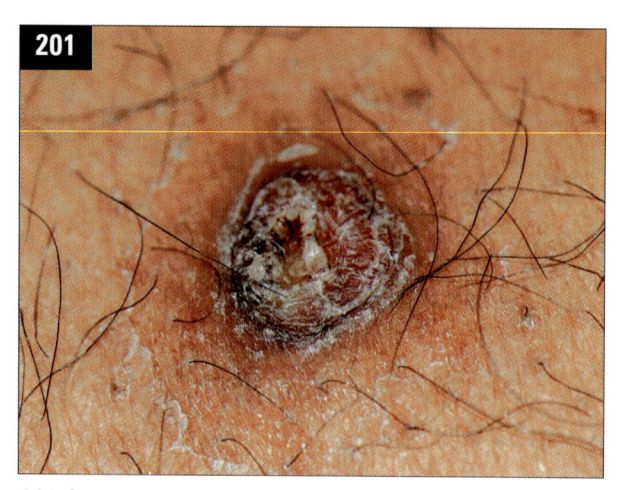

201 Cytomegalovirus infection. Verrucous nodule.

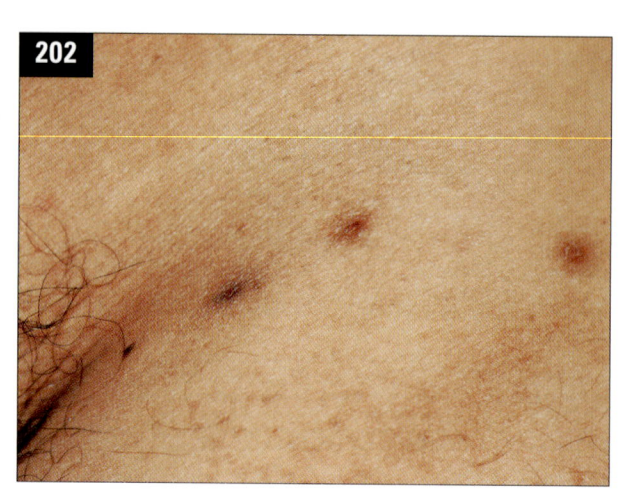

202 Cytomegalovirus infection. Lesions follow skin tension lines.

CYTOMEGALOVIRUS INFECTION

Most cases of cytomegalovirus (CMV) infection are subclinical (>90%), and a mononucleosis-like syndrome similar to one induced by EBV is the most common CMV disease in immunocompetent persons. CMV infection is a leading cause of congenital illness and disability, including hearing loss and mental retardation (Staras et al., 2006).

In the normal host, cutaneous manifestations of CMV are uncommon. Cutaneous manifestations include blueberry muffin lesions, which represent dermal erythropoiesis (Bowden et al., 1989), petechiae and purpura (Lesher, 1988), cutaneous vesicle (Blatt et al., 1978), and ichthyosis of the skin found concomitantly with keratitis and deafness (Helm et al., 1990). There have also been reports of rashes associated with CMV mononucleosis syndrome which include the maculopapular rubelliform rash caused by ampicillin (Spear et al., 1988). Further cutaneous vasculitis has been reported as a presenting sign of acute CMV infection in a 4-month old child (Sandler & Snedeker, 1987).

CMV-associated skin lesions in the immunocompromised individual are uncommon compared with the prevalence of CMV infection of other organs. Those with cutaneous manifestations usually have concurrent systemic CMV disease (Sandler & Snedeker, 1987; Lee, 1989). The majority of the cutaneous lesions are comprised of ulcers and occur most frequently over the perianal area and buttocks (Lesher, 1988; Lee, 1989; Colsky et al., 1998). Other less frequently reported cutaneous lesions include purpura, petechiae, morbilliform and maculopapular rash, vesicles, and verrucous or indurated plaques and nodules (**201, 202**).

CMV-associated ulcers and nodules appear to arise from infection of the endothelium of cutaneous blood vessels during the viremic phase of illness. Progression to vasculitis may occur (Homsy et al., 1989), with the appearance of purpuric nodules that can infarct and slough off the overlying epidermis.

A variety of methods are used for diagnosis of CMV infection. The gold standard for diagnosis is culture of CMV in human fibroblasts; however, several weeks are needed for confirmation. Culture for detection of CMV can also be done with results within 24–48 hours. Direct detection of virus and CMV-infected cells can be performed with a urine sample. Other methods to diagnose CMV infection include immunofluorescence, PCR, and detection of CMV-specific serologies (Colsky et al., 1998).

CMV, human herpesvirus-5 (HHV-5) is a cytotoxic virus that causes cell enlargement (cytomegaly) and nuclear condensation (nuclear inclusion). The virus typically infects endothelial cells and contains purplish, crystalline, intranuclear inclusion bodies surrounded by a clear halo giving them the pathognomonic 'owl's eye appearance'. It uses blood leukocytes as a transport medium to disseminate throughout the body, infecting various organs. Transmission of CMV is through bodily fluids including saliva, blood, urine, semen, breast milk, cervical and vaginal secretions, and transplanted organs, and further with contaminated fomites.

CMV infection can be primary or recurrent. Following primary infection, CMV persists in a latent condition and rarely induces disease. Reactivation of latent virus often occurs in immunocompromised individuals.

Controlling CMV infection involves prevention, immunoprophylaxis, and therapy with antiviral drugs. Preventative therapy is useful for immunocompromised individuals who are not yet infected but are at risk of infection from an event such as blood transfusion or organ transplantation. CMV antibody-negative tissues and blood are used for this specific population. Pre- and post-transplant CMV prophylaxis includes interferon, ganciclovir, and the use of intravenous immunoglobulins, particularly high-titer CMV immunoglobulins (Meyers, 1991; Baldanti et al., 1998).

For the treatment of CMV infection in immunocompromised individuals, currently approved antivirals including ganciclovir, valganciclovir, foscarnet, cidofovir, and fomivirsen have been used with variable success. Further, treatment of CMV-induced mononucleosis is symptomatic.

EXANTHEM SUBITUM INFECTION

Human herpesvirus type 6 (HHV-6) is the etiologic agent of exanthem subitum (roseola). Viral incubations lasts approximately 5–15 days and clinical manifestations of this disease occur in 30% of primary HHV-6 infections.

The classic presentation of exanthem subitum consists of rapid onset of high fever, with subsequent cutaneous eruption as the fever subsides. The cutaneous eruption lasts approximately 24–48 hours and can occur with concomitant fever or even up to 2 days after the temperature returns to normal. Characteristically, the lesions are discrete, circular, or elliptical, erythematous, 'rose-red' macules or maculopapules that are 2–5 mm in diameter with an occasional white halo surrounding them. Subsequent to the third day of fever, palpebral edema can occur.

Complications of exanthem subitum in children are not common, but can include seizures, increased intracranial pressure, pneumonitis, hepatitis, and encephalitis (Mancini, 1998). Immunocompromised patients can in addition develop other serious sequelae, including fever and cutaneous eruption, bone marrow suppression, and transplanted tissue rejection (Drago & Rebora, 1999).

The diagnosis is typically made clinically. Serology may be helpful in difficult situations; other potential diagnostic tools (during the febrile phase of disease course) include electron microscopy, PCR, and viral culture.

In most patients no treatment is necessary. Only in immunocompromised individuals, where serious sequelae can occur, is it necessary to consider treatment. Cidofovir, foscarnet, and ganciclovir have been shown to have a high antiviral activity against HHV-6 (De Clercq et al., 2001; Tokimasa et al., 2002), and recently new arylsulfone derivatives have demonstrated activity against HHV-6 (Naesens et al., 2006).

KAPOSI'S SARCOMA INFECTION

Human herpesvirus type 8 (HHV-8), also known as Kaposi's sarcoma-associated herpesvirus (KSHV), is a latent virus found in almost all types of Kaposi's sarcoma (KS) worldwide. Viral reactivation has been postulated to result in the associated diseases. The mechanisms of HHV-8 transmission are not well elucidated, although receptive anal intercourse appears to be a primary factor for transmission (Levy, 1997). Further, other studies have found mother-to-child transmission to occur in one-third of infected mothers in African countries (Bourboulia et al., 1998).

KS is an angioproliferative disease, varying from an indolent to fulminant disease with significant morbidity and mortality. The disease usually presents with disseminated and pigmented skin lesions, which can evolve from patches to plaques and eventually ulcerating tumors (203–206). Lesions are often associated with edema and lymph node and visceral involvement. There are four different types of KS: classic, human immunodeficiency virus/aquired immunodeficiency syndrome (HIV/AIDS)-related, immunosuppression-associated, and African endemic.

Classic KS

Lesions in this form of KS initially develop as purplish-red plaques, mostly on the lower legs of elderly men of Mediterranean descent. In later stages, they can become hyperkeratotic and/or eczematous. Progression to more advanced stages is slow.

HIV/AIDS-related KS

This form of KS generally presents as small macules, patches, or plaques, but can evolve into exophytic and ulcerative lesions. It is common to have involvement of the oral cavity and perioral area, and it often can signify the first sign of HIV infection (206). Other areas may be affected, such as the genital mucosa, lungs, and the gastrointestinal tract. Oral lesions can cause great discomfort and difficulty with oral intake and speech. The disease can worsen with the decline of the CD4+ count.

Immunosuppression-associated KS

The clinical course is comparable to HIV/AIDS-related KS, with rapid progression unless the offending immunosuppressive agent is terminated. KS is much more strongly associated with HIV infection than immunosuppression from other causes, such as in transplant recipients.

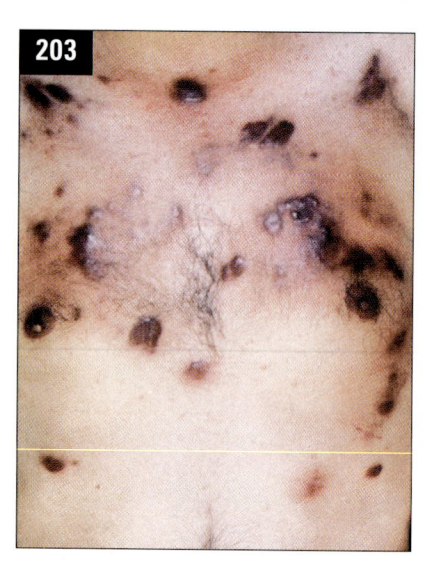

203 Kaposi's sarcoma in HIV infection. Lesions often follow skin tension lines.

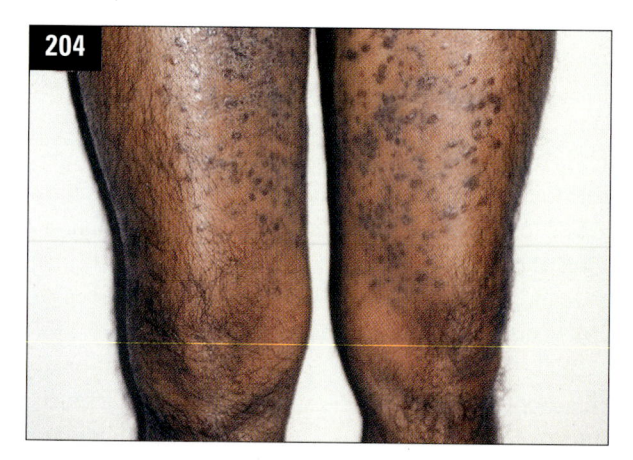

204 Kaposi's sarcoma in HIV infection. Widely disseminated lesions.

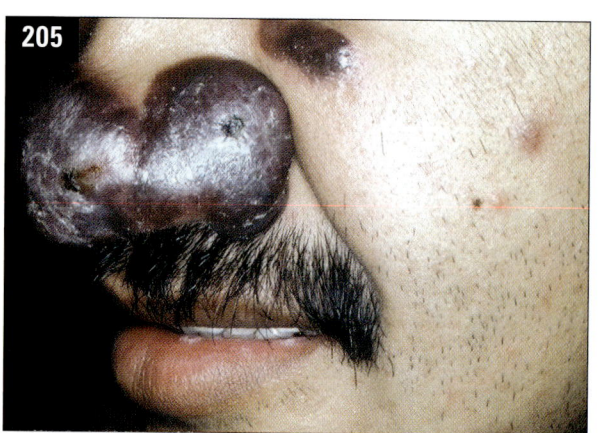

205 Kaposi's sarcoma in HIV infection. Lesions bordering mucosal surfaces.

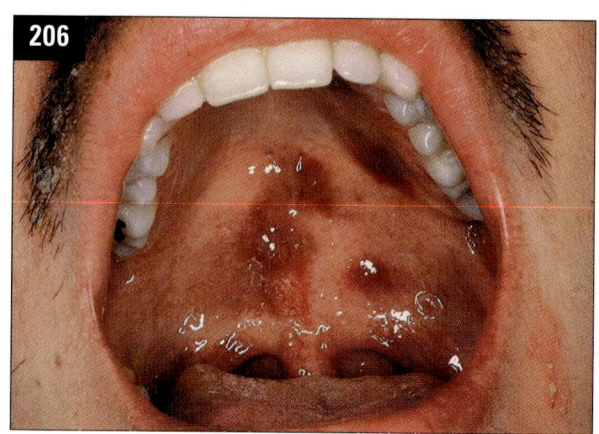

206 Kaposi's sarcoma in HIV infection. Mucosal lesions.

African-endemic KS

There are four subtypes of African-endemic KS: nodular, lymphoadenopathic, florid, and infiltrative. The nodular subtype is delineated by small, well-circumscribed nodules with a benign disease course. The second form generally affects lymph nodes, and it is more common in children and young adults. The florid and infiltrative forms typically have cutaneous lesions on the extremities and depict a very aggressive course. Skin biopsy of a suspected lesion confirms the diagnosis of KS, and serology for the virus is not indicated.

Treatment is guided by the extent of symptomatic and extracutaneous KS, immune system conditions, and concurrent complications of HIV infection, since KS is not considered curable by standard therapies. Localized KS lesions can be treated with alitretinoin gel, intra-lesional chemotherapy, radiation therapy, laser therapy, cryotherapy, and surgical excision (Berretta et al., 2003). Systemic chemotherapy is used in individuals with progressive, widespread disease and, in particular, with visceral involvement. Interferon has been used with favorable results in HIV-infected individuals with disseminated disease, but only those who have appropriate immune reconstitution (Tirelli et al., 2002). Highly active antiretroviral therapy (HAART) has significantly decreased the incidence of AIDS-associated KS, while other antivirals such as ganciclovir and cidofovir have produced variable results (Kedes & Ganem, 1997).

ERYTHEMA INFECTIOSUM (FIFTH DISEASE) INFECTION

Erythema infectiosum is the most common clinical presentation of infection by parvovirus B19, and is usually recognized as a childhood exanthem that appears as a 'slapped cheek' rash (207–209). The rash is a more generalized lacy, reticular pattern of erythema (Mortimer et al., 1983). Infection with parvovirus B19 occurs in a worldwide distribution (Young & Brown, 2004; Broliden et al., 2006). Parvovirus B19 infection is common in childhood and about 50% of adolescents have specific antiparvovirus B19 antibodies. Almost all elderly people are seropositive. The only known natural host cell of parvovirus B19 is the human erythroid progenitor (Mortimer et al., 1983; Broliden et al., 2006). Transmission is by respiratory droplets, and secondary infection rates among household contacts are very high (Chorba et al., 1986). After infection, the subject develops fever and influenza-like symptoms during the parvoviremia. The cutaneous eruption has a later onset as well as the rheumatic symptoms, 2 weeks later.

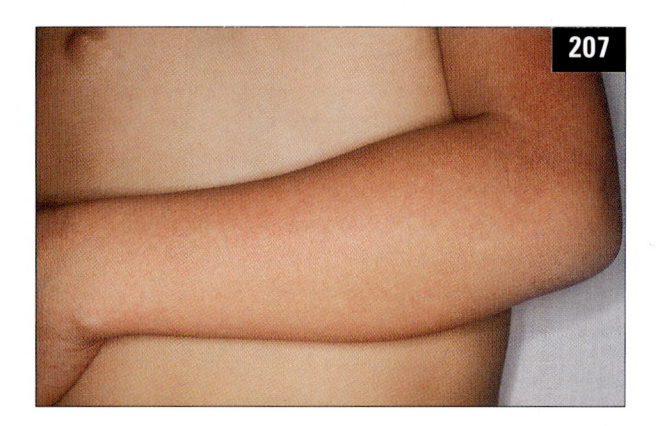

207 Erythema infectiosum. The erythema becomes more prominent with exertion.

208 Erythema infectiosum. The reticulated pattern of erythema on the trunk and extremities often persists in children for months after the acute infection.

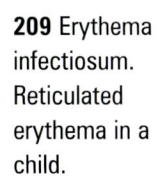

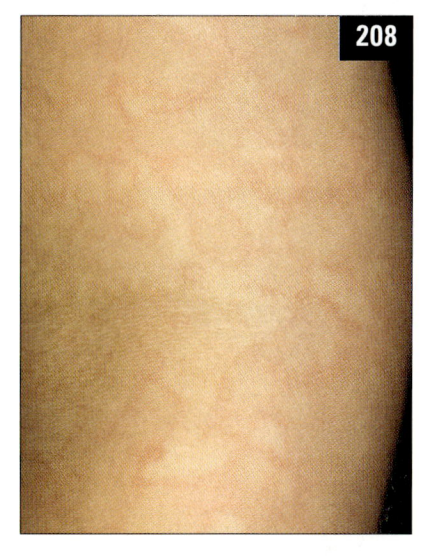

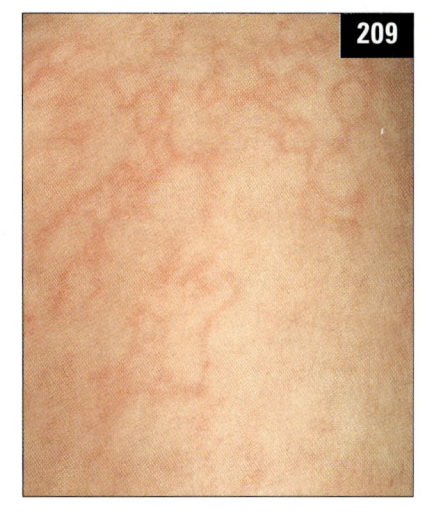

209 Erythema infectiosum. Reticulated erythema in a child.

Sometimes the rash can be provoked by exposure to sunlight, emotions, exercise, and heat (Young & Brown, 2004). Individuals are no longer contagious when the rash appears. Pregnant women exposed during the incubation period may miscarry. Children with chronic hemolytic anemia may develop aplastic crisis when exposed. Adults exposed to the virus may develop a syndrome of chronic arthralgias or the purpuric 'gloves and socks syndrome' (**210–213**).

Laboratory diagnosis of parvovirus B19 infection relies on serologic and deoxyribonecleic acid (DNA) detection in blood or tissue samples by measurement of B19 IgG and IgM antibodies (Anderson *et al.*, 1985; Broliden *et al.*, 2006) and PCR tests, respectively. The fifth disease in adults can be confused with rubella due to the characteristic presentation.

Most cases in children and adults do not require specific therapy. In severe cases, commercial immune globulins are used as a source of antibodies against parvovirus. Persistent B19 infection responds to a 5- or 10-day course of immune globulin at a dose of 0.4 g per kilogram of body weight (Broliden *et al.*, 2006).

HUMAN PAPILLOMAVIRUS INFECTION

Warts may occur on any cutaneous surface, and common warts are hyperkeratotic, epidermal proliferations most commonly found on the hands, periungual skin, elbows, knees, and plantar surfaces (**214–219**). Flat warts are flat-topped papules usually

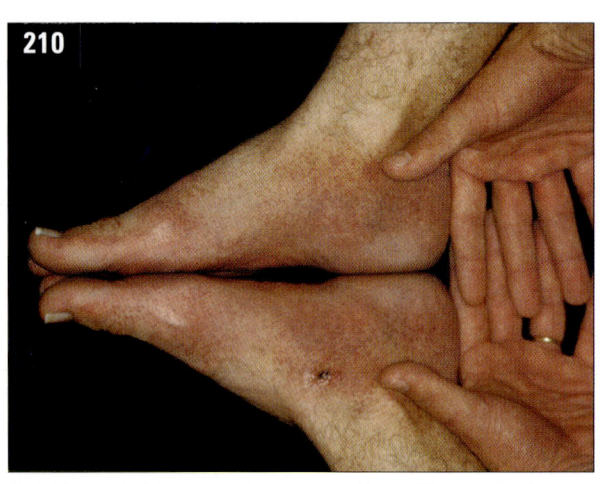

210 Purpuric 'gloves and socks syndrome' is a typical presentation in adults with Parvovirus B19.

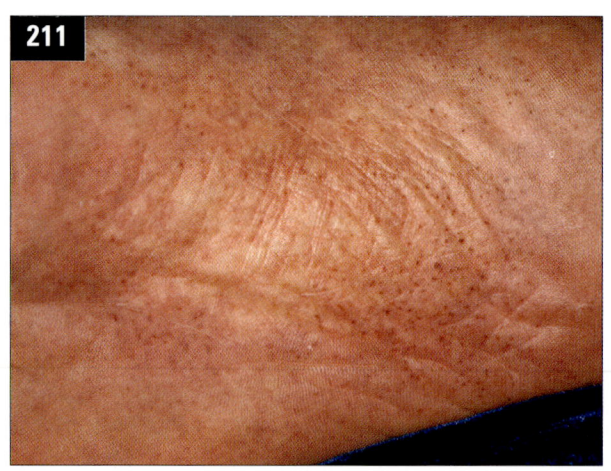

211 Purpuric 'gloves and socks syndrome'. Petechial lesions on the plantar aspect of the foot.

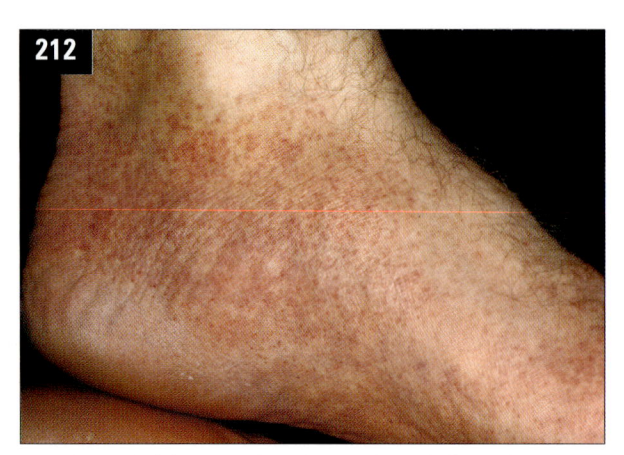

212 Purpuric 'gloves and socks syndrome'. Sharp 'sock-like' cut-off.

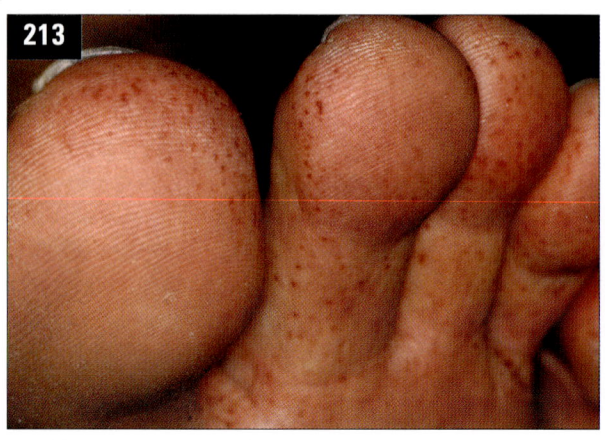

213 Purpuric 'gloves and socks syndrome'. Discrete petechial lesions.

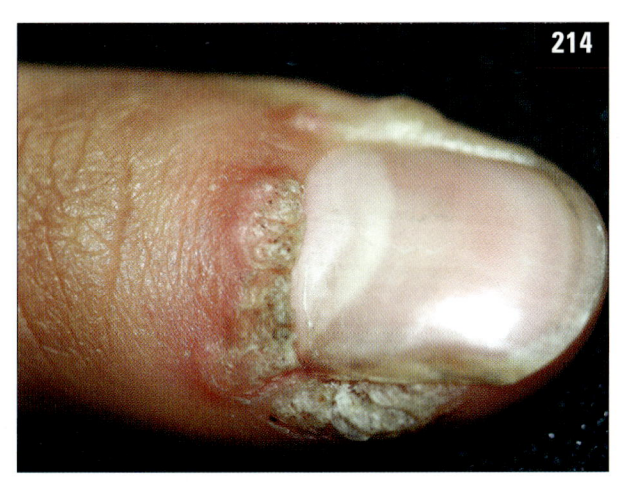

Viral Diseases

214 Human papillomavirus infection. Periungal warts are challenging to treat.

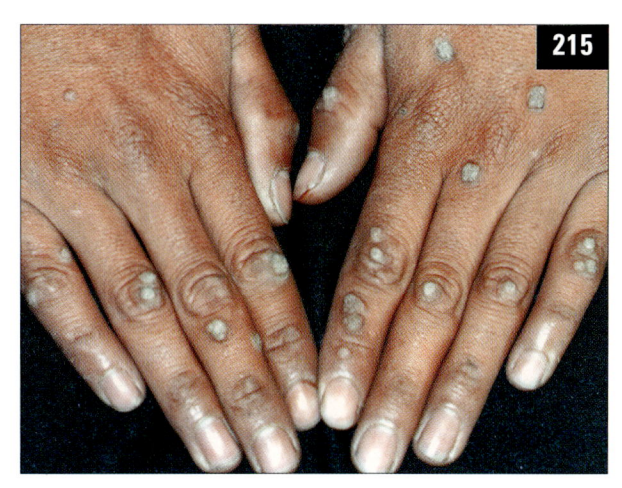

215 Human papillomavirus infection. Numerous warts on the hands.

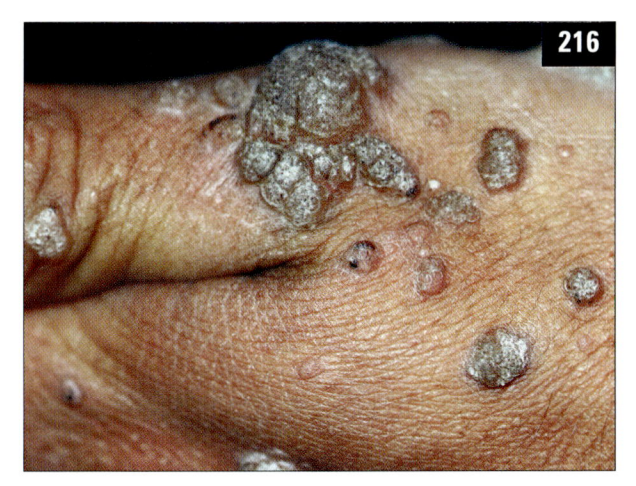

216 Human papillomavirus infection. Agminated warts.

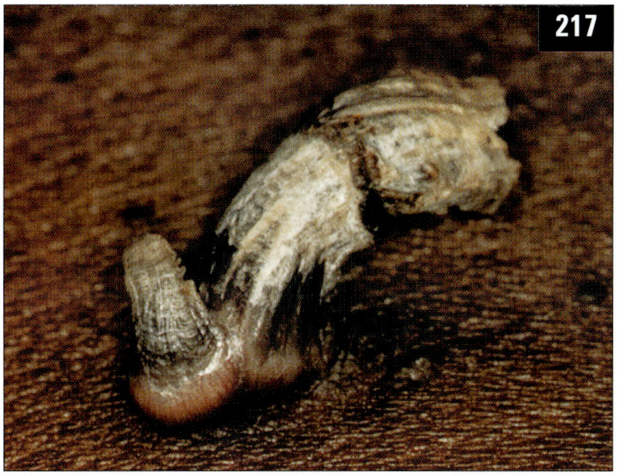

217 Human papillomavirus infection. Cutaneous horn arising from a common wart.

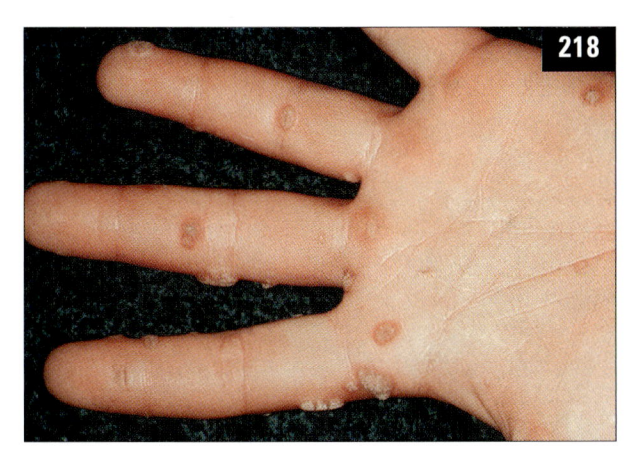

218 Human papillomavirus infection. Numerous warts involving the hand.

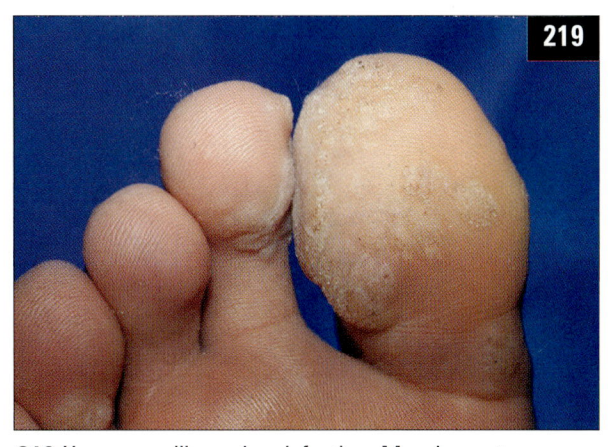

219 Human papillomavirus infection. Mosaic warts.

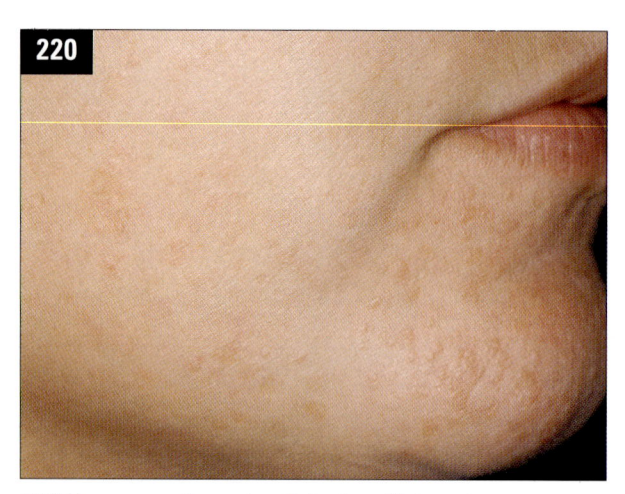

220 Human papillomavirus infection. Flat warts are typically caused by HPV type 3.

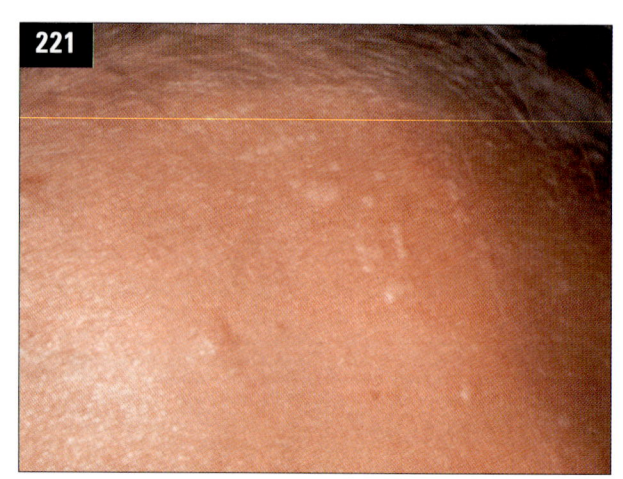

221 Flat warts on the forehead.

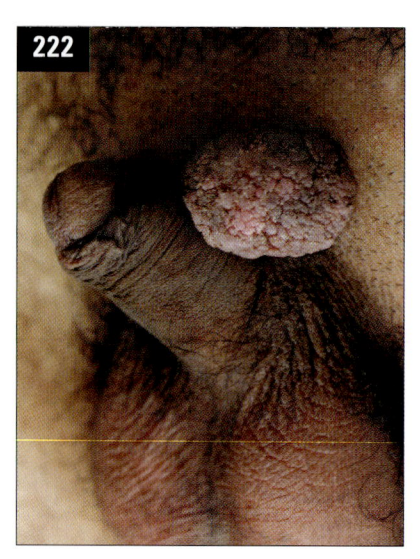

222 Condylomata acuminata. Large solitary lesions are best treated with simple excision.

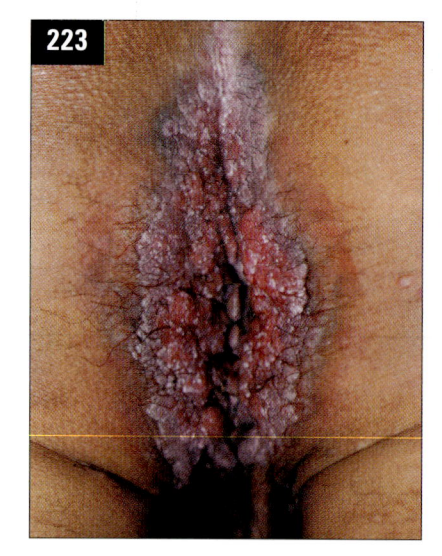

223 Condylomata acuminata. Involvement often extends into the anal canal.

found on the forehead, dorsal surface of the hands, chin, neck, and legs (**220, 221**). Condylomata acuminata refers to the clinical lesions found on the anogenital area (**222–227**). Their appearance ranges from small verrucous papules to discrete, sessile, smooth-topped papules or nodules to large exophytic masses, seen more commonly in immunocompromised individuals. The lesions are moist and fleshy and can turn friable with irritation. The skin color varies from skin-colored to reddish-brown (Wikstrom, 1995).

Small condylomas can be better visualized by application of 5% acetic acid soak, which can turn previously unnoticed lesions into whitish plaques. This method is neither sensitive nor specific and yields high false-positives and negatives. Diagnosis is usually based on clinical findings since the lesions have a straightforward appearance. Histological correlation can be done if necessary. Human

Viral Diseases

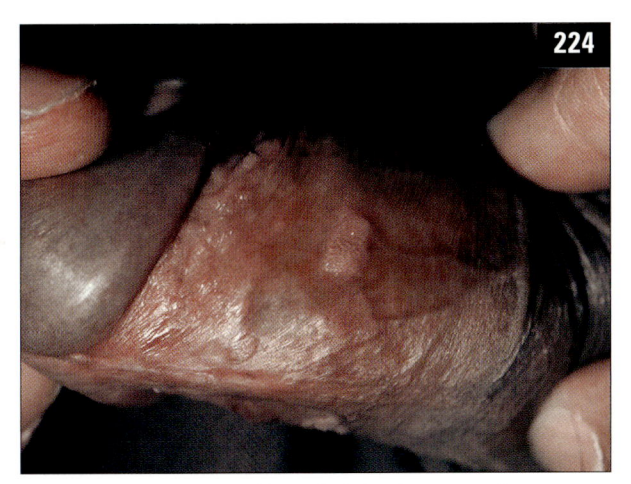

224 Condylomata acuminata. Subtle warts may be visualized with acetowhitening using 5% acetic acid.

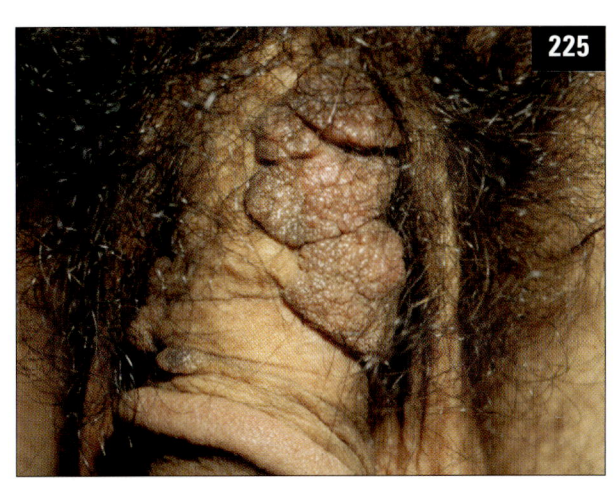

225 Condylomata acuminata. Extensive lesions often require more than a single treatment modality.

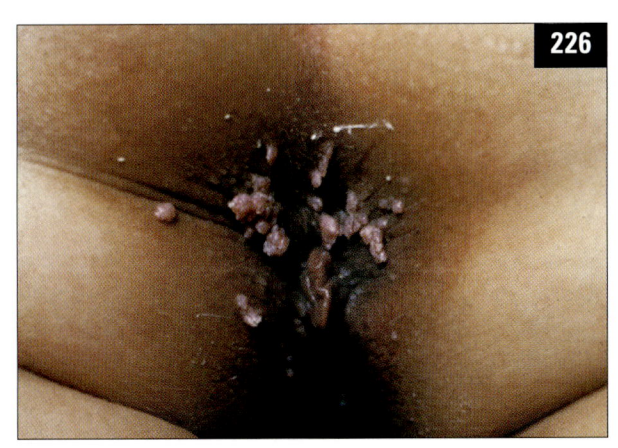

226 Condylomata acuminata. After treatment, patients should be monitored for recurrence and the development of carcinoma. Pap smears are being used in this setting.

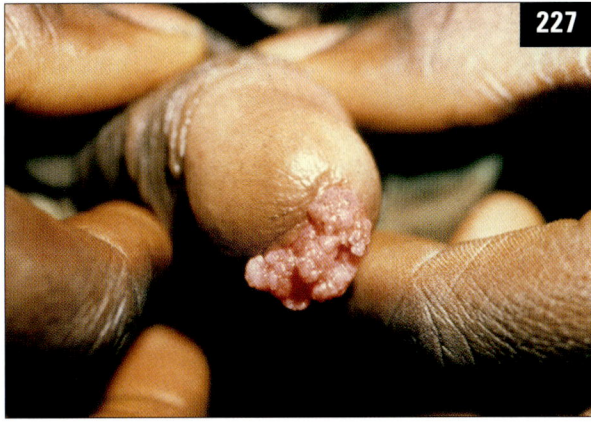

227 Condylomata acuminata. Urethral involvement may be treated with intraurethral 5-fluorouracil.

papillomavirus (HPV) DNA can also be detected by PCR, which is currently the most sensitive method for diagnosis. Further, cytologic smears serve as a screening tool for cervical dysplasia along with colposcopy and HPV DNA typing, pending abnormal smear results (Fazel et al., 1999; Kodner & Nasraty, 2004).

More than 100 different strains of HPV exist. Infection with HPV is highly contagious, and viral incubation is from 1–6 months. Transmission is through direct contact with lesions. Low-risk subtypes, such as HPV-2, result in verruca vulgaris (common warts), HPV-1, -2 and -4 cause flat warts, and HPV-3 and -10, plantar warts. HPV-6 and -11 are responsible for condyloma acuminatum (genital warts). Cancerous lesions of the skin of the penis, vulva, and inner linings of the vagina, cervix, and rectum have been associated with types 16 and 18

(Bosch *et al.*, 1995; zur Hausen, 1996). Epidermodysplasia veruciformis (228–233) represents an inherited susceptibility to premalignant flat warts. The lesions resemble tinea versicolor, but progress to Bowen's disease and invasive carcinoma.

There are a multitude of treatments for warts; due to high rates of recurrence, several treatments are typically required over a course of weeks to months. Topical therapies are first-line therapy, and salicylic acid preparations and liquid nitrogen cryotherapy are most commonly used. Other modalities include podophyllin, bleomycin, interferon, cidofovir, imiquimod, and laser therapy. Surgical treatment with electrodesiccation and curettage may be indicated for resistant or severe cases. Immunocompromised patients may necessitate more aggressive therapy, such as combination treatment, due to the extent of their disease and resistance to therapy (Snoeck *et al.*, 1998).

The FDA approved a quadrivalent vaccine against HPV types 6, 11, 16 and 18 in June 2006. The vaccine targets the most common subtypes associated with condyloma acuminatum (6 and 11) and cervical cancer (16 and 18) and is approved for females aged 9–26 (Inglis *et al.*, 2006; Speck & Tyring, 2006).

MEASLES INFECTION

The measles virus is a paramyxovirus, and initiates replication in the epithelial cells of the respiratory tract, and then progresses to viremia through spread via lymphoid tissue and blood. Dissemination to the lungs, liver, and gastrointestinal tract then occurs. Measles (234, 235) typically presents with a prodrome of fever, cough, nasal congestion, and rhinoconjunctivitis. Koplik spots, which are pathognomonic for this disease, appear during the prodrome and are clinically gray-white papules on the buccal mucosa. The exanthem appears over 2–4 days and are characterized by erythematous macules and papules that begin on the forehead, hairline, and behind the ears and then progress in a cephalocaudal fashion. The exanthema begin to fade on the fifth day in the same fashion it appeared.

Complications of measles include otitis, pneumonia, encephalitis, and myocarditis. Subacute sclerosing panencephalitis, a delayed neurodegenerative disorder, can occur years after the primary acute disease.

Clinical diagnosis is usually sufficient, but if laboratory diagnosis is needed, it can be accomplished by virus isolation from nasopharyngeal secretions, immunofluorescent examination, or serologic assay for measles-specific antibodies.

There is no recommended therapy for measles. In children residing in communities where vitamin A deficiency is common and mortality is greater than 1%, vitamin A is recommended by the World Health Organization (WHO). Prevention of measles by vaccination is the most effective way to decrease the incidence of measles morbidity and mortality (Mancini & Shani-Adir, 2003).

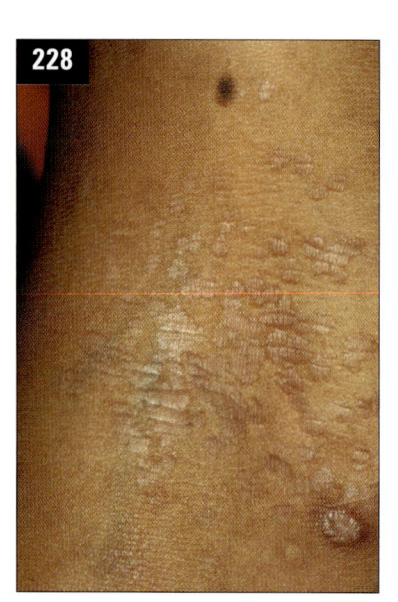

228 Epidermodysplasia veruciformis. The disorder is inherited in an autosomal recessive manner.

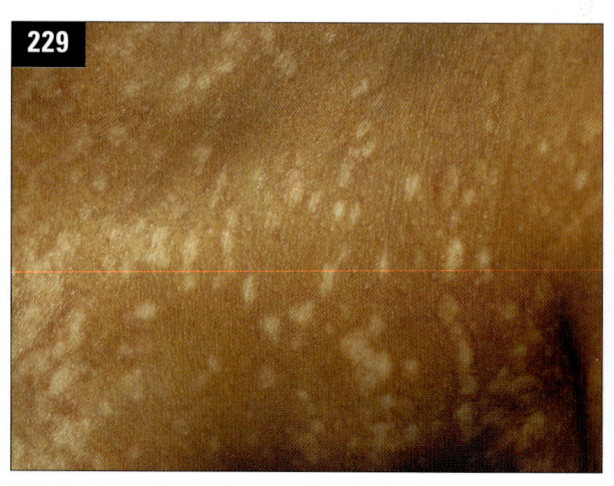

229 Epidermodysplasia veruciformis. Lesions may resemble tinea versicolor.

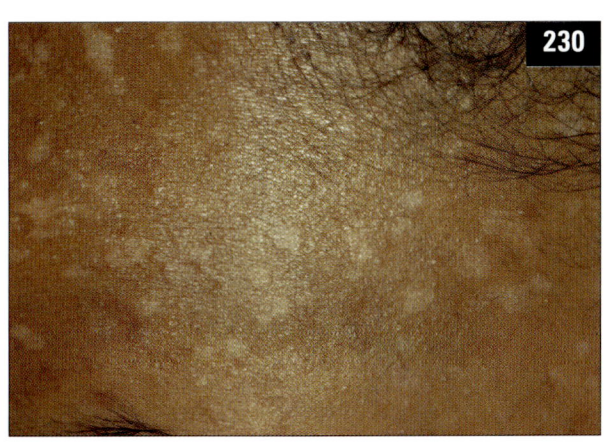

Viral Diseases

230 Epidermodysplasia veruciformis. Lesions may be hyper- or hypopigmented.

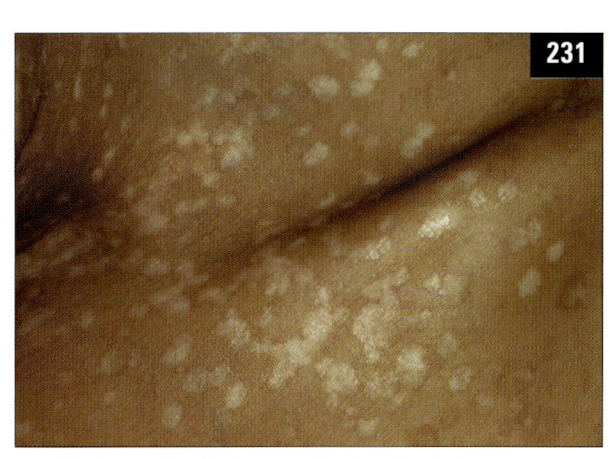

231 Epidermodysplasia veruciformis. The lesions are typically refractory to treatment.

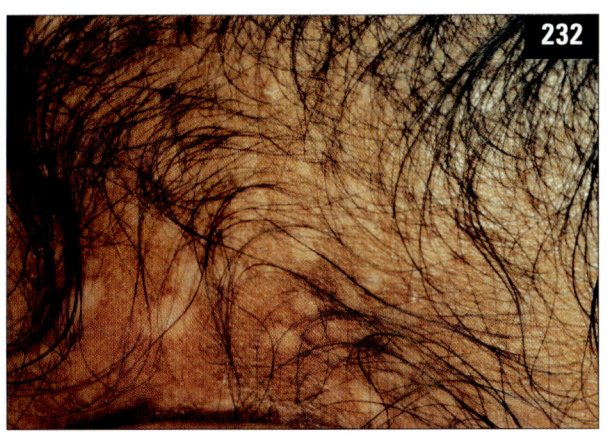

232 Epidermodysplasia veruciformis. Patients are infected with a wide variety of warts.

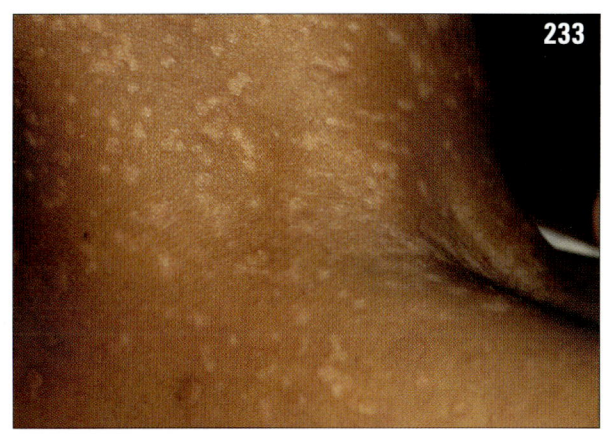

233 Epidermodysplasia veruciformis. Lesions in sun-exposed areas are most likely to become malignant.

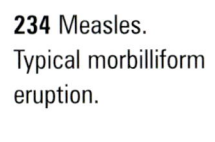

234 Measles. Typical morbilliform eruption.

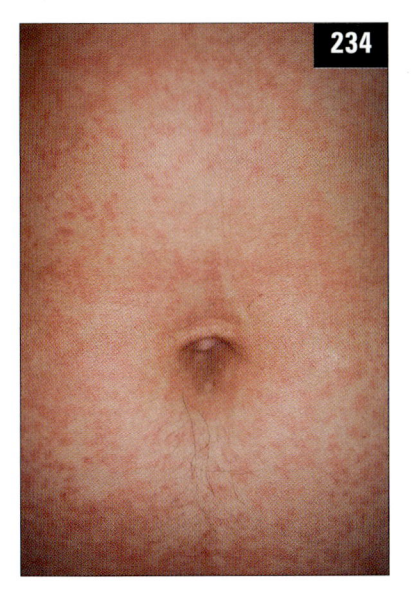

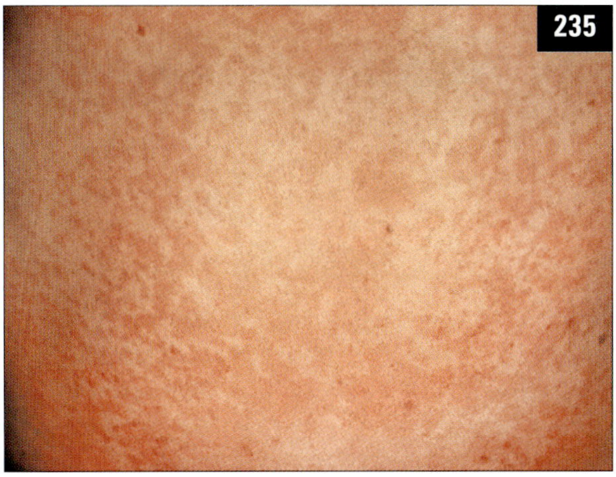

235 Measles. Patients typically have a rash with cough, coryza, or conjunctivitis.

Viral Diseases

RUBELLA INFECTION

Rubella is a viral infection that affects children and young adults. Transmission is due to inhalation of droplets and the disease is moderately contagious. It affects the population worldwide, but the incidence has been reduced in the developed countries. It usually presents with an exanthem and lymphadenopathy. However, many infections are subclinical. The skin lesions are characterized by pink macules and papules initially on the forehead spreading inferiorly to the face, trunk and extremities. The exanthem disappears by the second day. The lesions on the trunk become confluent forming a scarlatiniform eruption. Mucous membranes are involved during the prodromal phase with petechiae on the soft palate (Forchheimer's sign). The lymph nodes become enlarged concomitantly with the mucosal involvement. The most common lymph node locations affected are the suboccipital and posterior cervical areas. Generalized and postauricular lymphadenopathy may also occur. The enlarged lymph nodes can last for several weeks to months. Sometimes the spleen and the joints can be affected (Mosquera *et al.*, 2005). If infection occurs in the third trimester of pregnancy, the chance of acquiring congenital rubella syndrome (congenital heart defects, cataracts, deafness, microcephaly and hydrocephaly) is almost 50% (Kirkham *et al.*, 2005). The diagnosis is clinical and can be confirmed by serology, PCR, and culture (Mosquera *et al.*, 2005). The treatment is symptomatic. This disease is preventable by immunization.

POXVIRUS INFECTION
MOLLUSCUM CONTAGIOSUM

Molluscum contagiosum (236–245) is a superficial skin infection which occurs most commonly on the exposed skin of children and some sexually active adults in the genital area (Brown *et al.*, 2006).

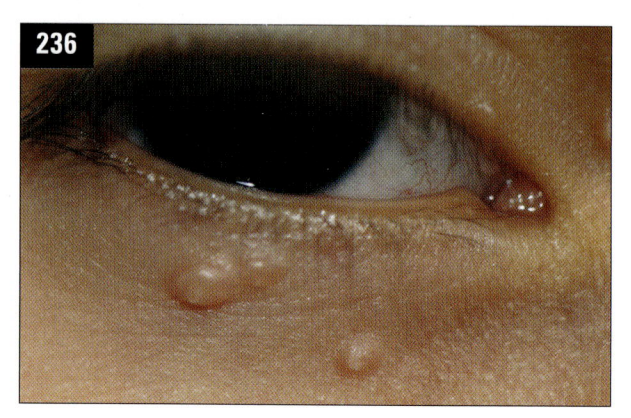

236 Molluscum contagiosum. Translucent umbilicated papules.

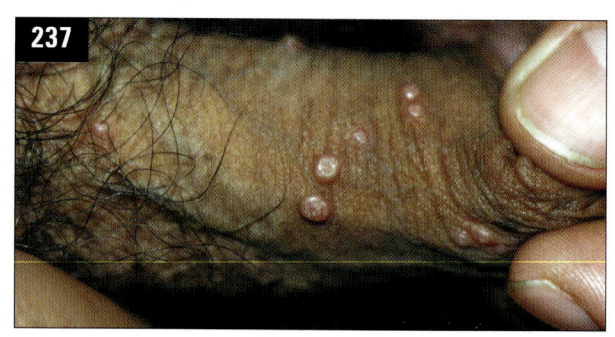

237 Molluscum contagiosum. Genital lesions are spread sexually.

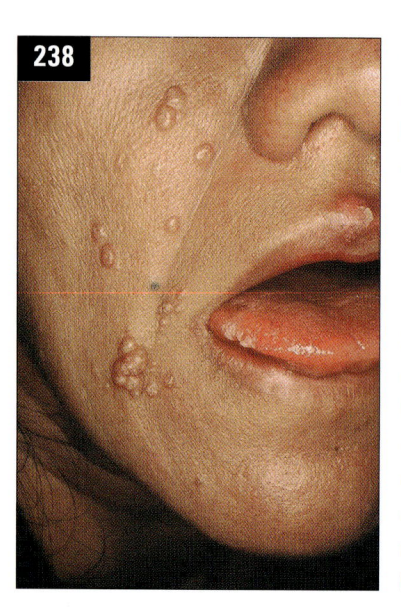

238 Molluscum contagiosum. Lesions often cluster.

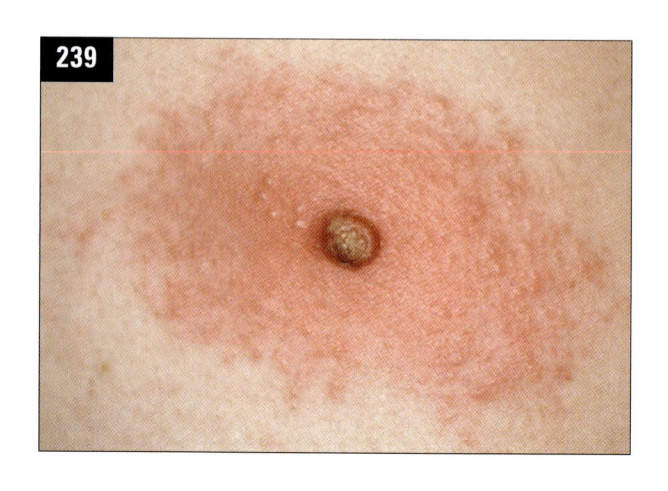

239 Molluscum contagiosum. Molluscum dermatitis does not respond well to corticosteroids, but resolves once the lesions are treated.

Viral Diseases

240 Molluscum contagiosum. Scratching spreads the lesions.

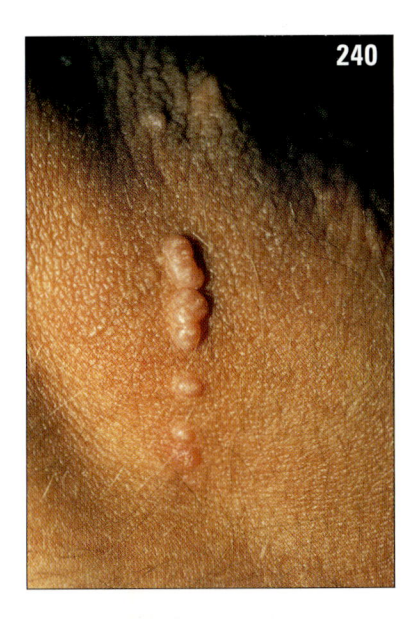

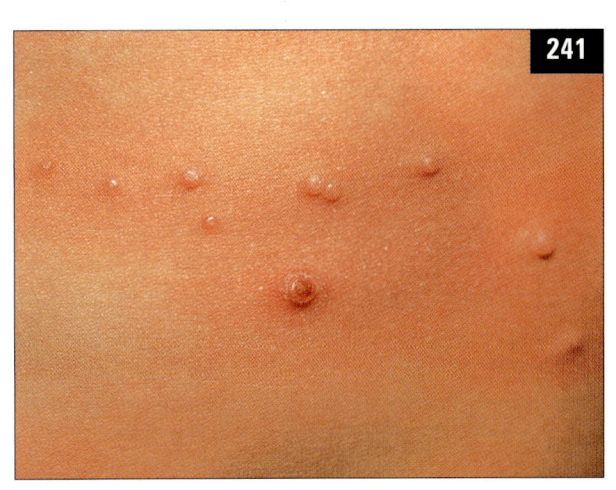

241 Molluscum contagiosum. Note surrounding dermatitis.

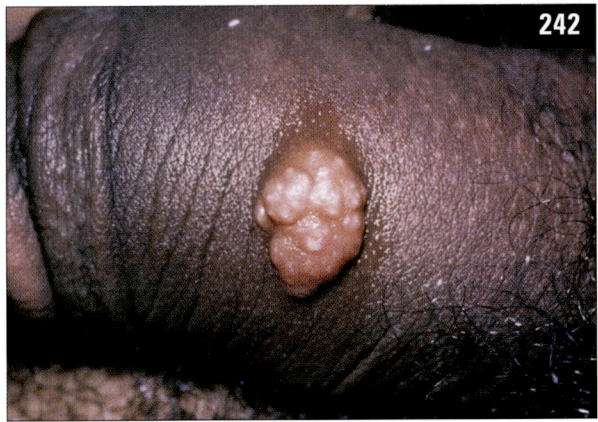

242 Molluscum contagiosum. Clustering of lesions on the penile shaft.

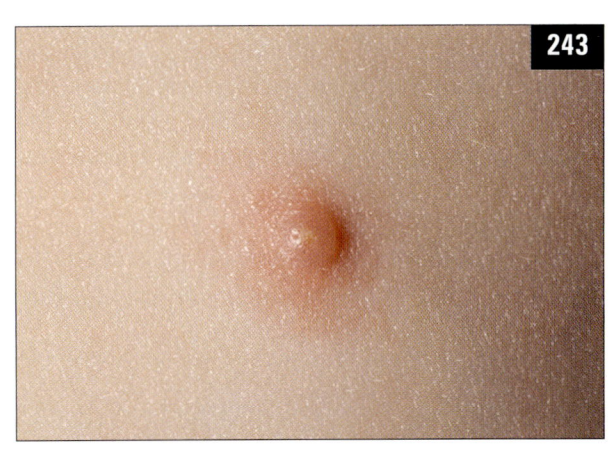

243 Molluscum contagiosum with surrounding inflammatory response.

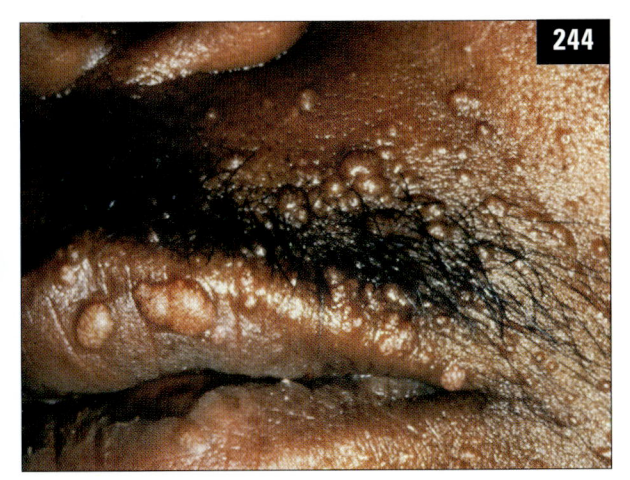

244 Molluscum contagiosum. In immunosuppressed patients, widespread lesions are often present.

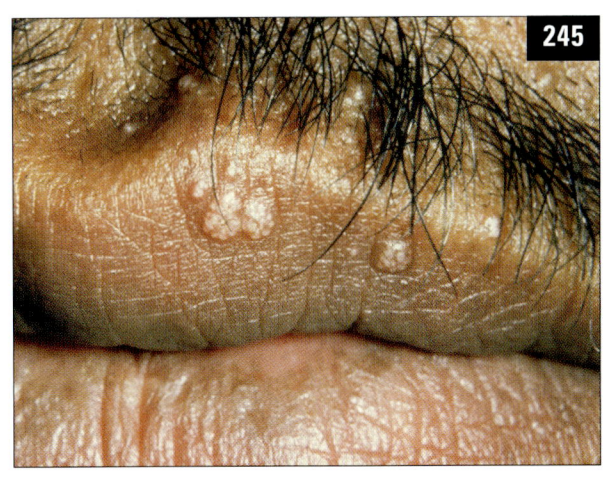

245 Molluscum contagiosum. Molluscum preparations or biopsy will confirm the diagnosis.

The transmission is by direct contact. HIV-infected individuals exhibit giant lesions commonly seen on the face, but are more likely to develop extensive disease (Cotton *et al.*, 1987). Spontaneous resolution is rarely seen.

The lesions are characterized by whitish (or flesh-colored) rounded, umbilicated papules (1–2 mm) or nodules (5–10 mm). The lesions can be isolated or present in clusters. The immune response to the infection causes the 'molluscum contagiosum' dermatitis, which is an erythematous halo with desquamation around the lesion (Brown *et al.*, 2006). In HIV-infected individuals, the lesions are bigger and can present in high numbers (as high as 100 lesions) (Cotton *et al.*, 1987).

The diagnosis is based on the clinical appearance, although in some patients it may be a challenge. Biopsy is performed in HIV patients to rule out invasive fungal infection such as cryptococcosis, histoplasmosis, coccidioidomycosis, and so on. Microscopy displays a typical pattern of numerous discrete ovoid intracytoplasmic inclusion bodies, called molluscum bodies (Brown *et al.*, 2006).

The etiologic agent is the molluscum contagiosum virus (MCV), a poxvirus (Thompson, 1998). MCV has four major viral types based upon DNA analysis: MCV-1, MCV-1v, MCV-2, and MCV-3. MCV-1 is more prevalent than MCV-2, and it is commonly the cause of molluscum contagiosum in children, while MCV-2 tends to be more sexually transmitted (Porter *et al.*, 1989).

The treatment depends on the age of the patient; it ranges from topical application to a procedure. Sometimes, reassurance alone is the best treatment. Topical treatments include: vitamin A derivatives, alpha-hydroxy (lactic) and beta-hydroxy (salicylic) acids (Thomas & Doyle, 1981; Ohkuma, 1990) and cantharidin (Brown *et al.*, 2006). Many procedures are used as treatment for molluscum contagiosum. These procedures include cryotherapy, curettage, electrodessication, and direct extraction in the office (Brown *et al.*, 2006).

ORF AND MILKER'S NODULE

A parapox virus is the etiologic agent in orf and milker's nodule. This virus is a complex double-stranded DNA virus that is a subgroup of Poxviridae (Dellamonica *et al.*, 1983; Buttner & Rziha, 2002). These diseases cannot be distinguished from one another based on morphology alone. Sheep are the

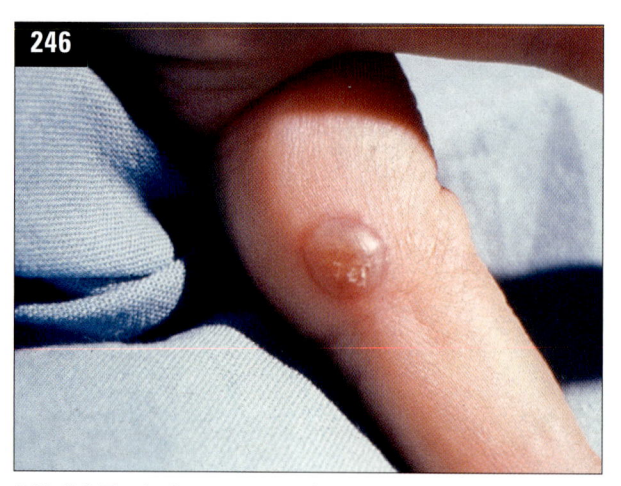

246 Orf. The lesions progress from edematous to verrucous phases.

natural hosts of orf, and cows are the natural hosts of milker's nodule. Both diseases can be acquired through direct contact with infected animals. Orf may also be acquired through contact with contaminated objects. Organ transplant recipients may be at increased risk for infection (Ballanger *et al.*, 2006).

A well-circumscribed solitary ulcerated papule or nodule on the fingers or hands after contact with an infected animal is the most common clinical presentation of orf (**246**) (Huerter *et al.*, 1991). Cases involving the head, neck, and perineum have also been described. Multiple lesions are more commonly seen with milker's nodule. Patients may also experience fever, malaise, erythema multiforme, or Stevens–Johnson syndrome (Erbagci *et al.*, 2005; Schmidt *et al.*, 2006).

Most diagnoses can be made based on clinical presentation and a history of occupational exposure. On microscopic examination, fully developed lesions show a zoned appearance. Parakeratosis, papillomatosis, acanthosis, and viral cytopathic changes consisting of cytoplasmic and nuclear vacuolation, and cytoplasmic inclusion bodies are present in the epidermis (**247**). The cytoplasmic inclusions generally occur in the upper epidermis, where they can be seen as deeply eosinophilic homogeneous bodies measuring 3–5 μm, often with a surrounding pale halo (**248**). The keratohyalin located in areas of viral cytopathic changes often has an inky, clumped appearance. Cytoplasmic vacuolation (ballooning) can be so extreme that it produces vesicles. In some instances, necrosis of epidermis and adnexal epithelium is present. The papillary dermis contains edema and an underlying perivascular inflammatory infiltrate, composed mainly of lymphocytes. The lymphocytic infiltrate may affect the epidermis. Newly formed dilated capillaries may be also seen within the dermis. The clinical differential diagnosis of these skin lesions is with potentially life-threatening zoonotic infections such as tularemia, cutaneous anthrax, and erysipeloid (Huerter *et al.*, 1991).

These diseases are self-limiting and usually spontaneously resolve. Surgical excision, surgical debulking, or cryotherapy can be curative for persistent lesions (Tan *et al.*, 1991; Degraeve *et al.*, 1999; Ballanger *et al.*, 2006). Some success has been seen using topical agents such as imiquimod or cidofovir in complicated cases (De Clercq & Neyts, 2004; Erbagci *et al.*, 2005; Dal Pozzo *et al.*, 2007; Lederman *et al.*, 2007).

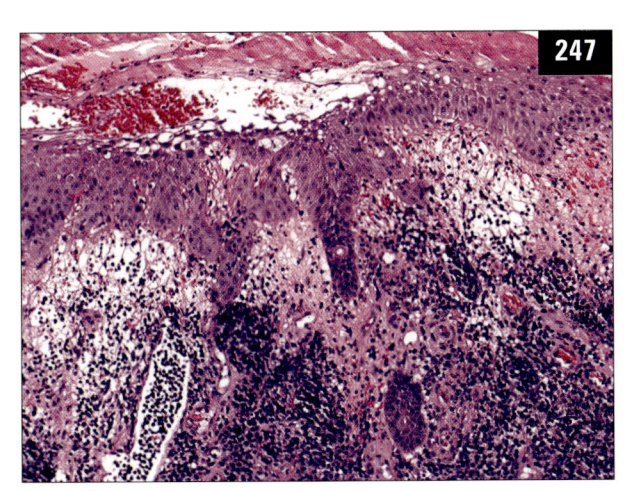

247 Orf. Pseudoepitheliomatous hyperplasia.

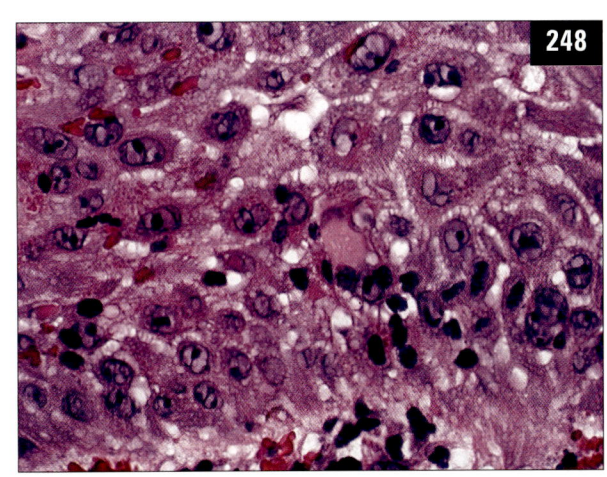

248 Cytoplasmic inclusions (orf). Cytoplasmic inclusion bodies.

CHAPTER 4

TROPICAL AND EXOTIC INFECTIOUS DISEASES

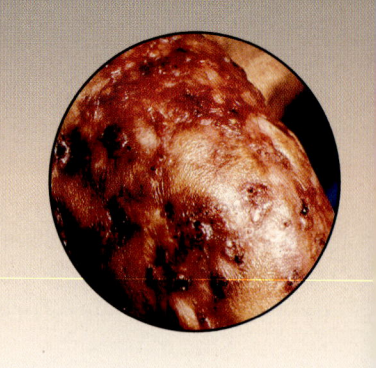

Omar P Sangüeza   Daniel J Sheehan   Gary Goldenberg

INTRODUCTION

During the past few years we have witnessed an increase in the incidence of infectious diseases. Two contributing factors are an increase in international travel and population migration. Diseases once considered to be exotic or indigenous to certain parts of the world are now seen on every continent and with an increased frequency. This chapter will provide an overview of tropical and exotic infectious diseases that present in the skin. It should be noted that the most common infectious diseases in tropical environments are impetigo, tinea, scabies, and louse infestation, conditions that are prevalent in temperate climates as well. Impetigo in tropical environments is often secondary to scabies infestation.

RHINOSCLEROMA

Rhinoscleroma is a chronic granulomatous disease that affects the oral and nasal mucosa and the upper respiratory tract and is caused by the encapsulated Gram-negative diplobacillus *Klebsiella rhinoscleromatis* (Boggino *et al.*, 2001; Iyengar *et al.*, 2005). In advanced cases, the disease can disseminate and compromise the trachea, larynx, and bronchi (Iyengar *et al.*, 2005). The mechanism of infection is unknown, but altered T-cell immunity has been implicated in cases of infection in the setting of human immunodeficiency virus (HIV) (Paul *et al.*, 1993). The incubation period is variable, lasting up to 6 months.

Artifacts from the Mayan culture dating to AD300 to 600 depict facial deformities thought to represent the earliest known evidence of rhinoscleroma (Goldman, 1979). Although traditionally a disease seen in developing countries, there are increasing numbers of cases being reported in the United States (Andraca *et al.*, 1993).

Initially, in the catarrhal stage, there is a nonspecific rhinitis with edema and inflammation of the mucosa (Boggino *et al.*, 2001; Verma *et al.*, 2005). Ulceration, with progression to nodules that infiltrate the nasal tissue and produce obstruction and deformation, can be seen in the granulomatous stage (Boggino *et al.*, 2001). In the final stage, there is scarring and further deformation with possible obstruction (Robbins *et al.*, 2004).

In the initial stage, the mucosa demonstrates granulation tissue with neutrophils. In the granulomatous phase, the epithelium shows pseudoepitheliomatous hyperplasia and the dermis contains dense infiltrates with plasma cells containing numerous Russell bodies with histiocytes known as Mikulicz cells that have ample cytoplasm loaded with bacilli (**249**) (Boggino *et al.*, 2001; Iyengar *et al.*, 2005). The bacilli are often visible with hematoxylin–eosin staining but can be highlighted with silver, Giemsa, Gram, or periodic acid-Schiff (PAS) stains (Boggino *et al.*, 2001). Under the electron microscope, these bacilli show long structures wrapped with phagosomes. The differential diagnosis includes leishmaniasis, leprosy, plasmacytoma, and squamous cellular carcinoma.

Treatment is often very difficult but may include fluoroquinolones, trimethoprim–sulfamethoxazole, tetracycline, chlortetracycline, chloramphenicol, cephaloridine, and rifampin (Boggino *et al.*, 2001; Fernandez-Vozmediano *et al.*, 2004). Months to years of antimicrobial therapy may be needed to prevent recurrence, which is common (Iyengar *et al.*, 2005; Robbins *et al.*, 2004). Surgical intervention is used to relieve airway compromise or for cosmesis (Robbins *et al.*, 2004).

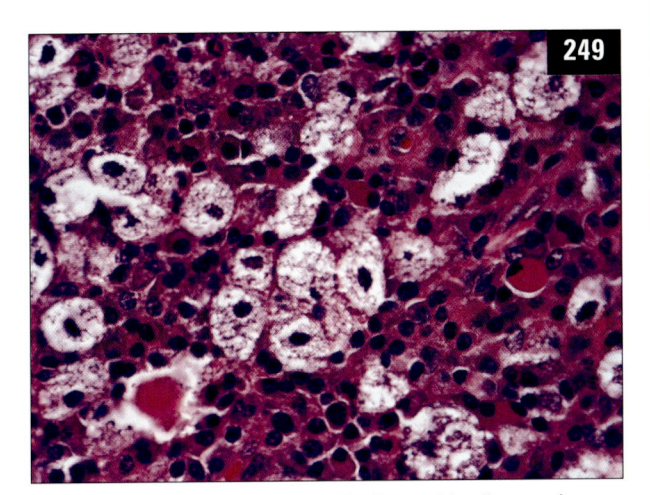

249 Rhinoscleroma. Plasma cells, Russell bodies, and parasitized histiocytes.

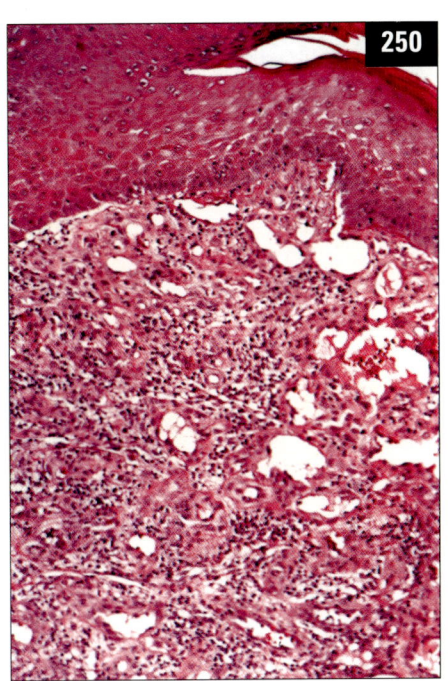

250 Bacillary angiomatosis. Proliferation of capillary-sized vessels.

BACILLARY ANGIOMATOSIS

Bacillary angiomatosis (BA) is a recently described systemic disorder that is usually associated with advanced immunosuppression, with CD4 counts below 200/µL, often in the setting of HIV (Jung & Paauw, 1998). It is usually seen in tropical areas where the prevalence of HIV is high and many patients go untreated. It is caused by two closely related Gram-negative coccobacilli, *Bartonella henselae* and *B. quintana* (Slater *et al.*, 1992). Recently reported cases describe infection in liver transplantation patients with cat exposure and in patients on long-term immunosuppressive agents such as methotrexate (Bonatti *et al.*, 2006; Kreitzer & Saoud, 2006). In addition, *B. henselae* causes cat-scratch disease and *B. quintana* can cause bacteremia and endocarditis in immunocompetent persons.

Clinically, these lesions resemble vascular proliferations and can affect any organ including the skin. Lesions vary in size and appearance, and may occur singly or be multiple depending on the immunologic status of the patient (Spach & Koehler, 1998). Typical cutaneous lesions are cherry to dusky-red papules or nodules surrounded by a rim of scale and may be pedunculated or ulcerative. Cutaneous lesions can mimic Kaposi's sarcoma. Subcutaneous lesions tend to be skin-colored and can be mistaken for soft tissue neoplasms (Schwartz *et al.*, 1997). Differential diagnosis includes pyogenic granuloma, angiolymphoid hyperplasia with eosinophilia, angiosarcoma, Kaposi's sarcoma, and verruga peruana.

Histopathologically, lesions of BA present with a vascular proliferation that occupies the dermis and can extend into the subcutaneous tissue (**250**). There may be prominent pseudoepitheliomatous hyperplasia in rare cases (Amsbaugh *et al.*, 2006). Numerous inflammatory cells, including lymphocytes, histiocytes, and neutrophils are present within the vessels. The endothelial cells lining the vascular spaces are prominent and may be pleomorphic, simulating a malignant vascular neoplasm. The cytoplasm of the endothelial cells shows a characteristic bluish granular material, which in sections stained with

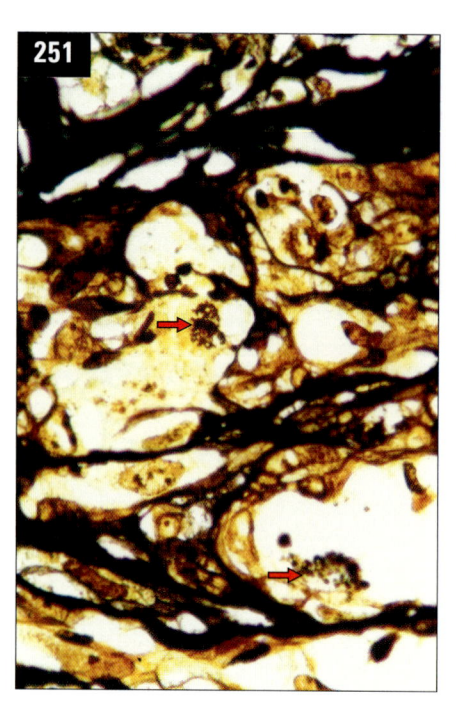

251 Bacillary angiomatosis. Silver stains demonstrate clusters of organisms.

Warthin–Starry or Grocott-methenamine silver, demonstrate bacilli (**251**) (Schwartz et al., 1997). Extraction, amplification by polymerase chain reaction (PCR), and sequencing of *Bartonella henselae* deoxyribonucleic acid (DNA) has been used successfully for diagnostic purposes as well as for monitoring treatment efficacy (Schlupen et al., 1997; Warren et al., 1998).

It is important to establish a quick and definitive diagnosis in cases of BA, since it responds to antibiotic therapy and may be life threatening (Rigopoulos et al., 2004). Treatment options include oral erythromycin or doxycycline. Recent evidence suggests erythromycin has potent antiangiogenic properties that contribute to therapeutic success (Meghari et al., 2006). Some patients require combination therapies such as azithromycin and doxycycline (Bonatti et al., 2006).

CUTANEOUS TUBERCULOSIS

Mycobacterium tuberculosis is an obligate intracellular, acid-fast bacillus that primarily causes pulmonary infections, and it is currently estimated to infect nearly one-third of the world's population, especially in tropical areas and the Indian subcontinent (Potter et al., 2005). Cutaneous tuberculosis (TB) represents 1.5% of all cases of extrapulmonary TB and occurs by exogenous inoculation, endogenous spread, and lymphatic or hematogenous dissemination. Cutaneous TB is still a common disease in India, and scrofuloderma and lupus vulgaris are the most common forms of cutaneous TB (Kumar & Muralidhar, 1999; Kumar et al., 2001).

Primary inoculation TB, or TB chancre, results from percutaneous inoculation or, rarely, mucosal inoculation of mycobacterium in patients without previous exposure (Sehgal & Wagh, 1990). Clinically, a nodule develops within 2–4 weeks at the site of inoculation. It then becomes a well-demarcated ulcer that heals with scarring. Associated lymphadenitis is common.

Acute miliary tuberculosis (AMTB), or TB cutis miliaris disseminata, is a usually fatal infection that is rare in adults and occurs more commonly in infants and children. It results from hematogenous dissemination from a pulmonary or meningeal source. Recently, the incidence of AMTB has been increasing, especially in adult patients with acquired immunodeficiency syndrome (AIDS) (Libraty & Byrd, 1996). Lesions may be located anywhere, but are frequently on the trunk, buttocks, genitalia, and thighs. Clinically, they are small papules capped with vesicles that rupture, crust over, and heal with scarring.

Lupus vulgaris (LV) may occur as a result of TB reinfection at sites distant to the primary disease, or as a result of direct inoculation, such as from a bacille Calmette–Guérin (BCG) vaccine (Mlika et al., 2006). It presents with several clinical variants, including plaque, hypertrophic, ulcerative, vegetating, and papulonodular forms. The plaque presentation may mimic other papulosquamous diseases (**252**) (Reich et al., 2006). Classically, LV presents as a plaque composed of multiple small, soft, brownish papules that have a characteristic 'apple-jelly' color when seen with diascopy (Bhardwaj & Mahajan, 2003). The papules enlarge and become infiltrative with central atrophy. Infiltration of mucous membranes may occur and cause destruction of cartilage.

TB verrucosa cutis is paucibacillary inoculation TB that occurs at sites of trauma in previously sensitized patients (Sethuraman et al., 2006). Clinically, patients may present with asymptomatic, erythematous papules that develop into a verrucous

Tropical and Exotic Infectious Diseases

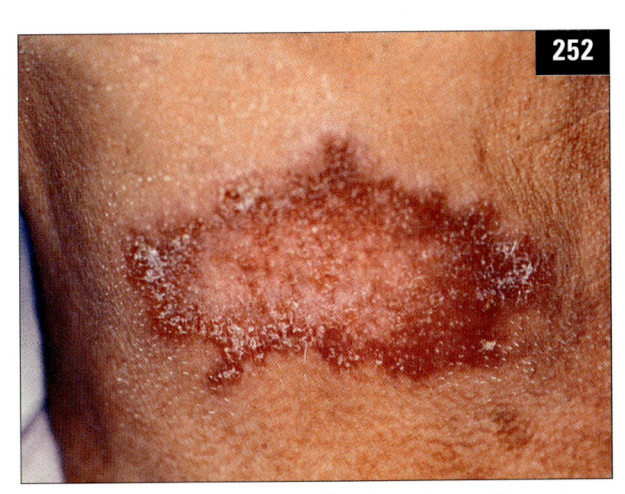

252 Lupus vulgaris. Verrucous border and atrophic center.

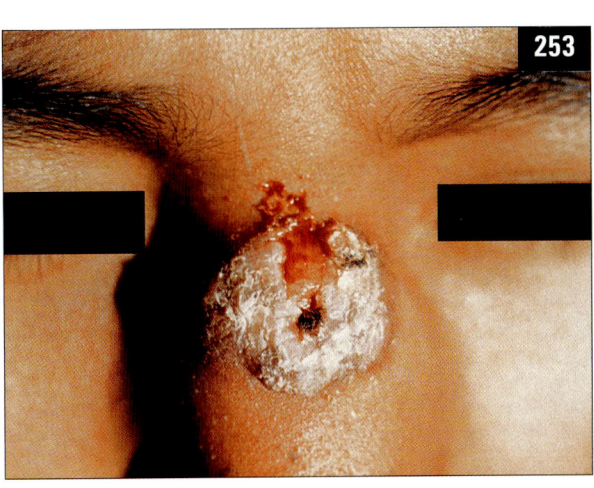

253 TB verrucosa cutis. These patients have a high degree of immunity.

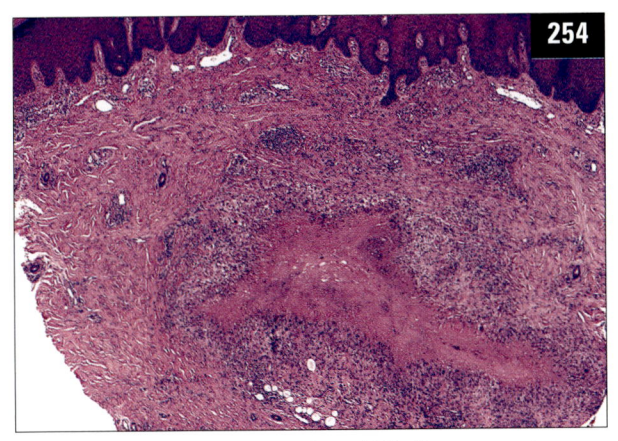

254 Histopathologic examination of TB. Note central caseous necrosis.

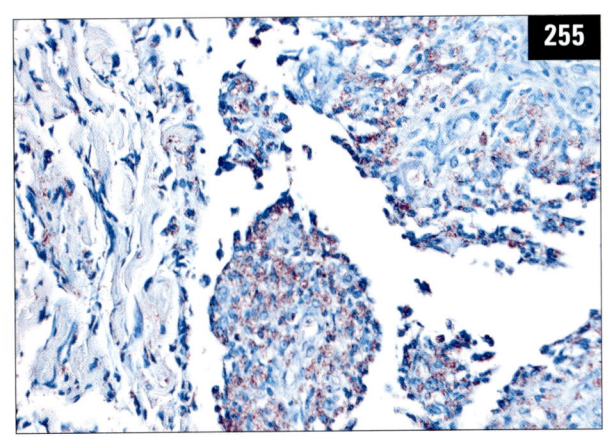

255 Ziehl–Neelsen stain of TB. Solidly acid-fast organisms resist decolorization.

plaque that may fissure and discharge purulent or keratinous material (**253**). Lymphadenopathy is usually not seen.

Scrofuloderma, or TB colliquativa cutis, is a direct extension of TB onto the overlying skin, usually from underlying infected lymph node, bone, or joint (Rai *et al.*, 2005). It is a reactivation form of TB that forms a sinus tract in the subcutaneous tissue overlying an infection focus, usually a cervical lymph node. The lesions begin as firm, mobile nodules that become attached to the skin, ulcerate, and develop draining sinus tracts. Healing usually produces characteristic chord-like scars.

Histopathologically, all forms of cutaneous TB show granulomas formed by histiocytes, some of them multinucleated, and collections of lymphocytes at the periphery (**254**). Areas of central necrosis may be present in some cases. Depending on the clinical form of TB, pseudoepitheliomatous hyperplasia may be present. In scrofuloderma, there are sinus tracts that connect the lymph node to the overlying epidermis. A Ziehl–Neelsen stain may help to identify the organisms (**255**); however, in skin biopsies organisms are usually very difficult to identify (Lee *et al.*, 2000). In one large case series, tissue culture revealed positive results in 9% of patients with cutaneous TB (Zouhair *et al.*, 2007). If available, PCR may be used as a very sensitive test to confirm infection rapidly from tissue samples (Negi *et al.*, 2005; Reich *et al.*, 2006). Purified protein derivative (PPD) skin-testing may be falsely negative in immunosuppressed patients (Lee et al., 2000).

Even patients with a history of BCG should be treated as if they have TB in the presence of a positive skin test (Rowland et al., 2006). Polychemotherapeutic regimens utilizing isoniazid, rifampin, ethambutol, and pyrazinamide are used to combat resistant organisms (Aliagaoglu et al., 2006; Reich et al., 2006; Zouhair et al., 2007). The World Health Organization (WHO) provides updated versions of recommended treatment regimens in an effort to minimize the propagation of multidrug-resistant organisms (WHOa).

LEPROSY

Leprosy, also known as Hansen's disease, is a systemic infection that has a clinical and histological spectrum related to the immunologic status of the host (Britton & Lockwood, 2004). Leprosy is caused by *Mycobacterium leprae*, which is endemic to tropical and subtropical regions (Hartzell et al., 2004). In the United States, cases have been seen in Texas, Louisiana, Hawaii, and California. Exposure to nine-banded armadillos, which may harbor the organism, is one means of infection (Paige et al., 2002; Lane et al., 2006). The organism prefers cooler parts of the body with the skin and peripheral nerves being the tissues primarily affected (Wathen, 1996). The classification of the spectrum of disease ranges from tuberculoid leprosy at one pole to lepromatous leprosy at the opposite pole, with various forms in between. Polymorphisms in the Toll-like receptor 2 gene have been implicated in the poor cellular immune response that results in lepromatous leprosy (Kang et al., 2004).

Upon initial contact with the organisms, lesions may be minimal and difficult to classify. This situation is referred to as indeterminate leprosy. Patients typically have a few hypopigmented, scaly macules on the face and extremities that can resemble tinea versicolor. In tuberculoid leprosy, patients can mount an adequate immune response resulting in few organisms in the skin. Tuberculoid leprosy patients present with one to several well-demarcated hypesthetic or anesthetic plaques in an asymmetric distribution (**256**). Cutaneous nerves may be enlarged. Many organisms are found in the skin in lepromatous leprosy because an adequate immune response cannot be achieved. These individuals usually have numerous symmetrically distributed nodules with irregular borders. Patients with borderline leprosy have various lesions including poorly circumscribed macules, papules, and plaques (**257**).

Indeterminate leprosy demonstrates a non-specific superficial and deep lymphohisticytic infiltrate. Biopsy of tuberculoid leprosy reveals histiocytes and granulomas around cutaneous nerves, sometimes extending into the surrounding dermis or all the way up to the epidermis. Bacilli are usually not identified with special stains in tuberculoid leprosy, but S-100 staining may facilitate identifying nerve fragmentation (Gupta et al., 2006). The granulomas of lepromatous leprosy are not discrete or clearly associated with nerve, but they tend to spare the epidermis and create a prominent Grenz (**258**). The macrophages of lepromatous leprosy often have a grayish, vacuolated cytoplasm, and identification of organisms in the macrophages and nerves is possible using the modified Fite–Faraco stain (**259**). *M. leprae* cannot be cultured on artificial media, but an ELISA test for phenolic glycolipid-I of *M. leprae* is available for confirmation, particularly in the setting of non-specific histologic findings (Jardim et al., 2005). The sensitivity of this test for phenolic glycolipid-I has been questioned (Sinha et al., 2004).

The WHO recommends treating multibacillary leprosy with 12 months of rifampin 600 mg once a month, dapsone 100 mg once a day, and clofazamine 300 mg once a month and 50 mg daily. This organization recommends treating paucibacillary leprosy with 6 months of rifampin 600 mg once a month and dapsone 100 mg daily (WHOb). Monthly doses of rifampin, ofloxacin, and minocycline (ROM) have been proven to be an effective treatment of multibacillary leprosy that may have advantages over the multidrug regimen recommended by the WHO (Villahermosa et al., 2004; Lane et al., 2006). BCG vaccination may provide some protection from infection and can be given to people known to have been exposed to *M. leprae* (Setia et al., 2006).

Tropical and Exotic Infectious Diseases

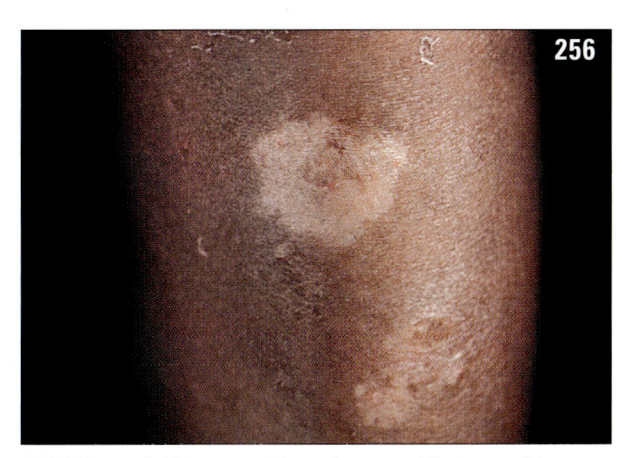

256 Tuberculoid leprosy. Hypopigmented lesions with subtle indurated border.

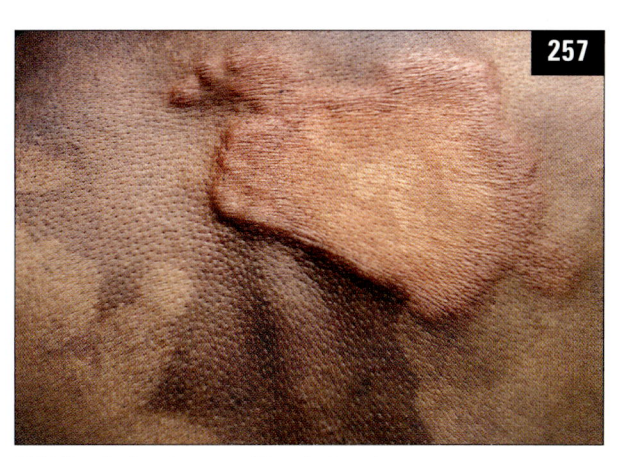

257 Borderline leprosy. Note induration.

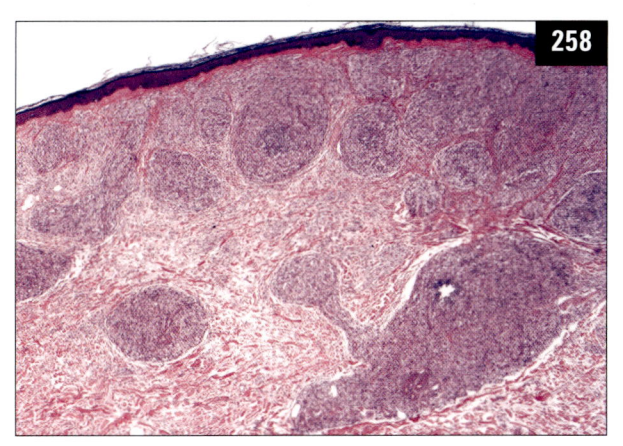

258 Granulomas of lepromatous leprosy. Granulomas are commonly parallel to the surface.

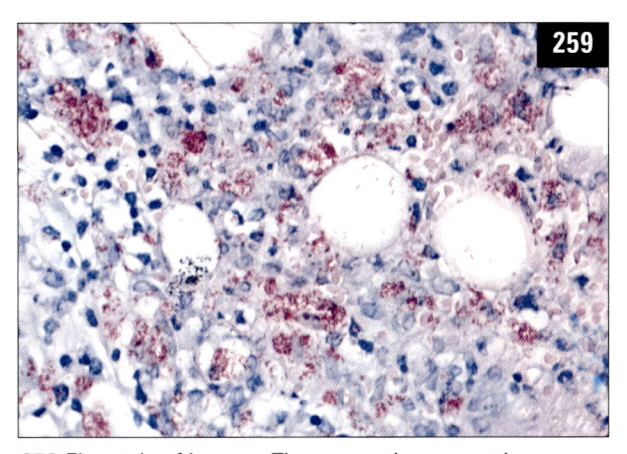

259 Fite stain of leprosy. These organisms must be decolorized gently.

MYCETOMA

Mycetomas are chronic, localized infections of the skin and subcutaneous tissue that may progress to involve muscle and bone. There is a strong male predominance (Maiti *et al.*, 2002). Infection often occurs on the extremities of people who work in rural areas and is usually secondary to traumatic inoculation of exposed skin (Saha S *et al.*, 2006). The highest incidence occurs in the tropics and subtropics secondary to the distribution of causative organisms, although some cases do occur in the southern United States. Mycetomas are classified as eumycotic (caused by fungi) or actinomycotic (caused by filamentous bacteria), with bacteria being responsible for the majority of infections (Lupi *et al.*, 2005). Bacterial causes include *Nocardia*, *Actinomyces*, and *Streptomyces*. The most common fungal causative organisms are *Madurella mycetoma*, *M. grisea*, and *Allescheria boydii* (McGinnis, 1996). The most common organism causing mycetoma in the United States is *Petrellidium boydii*.

The clinical manifestations of mycetoma include a triad of tumefaction, draining sinus tracts, and granule formation and extrusion (Lupi *et al.*, 2005). The affected skin is often indurated and hyperpigmented compared to the surrounding area (Fahal & Suliman, 1994). Lesions develop after a variable incubation period, and begin as a nodule that drains serosanguineous fluid. The lesions gradually progress and the extremity becomes edematous with multiple nodules and sinus tracts draining fluid and granules (260). The granules may be visible to the naked eye at times (Lupi *et al.*, 2005).

Diagnosis can be made clinically but identification of the etiologic organism is usually necessary. Microscopically, lesions of mycetoma contain areas of suppuration surrounded by histiocytes. The characteristic granules are located in the middle of the areas of suppuration (261). Special stains are important in differentiating between eumycotic and actinomycotic mycetomas, pseudomycetomas caused by the superficial dermatophytes, and the bacteria causing botryomycosis. Fungal mycetomas are Gomori methenamine-silver (GMS)- and PAS-positive, whereas actinomycotic mycetomas are Gram-positive (Lupi *et al.*, 2005). Fine needle aspiration (FNA) can facilitate diagnosis and differentiation between eumycetoma and actinomycetoma (El Haq *et al.*, 1996). Serologic tests exist but are complicated by cross reactions with mycobacteria (Lupi *et al.*, 2005). The causative organism may be determined based upon microscopic examination of granules and isolation of the organisms by culture (Zaias *et al.*, 1969). Bone involvement, which occurs late in the course of the disease, can be assessed by radiographs or magnetic resonance imaging (MRI) (De Palma *et al.*, 2006).

Actinomycetomas at all stages of involvement can be successfully treated with combination chemotherapy using regimens such as streptomycin and dapsone or trimethoprim–sulfamethoxazole and amikacin (Lupi *et al.*, 2005; De Palma *et al.*, 2006).

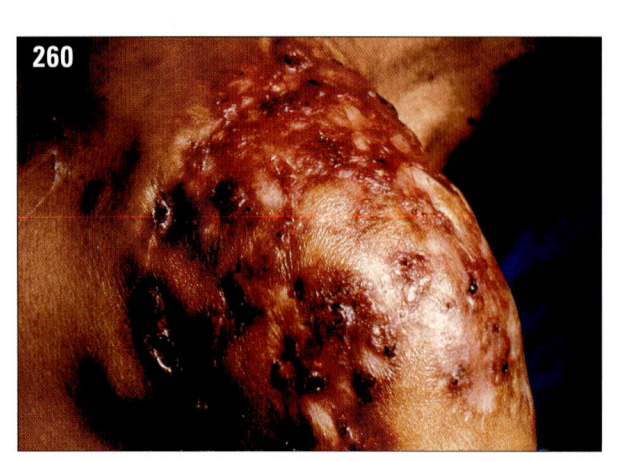

260 Mycetoma. Multiple draining sinus tracts.

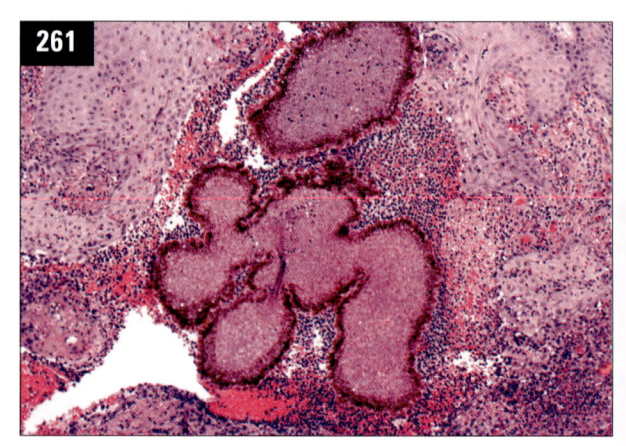

261 Characteristic granules of mycetoma. Pigmented grains of a eumycetoma.

Often, more than 1 year of therapy is needed (Lupi *et al.*, 2005). Surgical intervention, including excision or amputation, is reserved for cases refractory to chemotherapy (De Palma *et al.*, 2006).

Surgery is the most widely used treatment for eumycetomas, with care exercised to avoid disrupting the lesion's capsule and consequently releasing fungal elements into the operative field (Lupi *et al.*, 2005). Some cases of eumycetoma have been successfully treated with agents such as posaconazole (Negroni *et al.*, 2005).

CHROMOBLASTOMYCOSIS

Chromoblastomycosis, also known as chromomycosis, is caused by several different dematiaceous fungi that naturally inhabit soil and organic matter. This disease can occur worldwide but is seen most commonly in rural areas of Africa, Asia, and South America. The fungi are thought to gain access with minor skin trauma, as with walking barefoot. The most commonly isolated pathogen is *Fonsecaea pedrosoi* (Esterre *et al.*, 1996). Other associated organisms include *Phialophora verrucosa*, *Fonsecaea compacta*, *Cladophialophora carrionii*, and *Rhinocladiella aquaspersa* (Lupi *et al.*, 2005).

Skin-colored papules insidiously evolve into ulcerated, verrucous plaques or vegetations (**262, 263**) (Lupi *et al.*, 2005). The lesions may be very pruritic, and over time they may cause significant lymphedema (Sangüeza *et al.*, 2000).

Sclerotic bodies are easily seen in hematoxylin and eosin tissue staining, usually in the deeper portion of the tissue (Lupi *et al.*, 2005). These bodies consist of brown septate round cells (**264**). Often there is overlying pseudoepitheliomatous hyperplasia (Sangüeza *et al.*, 2000). Culture, with attention to sporulation patterns, is needed to identify the causative organism.

Excision is the most reliable treatment, as many different systemic antifungal agents have been utilized with mixed results (Iijima *et al.*, 1995; Poirriez *et al.*, 2000; Lupi *et al.*, 2005). Posaconazole has been advocated as a successful treatment for particularly challenging cases (Negroni *et al.*, 2005). Physical methods such as local heat or cryotherapy have also been advocated. Ultimately, amputation of the affected limb may become necessary.

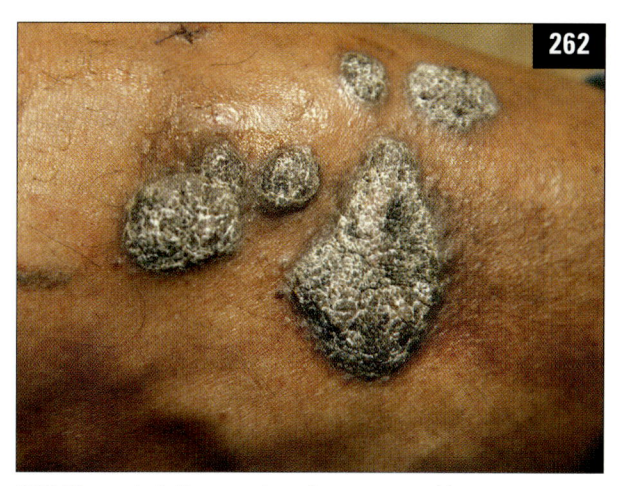

262 Characteristic granules of mycetoma. Verrucous plaques.

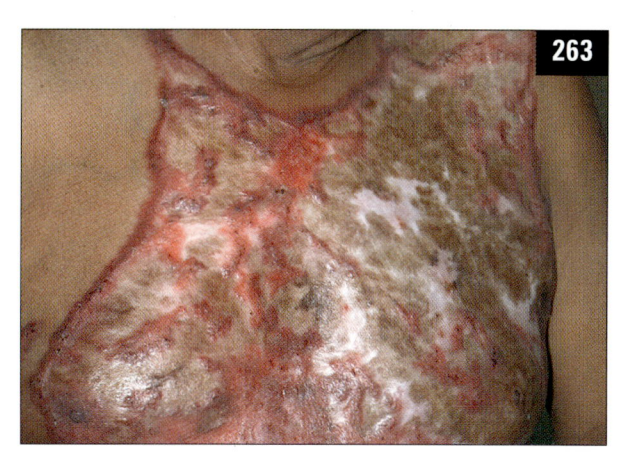

263 Chromoblastomycosis. Note raised border and central scarring.

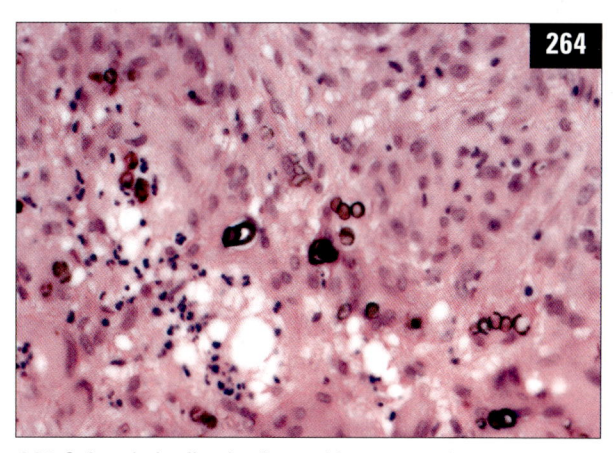

264 Sclerotic bodies in chromoblastomycosis. Characteristic 'copper pennies'.

LOBOMYCOSIS

Lacazia loboi causes chronic granulomatous skin infections known as lobomycosis, keloidal blastomycosis, or Lobo disease (Sangüeza *et al.*, 2000; Lupi *et al.*, 2005). Agricultural workers acquire the infection via percutaneous inoculation. Only rarely do cases occur outside of Central or South America (Burns *et al.*, 2000; Elsayed *et al.*, 2004). In some cases, there may be an incubation period lasting years (Burns *et al.*, 2000). The causative organism has never been cultured, but DNA evidence suggests it is a dimorphic fungus (Herr *et al.*, 2001). Dolphins can have lesions identical to those seen in humans, suggesting that an aquatic reservoir must exist (Lupi *et al.*, 2005; Norton, 2006). Certain bodies of water have been noted to have a dolphin population with a prevalence of lobomycosis approaching 30% (Reif *et al.*, 2006). One case report exists documenting transmission from an infected dolphin to a human (De Vries & Laarman, 1975).

Any cutaneous surface can be affected, although the mucous membranes are usually spared (Sangüeza *et al.*, 2000). Keloidal nodules, which may be pruritic or hypoesthetic, are the most common type of cutaneous lesion, but verrucous or ulcerative plaques may also be seen (**265**) (Sangüeza *et al.*, 2000). The earliest lesion may be a papule, pustule, or wart-like lesion which evolves over months or years to a keloidal nodule (Lupi *et al.*, 2005). The ears and the lower extremities are the most commonly affected areas (Lupi *et al.*, 2005).

Histologically, there is prominent fibrosis in the dermis and subcutaneous tissue, with a dense infiltrate of lymphocytes, histiocytes, and foamy macrophages (Sangüeza *et al.*, 2000). Multinucleated histiocytes or asteroid bodies may be present. The yeast are found within the histiocytes and are easily identified on hematoxylin and eosin staining due to the melanin content of their cell walls (**266**) (Lupi *et al.*, 2005). They are 6–12 μm round thick-walled cells with a double contour membrane, and they may appear as a chain (Sangüeza *et al.*, 2000; Lupi *et al.*, 2005). PAS or GMS stains may be used to help identify the organisms in more subtle cases (**267**). Serologic tests exist but lack specificity due to cross reaction with organisms such as *Paracoccidioides* (Camargo *et al.*, 1998; Lupi *et al.*, 2005).

Many traditional antifungal agents have been found to be ineffective (Lawrence & Ajello, 1986; Lupi *et al.*, 2005). Clofazimine has been used with some success at a dose of 300 mg/day (Fischer *et al.*, 2002; Lupi *et al.*, 2005). Wide surgical excision has been advocated to prevent relapse (Burns *et al.*, 2000; Lupi *et al.*, 2005).

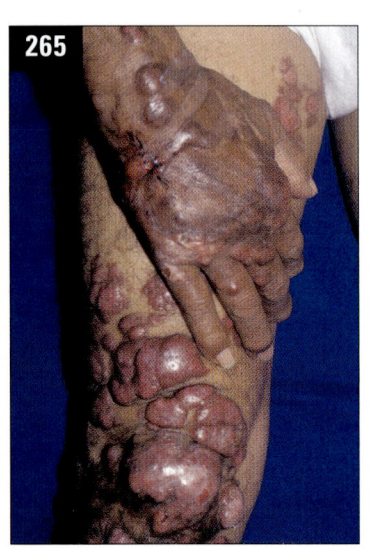

265 Nodular plaques in lobomycosis.

266 Hematoxylin and eosin staining of lobomycosis. Note chains of organisms.

267 PAS or GMS stain of lobomycosis.

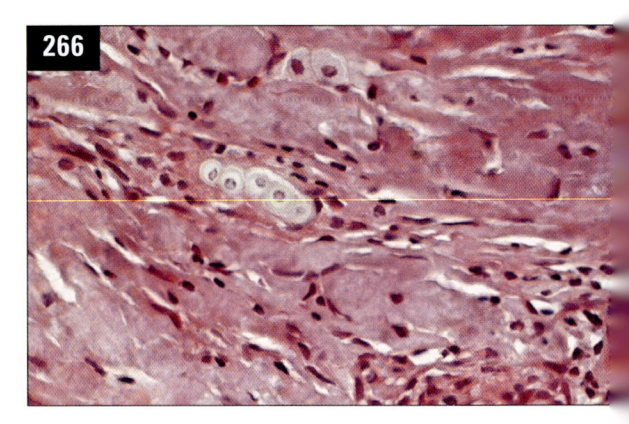

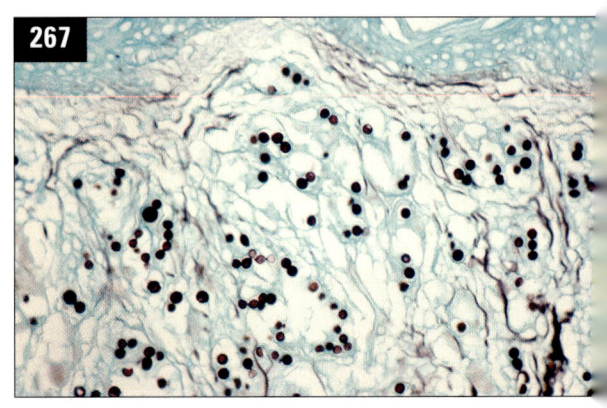

PARACOCCIDIOIDOMYCOSIS

Paracoccidioides brasiliensis causes a disease known as paracoccidioidomycosis, or South American blastomycosis, in Central and South America (Sangüeza *et al.*, 2000). The organism, a dimorphic fungus, is found in the soil and infection occurs via inhalation (Lupi *et al.*, 2005). The resulting infection can vary from a subclinical phenomenon to acute or chronic pulmonary and/or skin infection, depending upon the immune status of the host (Sangüeza *et al.*, 2000; Mamoni & Blotta, 2005). There are several postulated mechanisms by which the organisms evade or alter host immunity (Batista *et al.*, 2005; Lupi *et al.*, 2005). Young to middle-aged males who work outdoors are typically affected. Bats and small monkeys are possible natural reservoirs (Lupi *et al.*, 2005).

The incubation period for the acute infection can be several years (Lupi *et al.*, 2005). Acute disseminated infection presents with variable skin lesions sparing the mucous membranes, while chronic disseminated infection tends to involve the mucous membranes (**268**). Approximately half of the patients with the chronic disseminated infection will have punctate nasal and pharyngeal ulcers known as Aguiar–Pupo stomatitis (Lupi *et al.*, 2005). The central face is commonly affected by cutaneous lesions such as crusted papules, nodules, or verrucous lesions (Lupi *et al.*, 2005). The condition can be fatal due to pulmonary, central nervous system, or adrenal involvement (de Almeida, 2005; Lupi *et al.*, 2005).

Histologically, pseudoepitheliomatous hyperplasia is a common finding (Kaminagakura *et al.*, 2006). Mixed infiltrates are present in the dermis, including lymphocytes, neutrophils, and histiocytes. The organisms, which at times may assume a 'steering wheel' appearance, range in size from 5 to 9 μm (**269, 270**). Tissue culture and serology may help to confirm the diagnosis (Sangüeza *et al.*, 2000; da Silva *et al.*, 2005; Lupi *et al.*, 2005). However, positive serology results may not be specific to *Paracoccidioides brasiliensis* (Albuquerque *et al.*, 2005).

Sulfonamides such as sulfamethoxypyridazine and sulfadimethoxine have been touted by some as the 'drugs of choice' in treating this condition (Lupi *et al.*, 2005). However, itraconazole, fluconazole, ketoconazole, terbinafine, and amphotericin B have been shown to be of benefit as well (Visbal *et al.*, 2005). The necessary treatment duration may be 24 months given the tendency of this disease to be slowly evolving and lethal (Nogueira *et al.*, 2006).

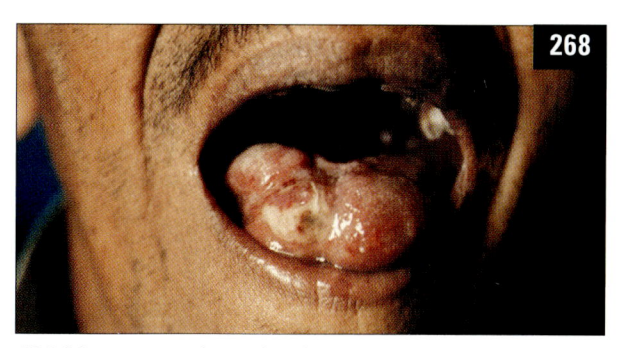

268 Mucous membrane involvement in *paracoccidioidomycosis*.

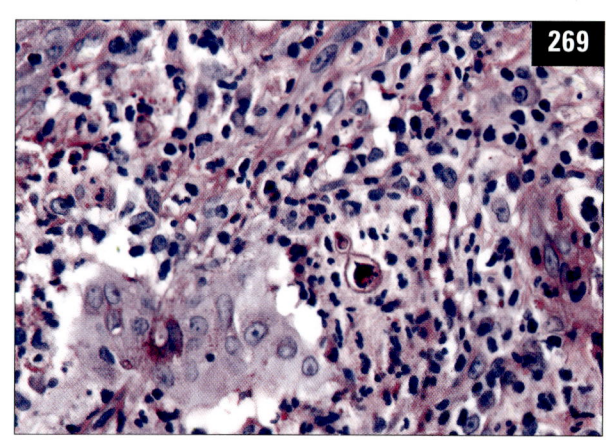

269 Narrow-based bud characteristic of *Paracoccidioides brasiliensis*.

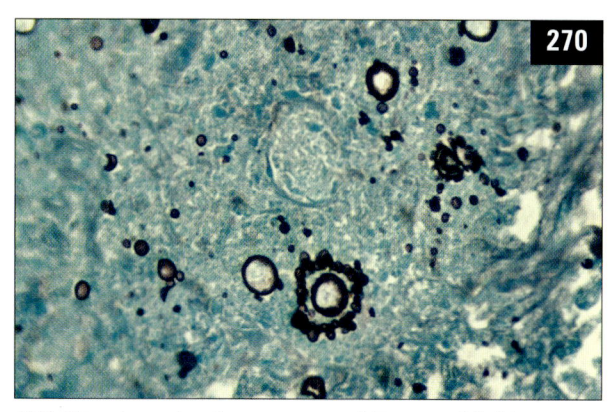

270 'Steering wheel' appearance of *Paracoccidioides brasiliensis*.

ACANTHAMEBIASIS

Species of the genus *Acanthamoeba* are ubiquitous, but rarely cause infections in humans (Steinberg *et al.*, 2002). Necrotizing keratitis is the most common infection produced by *Acanthamoeba*, and is usually not associated with cutaneous lesions or immunodeficiency (Vemuganti *et al.*, 2005). Cutaneous infections caused by *Acanthamoeba* are most common in patients with AIDS and may be primary, occurring as a result of direct inoculation, or secondary to dissemination from a pulmonary or central nervous system infection (Murakawa *et al.*, 1995; Marciano-Cabral & Cabral, 2003). Organ transplant recipients are also at risk (Steinberg *et al.*, 2002).

Cutaneous lesions are a common initial sign of infection in immunocompromised patients (Steinberg *et al.*, 2002). Erythematous papules or nodules appear, drain purulent material, and ulcerate (Marciano-Cabral & Cabral, 2003). The skin lesions, often on the extremities, can progress to life-threatening central nervous system involvement (Rosenberg & Morgan, 2001). Unusual clinical scenarios have involved osteomyelitis or lobular panniculitis with vasculitis as the initial sign of infection (Rosenberg & Morgan, 2001; Steinberg *et al.*, 2002).

When performing a skin biopsy, it is important to biopsy the raised advancing margin, where the organisms are usually concentrated. The histopathologic features depend on the immune status of the patient. Lesions in immunocompetent hosts show granulomas with only a few organisms, while lesions in immunosupressed patients have areas of necrosis in the dermis and subcutaneous tissue mixed with foci of suppuration. In some cases, deposits of fibrin in the vessel walls and nuclear dust may be present. This pattern resembles a vasculitis. The trophozoites, in these cases, are easily identified within the areas of suppuration and around the vessels. They have a centrally located nucleus, a single nucleolus, and prominent perinucleolar clearing (**271**) (Rosenberg & Morgan, 2001; Steinberg *et al.*, 2002). Trophozoites are often mistaken for macrophages, and may also be confused with the yeasts of *Blastomyces dermatitides* (Steinberg *et al.*, 2002). GMS and PAS help differentiate between the cysts of *Acanthamoeba* and *Entameba histolytica*. The cysts of *Acanthamoeba*, which measure 15–20 μm,

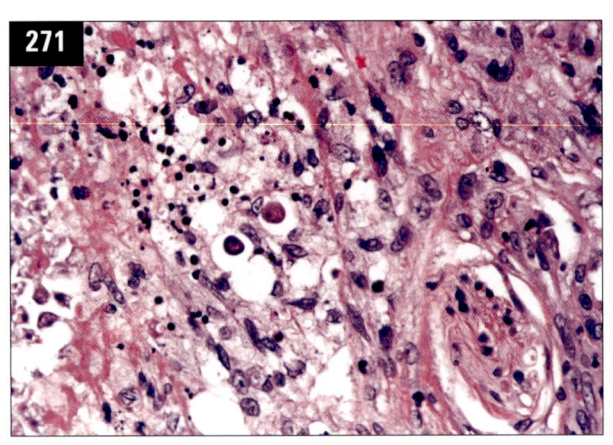

271 Acanthamebiasis. The vasculotropic organisms are best cultured on a lawn of *E. coli*.

have a double cell wall which is highlighted by both GMS and PAS (Rosenberg & Morgan, 2001; Steinberg *et al.*, 2002). The ectocyst has a wavy, wrinkled appearance while the endocyst is described as scalloped (Rosenberg & Morgan, 2001). Culture and immunochemistry can confirm the diagnosis.

Combination medical therapies are used as adjunctive treatments to surgical debridement. One patient was successfully treated with itraconazole, azithromycin, 5-flucytosine, and rifampin (Rosenberg & Morgan, 2001). Pentamidine has also been used in combination with 5-flucytosine (Steinberg *et al.*, 2002). Patients with central nervous system involvement typically do not respond to medical therapy (Steinberg *et al.*, 2002).

AMEBIASIS

Amebiasis is a gastrointestinal infection caused by *Entamoeba histolytica*, the only species of entameba that is typically pathogenic for humans (Magana *et al.*, 2004). The cyst, which measures 10–25 μm, starts the infective stage once ingested. The trophozoites are responsible for tissue invasion (Magana *et al.*, 2004). Cutaneous involvement is very rare, but may occur secondary to extension of rectal amebiasis to the anus, perianal skin, and the vulva, extension of a liver abscess to the skin of the abdominal wall, sexual transmission, or by primary infection (Magana *et al.*, 2004). Anogenital involvement in young children is thought to be due to prolonged contact between skin and feces in the diaper in the setting of diarrhea or dysentery (Kenner & Rosen, 2006). Mexico has the

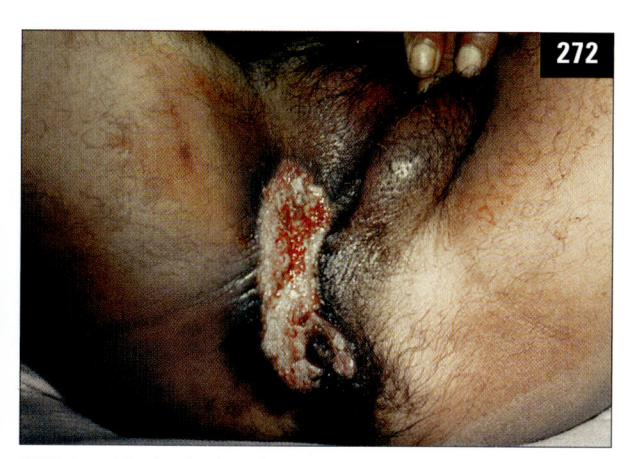

272 Amebiasis. Peri-anal verrucous lesions and fistulas occur.

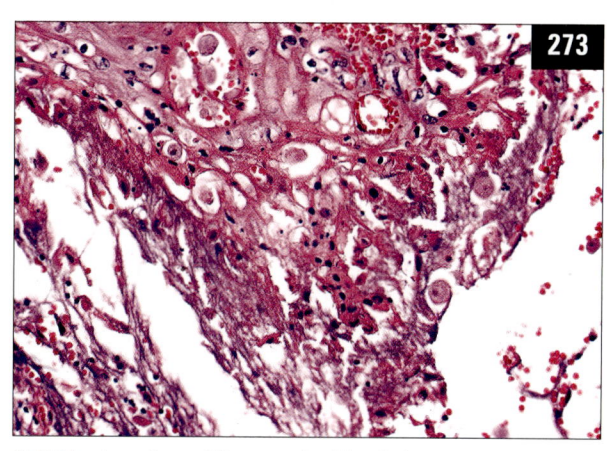

273 Trophozoites of *Entamoeba histolytica*.

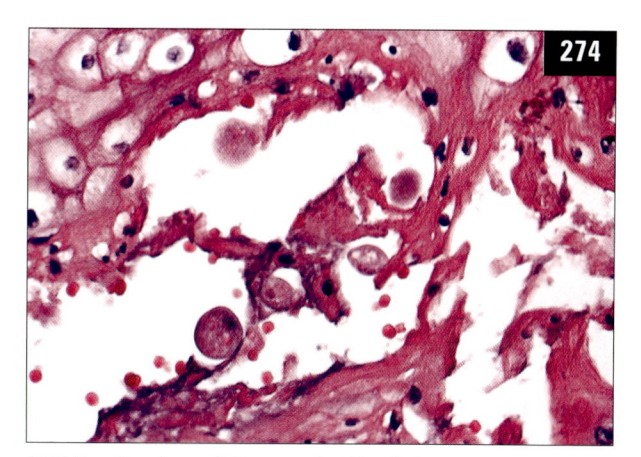

274 Trophozoites of *Entamoeba histolytica*.

highest known incidence of cutaneous amebiasis. Only two cases have been reported in the United States (Kenner & Rosen, 2006).

Cutaneous lesions are usually tender, oval ulcers with irregular borders and a gray-white necrotic base (**272**). The lesions may bleed easily (Kenner & Rosen, 2006). Skin involvement can be both painful and rapidly progressive, resulting in significant tissue destruction (Magana *et al.*, 2004). The verrucous lesions in the genital area may be confused with squamous cell carcinoma or condylomata acuminata. One case report of *Balamuthia mandrillaris* infection describes the slow progression over 18 months of cutaneous lesions, evolving to fatal central nervous system involvement (granulomatous amebic encephalitis) in an immunocompetent patient (Pritzker *et al.*, 2004).

Serologic tests are sensitive and specific but cannot distinguish between current and past infection (Kenner & Rosen, 2006). Histopathologically, ulcerated lesions of cutaneous amebiasis demonstrate ulceration and necrosis covered by cellular debris and crust. Adjacent to these areas is prominent pseudoepitheliomatous hyperplasia. Mixed inflammatory infiltrates are present in the dermis, and can extend into the subcutaneous tissue (Magana *et al.*, 2004). Within the ulcerated and necrotic areas, it is possible to identify the trophozoites of *E. histolytica*. They measure 20–50 µm and have ample finely granular eosinophilic cytoplasm, excentric nuclei, and prominent nucleoli (**273, 274**) (Magana *et al.*, 2004). The trophozoites often contain erythrocytes within their cytoplasm (Magana *et al.*, 2004). Motile trophozoites may also be seen in a scraping from the edge of an ulcer (Kenner & Rosen, 2006). Verrucous lesions show prominent irregular hyperplasia and inflammatory infiltrates, with few organisms present.

Metronidazole in combination with dehydroemetine, chloroquine, or iodoquinol has proved to be a successful regimen in treating intestinal amebiasis (Kenner & Rosen, 2006). Cutaneous infection can be treated with dehydroemetine in combination with diiodohydroxyquinolone, iodoquinol, or metronidazole (Magana *et al.*, 2004; Kenner & Rosen, 2006). Metronidazole at a dose of 40 mg/kg and iodoquinol 40 mg/kg were used to successfully treat one case (Kenner & Rosen, 2006). Surgical debridement may also be necessary. Pentamidine has *in vitro* evidence for effectiveness against *Balamuthia mandrillaris* (Pritzker *et al.*, 2004).

LEISHMANIASIS

Leishmaniasis is a parasitic infection transmitted by sandflies endemic to South America and areas of Asia and Africa. Leishmania are obligate intracellular parasites that exist in two forms. After inoculation with the promastigotes, transformation into amastigotes in the cells of the reticuloendothelial system in the human host occurs (Herwaldt, 1999). Sandflies transmit the organism between humans, dogs, and rodents. Humans are an accidental host and contract leishmaniasis when they venture into endemic habitats. There are three clinical variants of leishmaniasis: localized cutaneous leishmaniasis caused by *L. tropica*, visceral leishmaniasis caused by *L. donovani*, and mucocutaneous leishmaniasis caused by *L. brasiliensis*. Cutaneous leishmaniasis is known by the synonyms oriental sore and Baghdad sore, while mucocutaneous leishmaniasis is also known as Chiclero's ulcer, Uta, espundia, and forest yaws. Visceral leishmaniasis, which has been associated with tourism to Mediterranean countries and HIV infection, is also referred to by the term kala-azar (Malik et al., 2006). Although rare, cases of leishmaniasis have been linked to transfusion of infected blood products (Cardo, 2006).

Cutaneous leishmaniasis presents as small, well-demarcated papules that may progress to nodules that become ulcerative or verrucous plaques (**275, 276**). They are usually solitary but may be multiple, following lymphatic chains. They may heal leaving significant milia (Walker et al., 2006). Most acute infections resolve spontaneously but may become chronic or disseminated, especially in patients with deficient cell-mediated immunity. Immunosuppression may result in atypical clinical presentations (Saha M et al., 2006).

The clinical lesions of mucocutaneous leishmaniasis may progress through three stages: cutaneous, cicatricial, and mucocutaneous (Sangüeza et al., 1993). In the cutaneous stage, patients present with small nodules or plaques that may ulcerate. Occasionally, verrucous lesions may be seen. In the majority of cases, these lesions resolve spontaneously with scars (cicatricial stage) and the only evidence of the previous infection is a positive Montenegro skin test. During this stage, inactive parasites may be present in the reticuloendothelial system, including bone marrow, lymph nodes, and spleen. Immunologically impaired patients may progress to the disseminated form of cutaneous leishmaniasis. After a variable period of time, ranging from months to more than 20 years, some patients develop the mucocutaneous stage (**277**). Mucosal lesions range from simple edema of the lips and nose to perforation of the nasal and laryngeal cartilage. The parasite has tropism for the nasal cartilage. In many cases, there is extensive loss of tissue in the mouth and nose and alteration in the phonation because of the destruction of the vocal cords.

Biopsy of cutaneous lesions shows areas of ulceration, pseudoepitheliomatous hyperplasia, and mixed inflammatory infiltrates composed of neutrophils, plasma cells, lymphocytes, and histiocytes. Amastigotes are present in dermal macrophages and are easy to identify (**278**). Over time, the lesions become granulomatous with an increasing number of giant cells and a declining number of parasites. Caseating necrosis in the dermis associated with chronic cutaneous leishmaniasis may be seen. In the cicatricial stage, the epidermis is atrophic and hyperpigmented with fibrosis and scarring in the dermis. Similar histopathologic changes are seen in mucosal lesions.

The diagnosis of leishmaniasis can be confirmed by demonstrating the presence of amastigotes in dermal macrophages by skin biopsy, dermal scrapings, or FNA. The Montenegro skin test uses leishmanial antigen to induce a cell-mediated response. This test has diagnostic value but cannot distinguish between past and present infections. False-negatives may occur in anergic patients with disseminated infections. The organisms can be cultured on specialized media. Serologic and immunologic tests are also available for confirmation. PCR testing may facilitate diagnosis, particularly in non-endemic areas (Willard et al., 2005; Boer et al., 2006).

Pentavalent antimony compounds have been the mainstay of treatment for cutaneous and visceral leishmaniasis since the 1940s. For localized cutaneous and mucocutaneous leishmaniasis, the drug of choice is meglumine antimonate, at a recommended dose of 15mg/kg/day for localized cutaneous leishmaniasis and 20 mg/kg/day for the mucocutaneous form, IM for 20–30 days. Adding pentoxifylline to the regimen may improve efficacy (Sadeghian & Nilforoushzadeh, 2006). Amphotericin B is often used when the antimonials prove ineffective, but has had particular success in treating visceral leishmaniasis (Bern *et al.*, 2006). Amphotericin B has also been shown to be safer during pregnancy than sodium stibogluconate (Mueller *et al.*, 2006). Pentamidine isothionate is an alternative treatment. The recommended dose is 4 mg/kg IM for 3 days. Alternative regimens using ketoconazole, itraconazole, terbinafine, and mefloquine have been used, but the results are controversial and they have yet to find a place in routine clinical practice. There is also increasing evidence that miltefosine may be as effective as traditional regimens in treating New World cutaneous leishmaniasis and visceral leishmaniasis, but it is contraindicated in pregnancy (Ritmeijer *et al.*, 2006; Sindermann & Engel, 2006; Soto & Berman, 2006). Local heat and cryotherapy have been reported to have some success in treating cutaneous leishmaniasis (Aram & Leibovici, 1987; Willard *et al.*, 2005; Stavropoulos *et al.*, 2006).

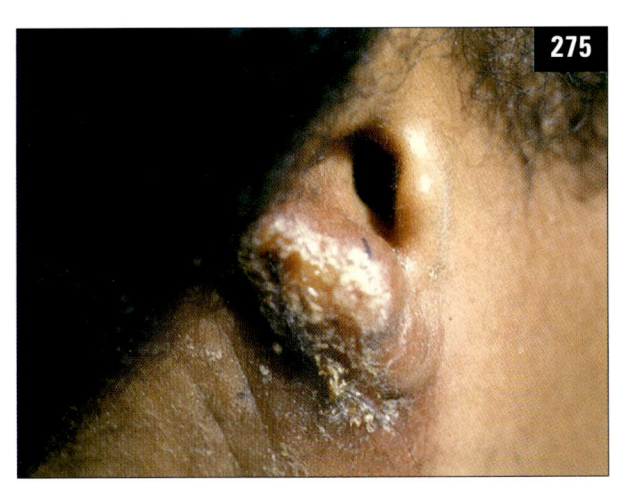

275 Cutaneous leishmaniasis. Typical involvement on the ear.

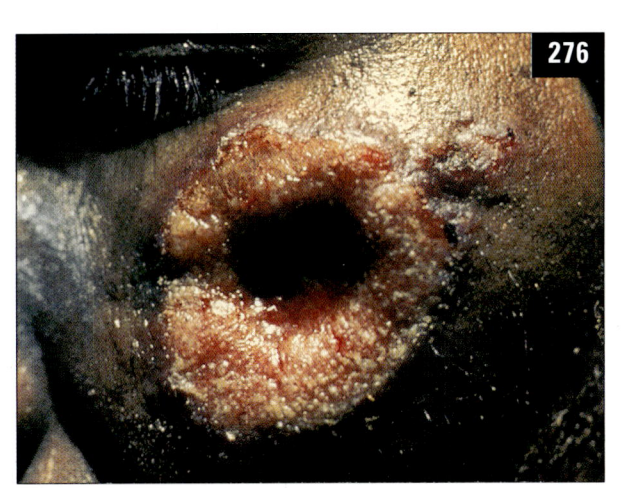

276 Cutaneous leishmaniasis. Indurated lesion.

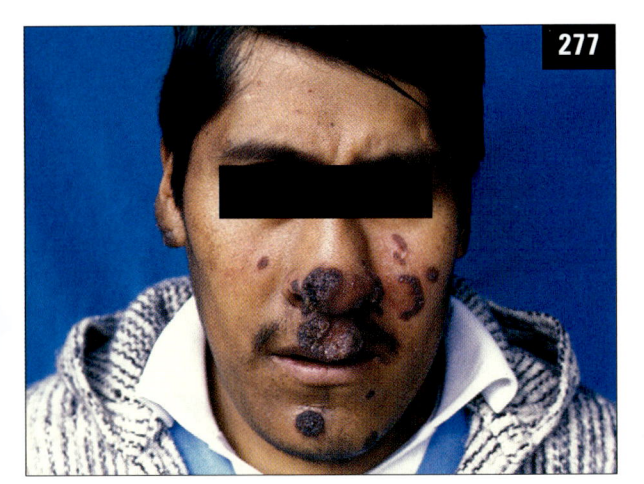

277 Mucocutaneous leishmaniasis. Nasal destruction may occur.

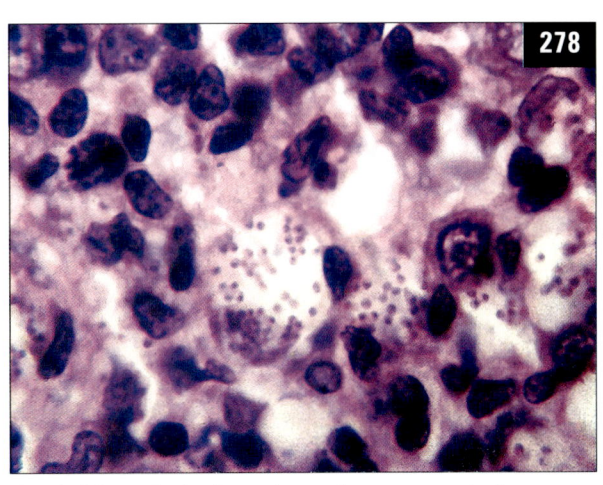

278 Leishmaniasis. Amastigotes in cutaneous lesions.

ONCHOCERCIASIS

Onchocerciasis is a filarial nematode infestation that predominantely affects cutaneous and ocular tissues and is caused by *Onchocerca volvulus*. It is common in Africa and Central and South America, and it is estimated that 17.7 million people are infected with *O. volvulus* (Hall & Pearlman, 1999). Infective larvae are transmitted by the bite of the black fly of the genus *Similium*, which is an obligate intermediate host of *O. volvulus* (Hall & Pearlman, 1999). These flies live near freely flowing bodies of water (Okulicz *et al.*, 2004). The larvae of *O. volvulus* develop into adults that aggregate into bundles to cause painless subcutaneous nodules called 'onchocercomas' (Okulicz *et al.*, 2004). These are located more frequently on the upper body in patients in Central and South America, and on the lower trunk in patients from Africa. Microfilariae are produced after copulation, and migrate and take residence in various tissues, including the skin.

Cutaneous lesions are the most common indication of infection (Nguyen *et al.*, 2005). Pruritus is the main symptom of cutaneous disease and is caused by an intense inflammatory reaction to degenerating microfilariae located in the skin or deep tissue (Stingl, 1997; Gardon *et al.*, 2002; Okulicz *et al.*, 2004). Abscesses may form when infected individuals are treated with diethylcarbamazine. In chronic disease, the skin becomes thickened, wrinkled, and atrophic. The back, thighs, and lower trunk are frequently affected, with pigmentary changes consisting of loss of pigment with sparing around hair follicles and subsequent repigmentation, so-called 'leopard skin' (Nguyen *et al.*, 2005). These changes are most notable on the shins. Chronic lymphatic obstruction can lead to 'hanging groin' and elephantiasis of the legs, feet, or genitalia (**279**) (Nguyen *et al.*, 2005). Travelers to endemic areas may present only with pruritus or unilateral limb edema (Wolfe *et al.*, 1974; Nguyen *et al.*, 2005). Clinical differential diagnosis includes leprosy and it may also be misdiagnosed if the skin snip is contaminated with blood filariae, especially *Mansonella perstans* and *Loa loa*. Blindness can occur as a result of chronic corneal inflammation, iridocyclitis, optic neuritis, or optic atrophy (Nguyen *et al.*, 2005).

Microscopic examination of a skin snip with normal saline is diagnostic when the microfilariae are visualized (Gardon *et al.*, 1997). Newer tests utilize PCR, enzyme-linked immunosorbent assay, or rapid antibody cards (Okulicz *et al.*, 2004; Nguyen *et al.*, 2005). The Mazzotti reaction, elicited by administration of diethylcarbamazine, is also diagnostic and can be seen with treatment of the infection (Awadzi *et al.*, 1995). The Mazzotti test is rarely used now because of the risk of sudden and often serious adverse effects (Okulicz *et al.*, 2004).

Histopathologically, in onchocercal dermatitis there is a mixed inflammatory infiltrate with a large number of eosinophils. Microfilariae can be seen in slits between collagen bundles in the upper dermis and measure 220–360 µm long and 5–9 µm wide (Okulicz *et al.*, 2004). The subcutaneous nodules are composed of dense hyaline fibrous tissue that surrounds the worms (**280, 281**). Associated with this fibrous tissue are inflammatory infiltrates composed of lymphocytes, histiocytes, and numerous eosinophils (Okulicz *et al.*, 2004). In older lesions, areas of fibrosis and calcification may be seen. The epidermis may show hyperplasia, with hyperkeratosis and parakeratosis as a consequence of the rubbing of the lesions later in the disease. In the dermis, there may also be pigment incontinence, tortuous vessels, and dilated lymphatics (Okulicz *et al.*, 2004).

Ivermectin has become the drug of choice in treatment with the standard dose being 150 µg/kg every 3–12 months (Stingl, 1997; Gardon *et al.*, 2002; Okulicz *et al.*, 2004; Nguyen *et al.*, 2005). Adverse reactions to the treatment can be addressed with topical or systemic steroids (Nguyen *et al.*, 2005). Amocarzine and suramin are also able to kill adult worms (Okulicz *et al.*, 2004). Onchocercomas can be excised (Okulicz *et al.*, 2004).

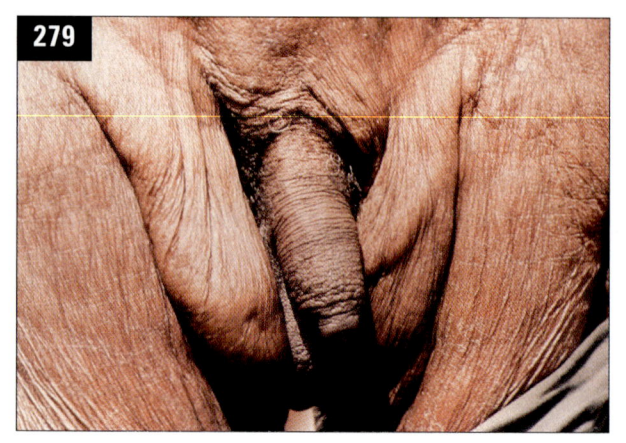

279 Chronic lymphatic obstruction in onchocerciasis (hanging groin sign).

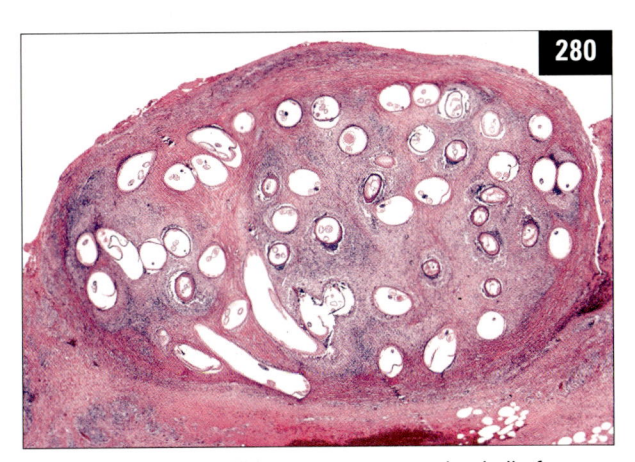

280 Onchocercoma. This represents a mating ball of numerous adult worms.

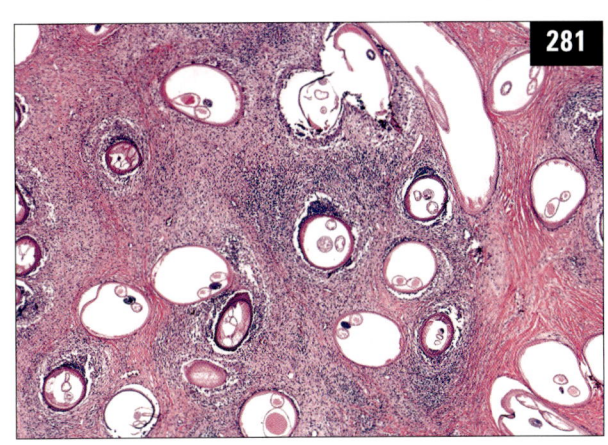

281 Onchocercoma. Females have paired uteri.

SCHISTOSOMIASIS

Schistosomiasis is a parasitic infection endemic to the tropics and subtropics caused by members of the genus *Schistosoma* (Amer, 1994). The three most common species that cause infection in humans are *S. haematobium*, which infects the urinary system, and *S. japonicum* and *S. mansoni*, which infect the gastrointestinal system (McKee *et al.*, 1983). All species are acquired after bathing in waters inhabited by the schistosomes (Leman *et al.*, 2001). Numerous cases of *S. haematobium* infection have been documented after swimming in Lake Malawi in Africa (Davis-Reed & Theis, 2000; Leman *et al.*, 2001). The cutaneous lesions may appear up to several years after the initial infection occurs (Davis-Reed & Theis, 2000; Payet *et al.*, 2006).

Several types of cutaneous involvement have been described. Cercarial dermatitis, or swimmer's itch, is a transient pruritic erythematous papular or urticarial eruption at the site of inoculation and is associated with cutaneous penetration by the cercariae (**282**) (Kullavanijaya & Wongwaisayawan, 1993). The reaction is relatively non-specific, and is more severe with *S. japonicum* and *S. mansoni*. Approximately 4–6 weeks later, patients may infrequently experience another transient cutaneous reaction secondary to dissemination of the cercariae. This reaction is also non-specific, ranging from urticarial or purpuric lesions to periorbital edema (Leman *et al.*, 2001). Bilharziasis cutanea tarda is characterized by papular, granulomatous, or verrucous lesions of the genital and perineal skin

282 Cercarial dermatitis in schistosomiasis.

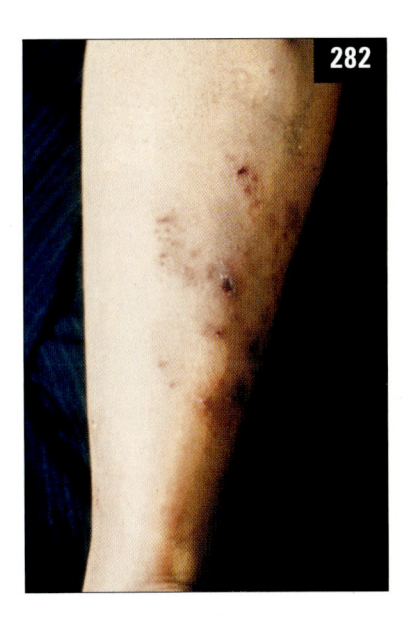

secondary to deposition of the ova in the dermal vessels (McKee *et al.*, 1983; Matz *et al.*, 2003). Ectopic cutaneous lesions have also been reported, often due to *S. haematobium*. These are rare, non-specific lesions, often appearing as clustered hyperpigmented papules in the periumbilical area or in a zosteriform distribution on the trunk (Matz *et al.*, 2003; Al-Karawi *et al.*, 2004).

Diagnosis by microscopic detection of eggs in the urine or feces is preferred. The ova of *S. haematobium* have a terminal spine and measure 112–170 μm long and 40–70 μm wide. The ova of *S. mansoni* measure 114–180 μm by 45–73 μm and have a lateral spine (Davis-Reed & Theis, 2000).

In *S. japonicum* and *S. mansoni*, mucosal snip and microscopic evaluation may provide the diagnosis. Serologic and immunologic tests are available (Davis-Reed & Theis, 2000; Leman *et al.*, 2001; Al-Karawi *et al.*, 2004). Skin biopsy is diagnostic when characteristic ova are observed. Ova of *S. haematobium* may be found in the urine in the setting of cutaneous disease, even in the absence of gross hematuria (Leman *et al.*, 2001).

Histopathologically, the cercarial dermatitis shows spongiosis and a mixed inflammatory infiltrate composed of histiocytes, lymphocytes, neutrophils, and eosinophils (Leman *et al.*, 2001). Edema is present in the dermis. Genital and perineal lesions show hyperkeratosis and acanthosis and, occasionally, prominent pseudoepitheliomatous hyperplasia (McKee *et al.*, 1983). The dermis may contain numerous ova, which may be in the lumen of veins or associated with a granulomatous reaction and mixed inflammatory infiltrate including neutrophils or eosinophils (McKee *et al.*, 1983; Leman *et al.*, 2001). Extragenital lesions contain ova in the superficial dermis associated with granulomas (**283**).

Praziquantel, 20–50 mg/kg by mouth divided into bid dosing, is the treatment of choice (Davis-Reed & Theis, 2000; Leman *et al.*, 2001; Al-Karawi *et al.*, 2004). This regimen has been effective even for immunosuppressed patients (Kallestrup *et al.*, 2006; Payet *et al.*, 2006). At this point in time, schistosomes have not yet demonstrated resistance to praziquantel (Doenhoff & Pica-Mattoccia, 2006).

STRONGYLOIDIASIS

Strongyloides stercoralis is a nematode endemic to tropical and subtropical areas of the world (Lam *et al.*, 2006). In the United States, it can be found in Tennessee and eastern Kentucky (Foreman *et al.*, 2006). The life cycle of the nematode begins when the filariform larvae enter the skin or mucous membranes, migrate to the lungs, and are subsequently swallowed to take up residence in the duodenum and jejunum (Lam *et al.*, 2006). Eggs and adult males are excreted in the feces (Foreman *et al.*, 2006). Intestinal infection in the normal host is mild, and many infected patients are asymptomatic while maintaining a low worm load (Foreman *et al.*, 2006). Immunosuppression is the main risk factor for dissemination, hyperinfection, and tissue invasion

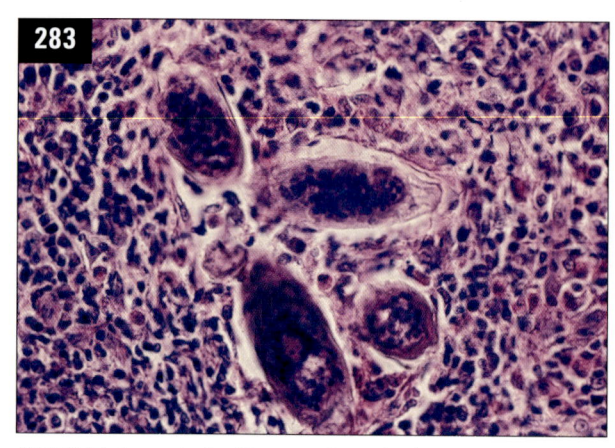

283 Schistosomiasis. Elongated ova in tissue.

(Foreman *et al.*, 2006; Lam *et al.*, 2006). The loss of cellular immunity allows previously asymptomatic patients to develop life-threatening infection many years after leaving an endemic area (Lam *et al.*, 2006). Screening for this disease is recommended before starting immunosuppressive treatment in patients from endemic areas (Johnston *et al.*, 2005; Lam *et al.*, 2006). Rare cases have been documented to be transmitted via kidney or pancreas transplants (Ben-Youssef *et al.*, 2005).

Pruritus, erythema, and edema are noted at the sites of cutaneous entry. Serpiginous and rapidly evolving urticarial tracts ('larva currens') may also be seen on the buttocks, thighs, and lower extremities (Foreman *et al.*, 2006). Presenting signs of disseminated infection include fever, abdominal pain, diarrhea, and respiratory distress (Lam *et al.*, 2006). The hyperinfection syndrome can involve many organ systems, but primarily the gastrointestinal system and lungs (Lam *et al.*, 2006). Systemic infection is frequently accompanied by Gram-negative septicemia, often with multiple enteric pathogens (Foreman *et al.*, 2006; Lam *et al.*, 2006). Eosinophilia is often seen in immunocompetent patients but is typically absent in the hyperinfection syndrome (Foreman *et al.*, 2006).

The diagnosis is made by the identification of larvae in the stool, body fluids, or other tissue by microscopy (**284**) (Foreman *et al.*, 2006; van Doorn *et al.*, 2007). Serial stool specimens may need to be examined as larval shedding can be sporadic (Johnston *et al.*, 2005; Foreman *et al.*, 2006). Several serologic methods are available and have been shown to be both

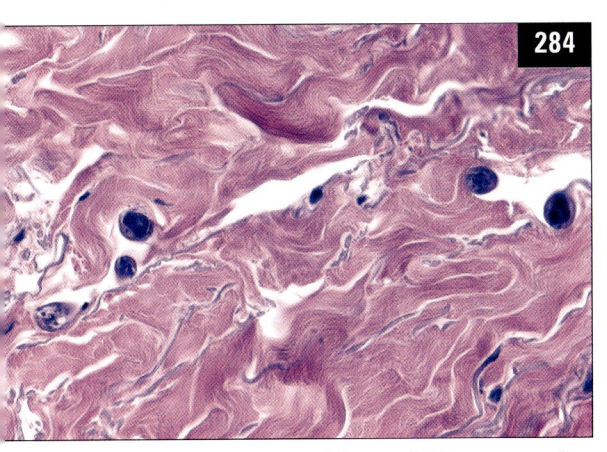

284 Microscopic identification of *Strongyloides stercoralis* in tissue.

sensitive and specific (van Doorn *et al.*, 2007).

Treatment options include thiabendazole at 25 mg/kg bid for 1–2 weeks, or ivermectin 25 µg/kg/day for one to two doses (Lam *et al.*, 2006). Ivermectin is more effective and better tolerated than thiabendazole. Ivermectin is also recommended by the WHO (Johnston *et al.*, 2005; Foreman *et al.*, 2006; Lam *et al.*, 2006). More prolonged treatment may be needed in disseminated cases (Lam *et al.*, 2006).

CUTANEOUS LARVA MIGRANS

Cutaneous larva migrans results from mammalian hookworm larvae, usually *Ancylostoma braziliense* or *A. caninum*, entering and migrating through the skin (O'Quinn & Dushin, 2005; Veraldi & Arancio, 2006). The organisms, which typically live in the intestines of dogs and cats, are endemic to the Caribbean, Africa, South America, southeast Asia, and the southeastern United States (Albanese *et al.*, 2001; O'Quinn & Dushin, 2005). This condition is not infrequently seen in travelers returning from endemic areas, often after exposure to beach sand or domestic animals (O'Quinn & Dushin, 2005; Ansart *et al.*, 2007). Within endemic areas, the prevalence of the disease varies with seasonal changes in rainfall (Heukelbach *et al.*, 2003).

The typical patient has one to several linear serpiginous erythematous plaques that migrate 2–5 cm per day (**285**) (Albanese *et al.*, 2001). Less commonly, exuberant vesiculobullous lesions may predominate over serpiginous tracks (Veraldi & Arancio, 2006). Pruritus is often severe (Heukelbach *et al.*, 2003). Some cases are accompanied by a folliculitis (Veraldi *et al.*, 2005).

The hookworm is often not seen on biopsy as its *in vivo* location is difficult to determine, but epiluminescent microscopy can facilitate location of the organism (Elsner *et al.*, 1997). The organism, when identified by histology, is almost always confined to the epidermis or papillary dermis (**286**) (O'Quinn & Dushin, 2005). Reports of serologic diagnosis do exist in the literature (Kwon *et al.*, 2003).

One to three 12 mg doses of oral ivermectin provides a cure rate approaching 100% and a rapid decrease in pruritus, which should resolve within 3 days (Dourmishev *et al.*, 2005; O'Quinn & Dushin, 2005). Albendazole 400 mg PO qday for 7 days represents an alternative regimen (Veraldi *et al.*, 2005; Veraldi & Arancio, 2006). Cryotherapy may be effective but is limited because the precise location of the organism is often difficult to determine (Albanese *et al.*, 2001).

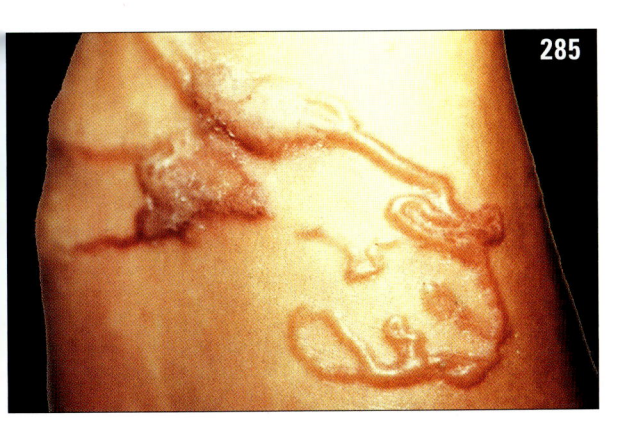

285 Linear serpiginous erythematous plaques in cutaneous larva migrans.

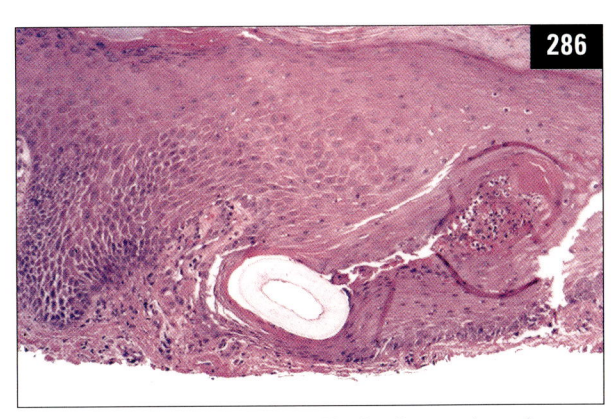

286 Cutaneous larva migrans. The hookworm larva is located in the epidermis.

CHAPTER 5

ARTHROPODS AND INFESTATIONS

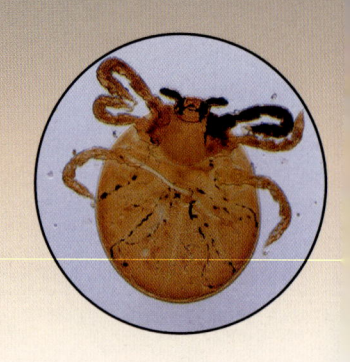

Dirk M Elston

INTRODUCTION
Insects and arachnids are common causes of bites, stings and infestations. Human infestation occurs in all societies and all socioeconomic groups. Arthropod vectors play a critical role in the spread of infectious diseases. Both common infestations and vector-borne illness are important to the practicing physician.

INSECTS

PEDICULOSIS
The lice that infest humans include the body louse, *Pediculus humanus humanus* (**287**), the head louse *Pediculus humanus capitis* (**288**), and the crab louse, *Pthirus pubis* (**289–292**). Body lice are important vectors of typhus, relapsing fever, and trench fever, while crab and head lice have not clearly been implicated as disease vectors. Head and body lice are similar in size and appearance, and differ by the location of their eggs. Head lice lay eggs on the hair shaft. Once the egg hatches, the empty egg case (nit) remains (**293**). Body lice lay eggs on clothing fibers. Crab lice lay eggs on pubic hair, as well as the hair of the legs, abdomen, chest, and back. Crab lice may also infest curly scalp hair.

The primary symptom associated with louse infestation is pruritus. Erythematous macules, papules, and bruise-like lesions may be found. The diagnosis can usually be made with the naked eye by identification of lice or nits. Hair casts (remnants of the inner root sheath) resemble nits clinically, but slide freely along the hair shaft and may be distinguished by microscopic examination (**294**).

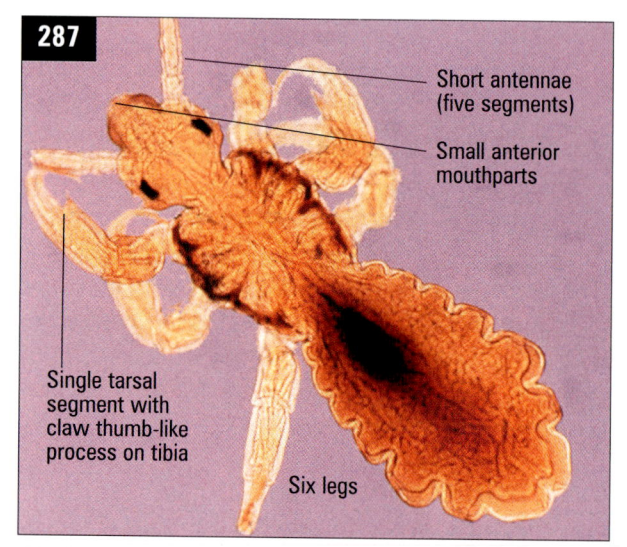

287 *Pediculus humanus humanus* (body louse). Body lice have three body segments, anterior piercing mouth parts, and a thumb-like process on the tibia.

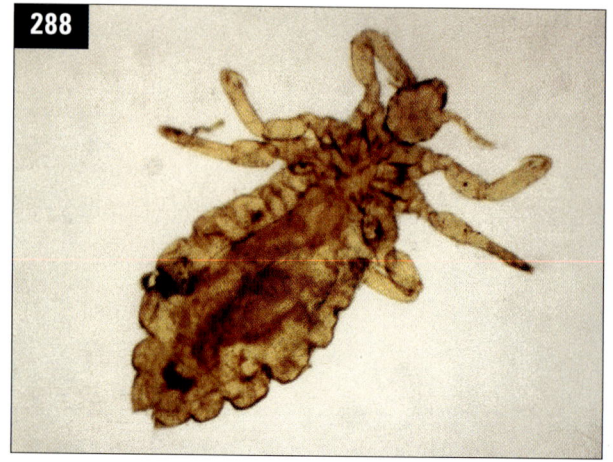

288 *Pediculus humanus capitis* (head louse). Head lice appear similar to body lice, but lay their eggs on hair fibers rather than clothing fibers.

Arthropods and Infestations

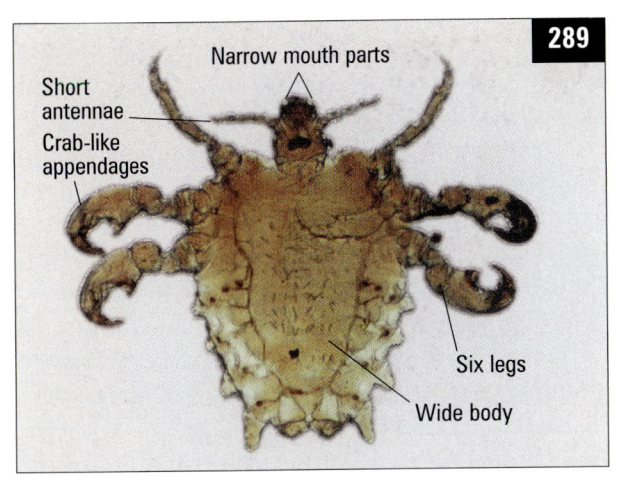

289 *Pthirus pubis* (crab louse). The crab louse has a broad thorax and widely spaced front legs suitable for navigating through areas of thick curly hair.

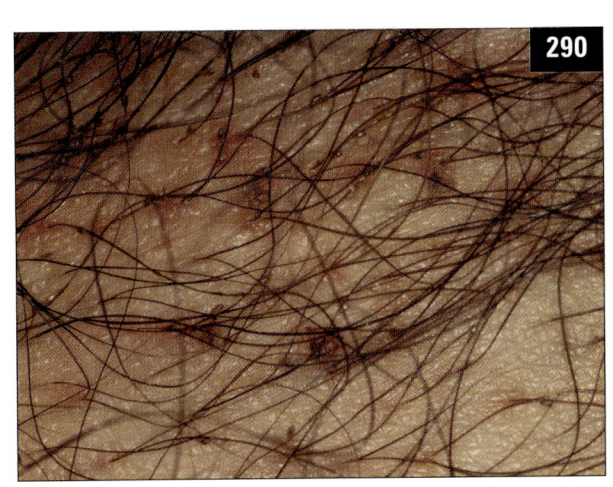

290 *Pthirus pubis* (crab louse). Crab lice may be found in pubic hair, but also infest leg, chest, and abdominal hair as well as eye lashes. They may also infest the scalp, especially in those with thick curly hair.

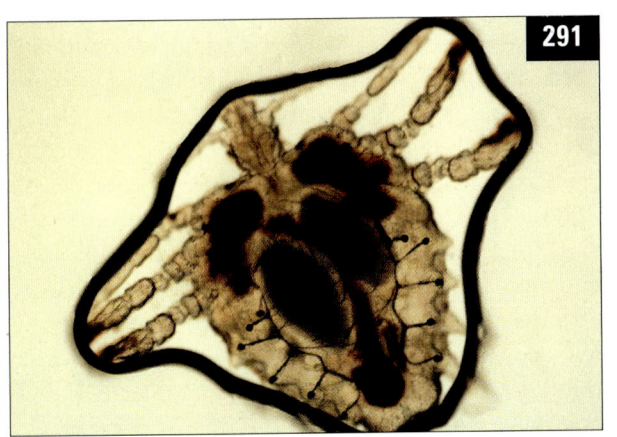

291 *Pthirus pubis* (crab louse). The quantity of blood found in head lice is sufficient for DNA identification. The tracheobronchial tree is noted as a system of tubules connected to respiratory spiracles. These may be occluded by newer pediculocides.

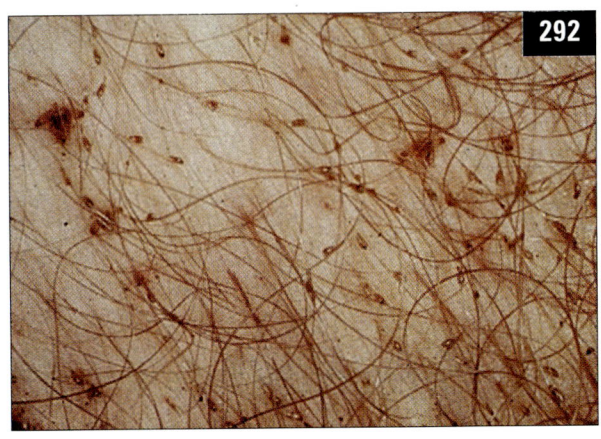

292 *Pthirus pubis* (crab louse). Many nit cases are present on the hairs. These are diagnostic of infection even when the adult lice are not seen.

293 Nit (empty egg case) on hair shaft. Empty nit cases my persist after successful treatment. Only the presence of living lice or viable ova are evidence of treatment failure.

294 Pseudonit (hair cast). Pseudonits are remnants of inner root sheath keratin that may be mistaken for nits. Unlike nits, they are freely moveable along the hair shaft.

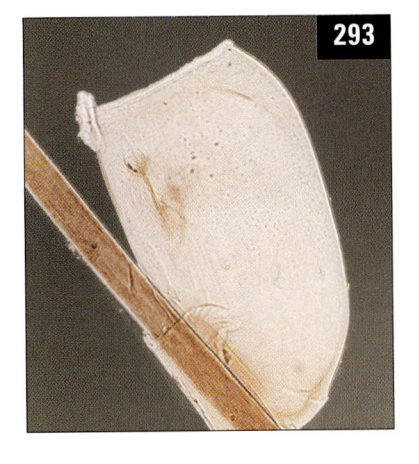

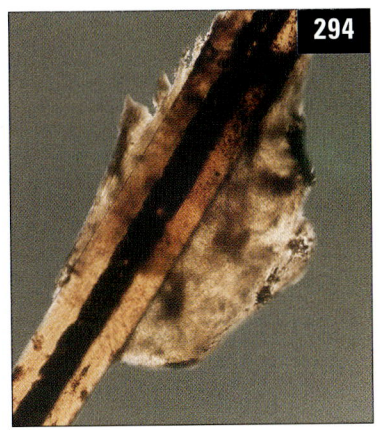

Maculae ceruleae (295) are bluish macules related to hemosiderin deposition from the bites (Ko & Elston, 2004). Lice must be distinguished from booklice (psocids) that are found in decaying vegetable matter and old books. Psocids (296) may occasionally infest the scalp.

The treatment of louse infestation can be difficult, as resistance is widespread in many parts of the world. Permethrin, lindane, pyrethrins, and malathion have all been used effectively. In the case of malathion, the vehicle contributes substantially to the efficacy of the product marketed in the United States. Unfortunately, the vehicle is also flammable and somewhat irritating. Each of these treatments appears relatively safe if used according to directions. In extremely high doses, permethrin can cause cleavage of the MLL gene, resulting in a chromosomal translocation that has been associated with leukemia (Borkhardt et al., 2003). Use of pediculicidal shampoos is a statistical risk factor for leukemia in children (Menegaux et al., 2006). Ivermectin has been used off-label, but safety and efficacy data are limited.

INSECT BITES

Papular urticaria (297) is a common manifestation of insect bites, and presents with solitary or disseminated 1–4 mm urticarial papules. The urticarial lesions may evolve into persistent pruritic papules or nodules. Vesiculobullous (298) reactions may occur, especially with flea bites. Exaggerated vesicular and nodular lesions (299–301) may occur in patients with chronic lymphocytic leukemia (CLL). Chigger (302) and flea bites tend to be clustered on the ankles. Chiggers also commonly affect the belt line and penis.

Treatment of insect bites depends on the clinical manifestations. Topical corticosteroids are useful for pruritic papules. Intra-lesional corticosteroid injections may be required for nodular lesions. Camphor and menthol or pramoxine lotion can be helpful in the control of pruritus.

Prevention of bites requires avoidance, protective clothing, or repellents. Anopheline mosquitoes carry malaria and tend to bite at night. In contrast, mosquitoes that carry dengue tend to bite during the day. Malaria chemoprophylaxis is recommended for travelers to endemic areas. Transmission can be reduced through judicious use of mosquito netting and repellents. N,N-diethyl-3-methylbenzamide (DEET) is the most widely used mosquito repellent in the United States, while picaridin is commonly used in other parts of the world. Although sunscreens have been shown to enhance DEET absorption, the effect may not be clinically significant at commonly used doses (Ross et al., 2004). High concentrations of DEET increase the risk of toxicity. As long-acting formulations containing 30% or lower concentrations are highly effective, higher concentrations should generally be avoided. In assays against *Aedes aegypti* and *Culex quinquefasciatus*, IR3535 is comparable to DEET and picaridin (Cilek et al., 2004; Naucke et al., 2007).

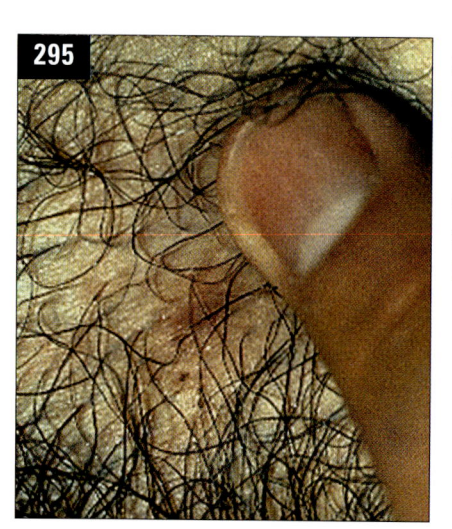

295 Maculae ceruleae represent hemosiderin staining at sites where lice have fed.

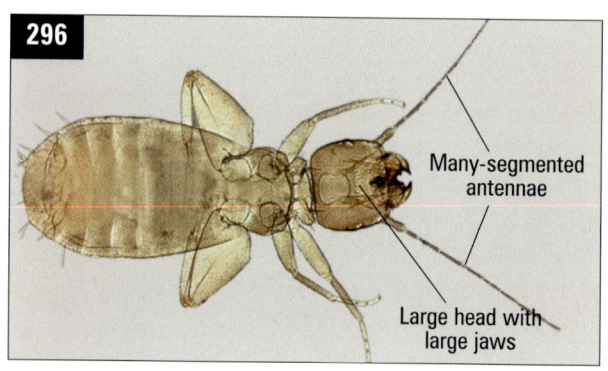

296 Psocid (booklouse). Psocids are primitive louse-like creatures that infest mildewed paper as well as the litter in pet habitats. Humans may be secondarily infested.

Arthropods and Infestations

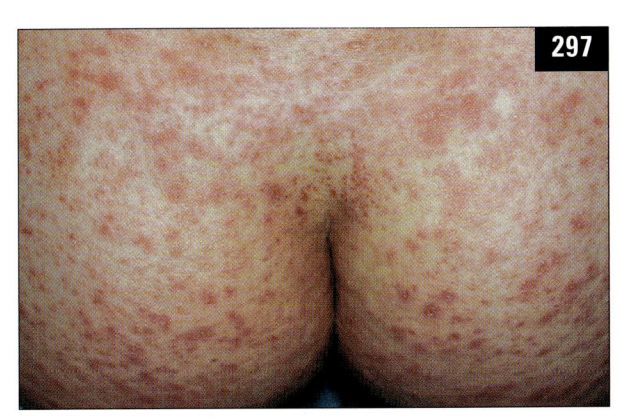

297 Papular urticaria occurs as a reaction to arthropod bites.

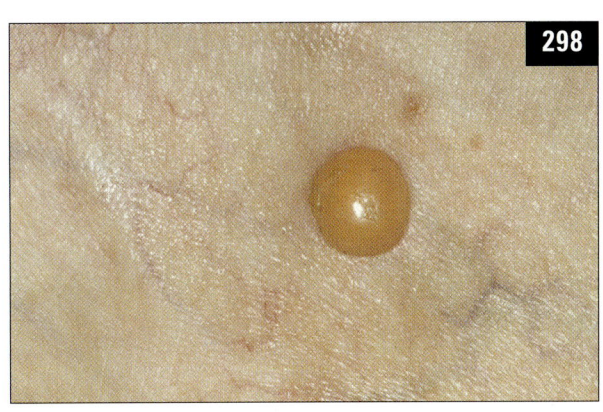

298 Bullous arthropod bite reaction. Bullous arthropod reactions are common. They tend to cluster on the distal extremities. Immunofluorescent studies may be positive, leading to a misdiagnosis of pemphigoid.

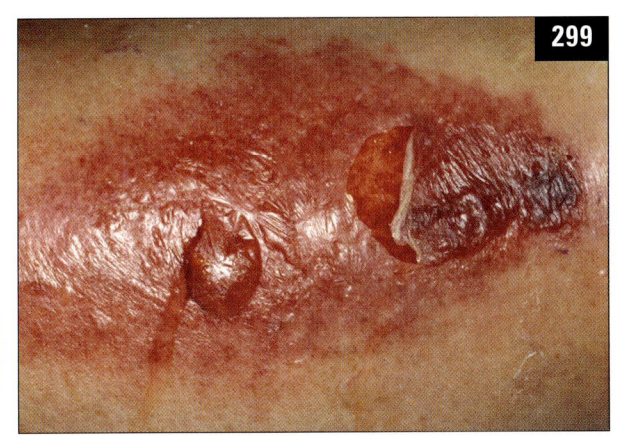

299 Bullous exaggerated arthropod responses in CLL. Patients with CLL may have bizarre and exaggerated reactions to arthropod bites. A screening blood count is reasonable in any patient with extreme bite reactions.

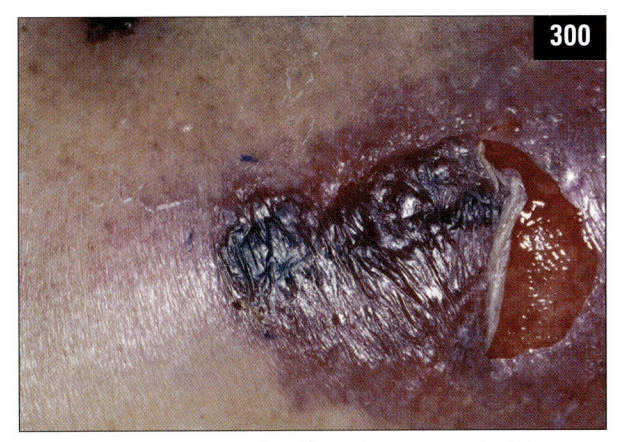

300 Bullous exaggerated arthropod responses in CLL. Extensive necrosis may be present. Such reactions commonly require intralesional corticosteroid injections.

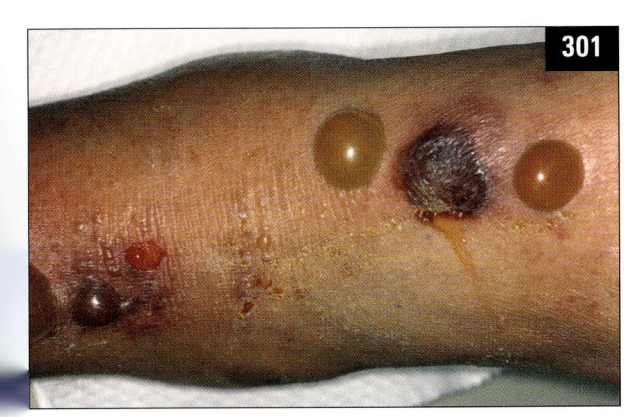

301 Bullous exaggerated arthropod responses in CLL. Bites reactions in CLL patients are frequently hemorrhagic and bullous.

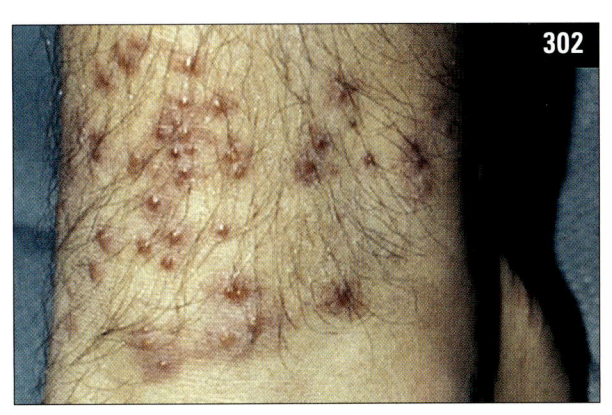

302 Chigger bites on the ankle. Chigger bites tend to be clustered on the lower legs, at the elastic rim of socks and underwear and on the penis.

HYMENOPTERIDS

The order Hymenoptera (303–310) contains wasps, hornets, bees, and ants. As a group, hymenopterids possess membranous wings and complex venoms that can contain proteinaceous allergens, formic acid, and kinins. Anaphylaxis is the most serious risk in individuals allergic to hymenopterid stings. Arrhythmia, myoglobinuria, or hemoglobinuria may also occur.

Anaphylaxis should be treated with epinephrine. Bee stingers should be removed as rapidly as possible. The exact method of removal is less important than the speed of removal. Venom immunotherapy improves the quality of life for patients with sting allergy and should be discussed with an allergist (Oude Elberink *et al.*, 2002).

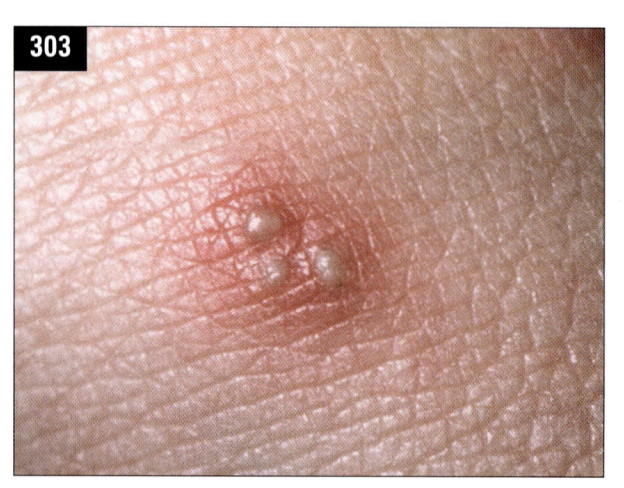

303 Fire ant stings. Fire ants grab the skin with their mandibles and rotate, inflicting multiple stings in a rosette pattern.

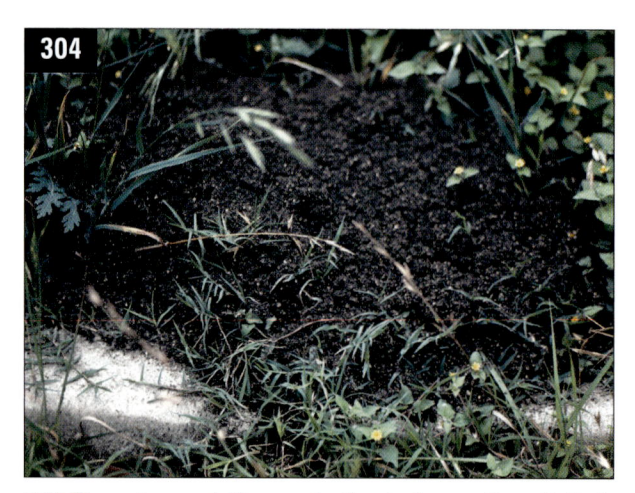

304 Fire ant mound. Those who live in the southern United States are familiar with fire ant mounds. During periods of drought, the mounds may be inconspicuous and the incidence of bites often increases.

Arthropods and Infestations

305 Fire ant. This image demonstrates the ant pivoting to inflict a rosette of stings.

306 Fire ant stings. At this stage, the lesions are characterized by intense pruritus. The lack of tenderness helps to exclude secondary infection.

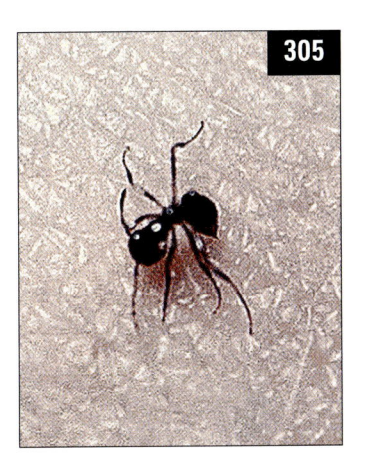

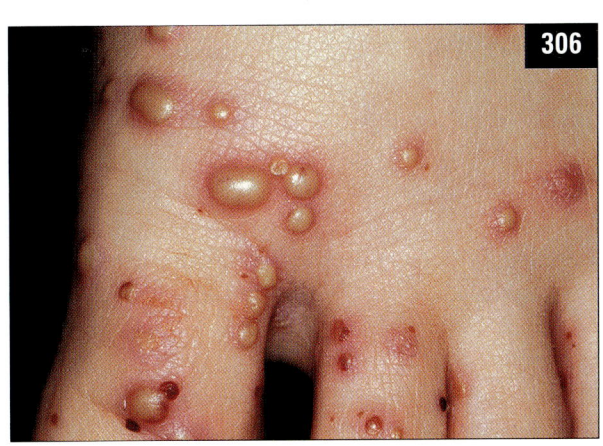

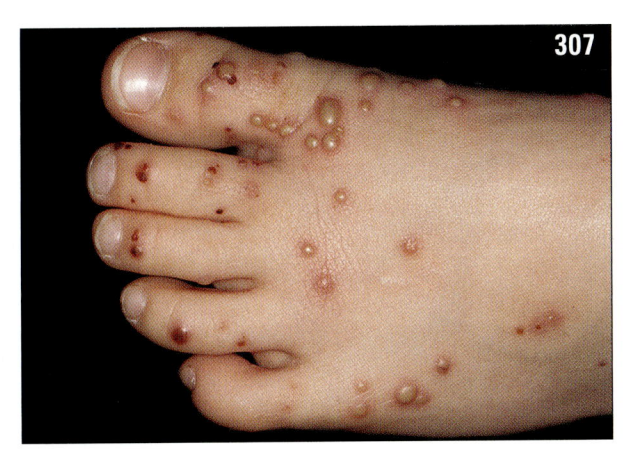

307 Fire ant stings. Fire ant stings are initially painful. The chronic phase is marked by intensely itchy vesicles and pustules.

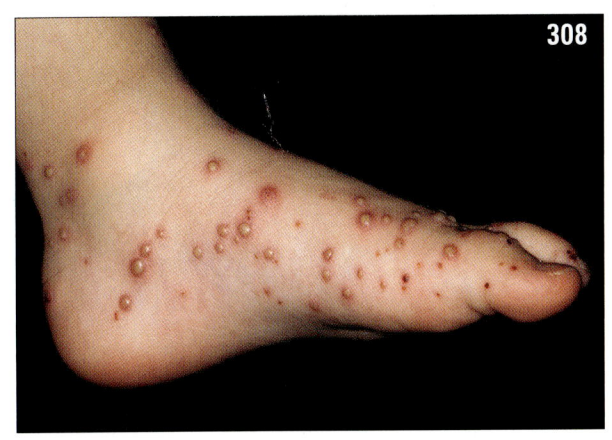

308 Fire ant stings. Fire ants swarm when their mound is disturbed. They are typically not noticed until they begin to sting simultaneously.

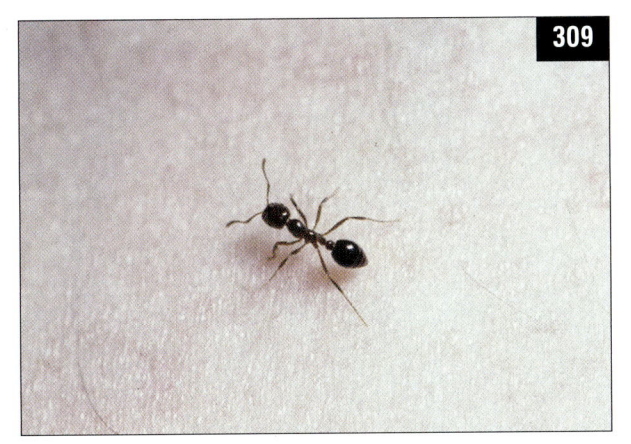

309 Fire ant. Fire ants are quite small (about the length of a sesame seed), have three body segments and six legs. Species vary from reddish brown to black.

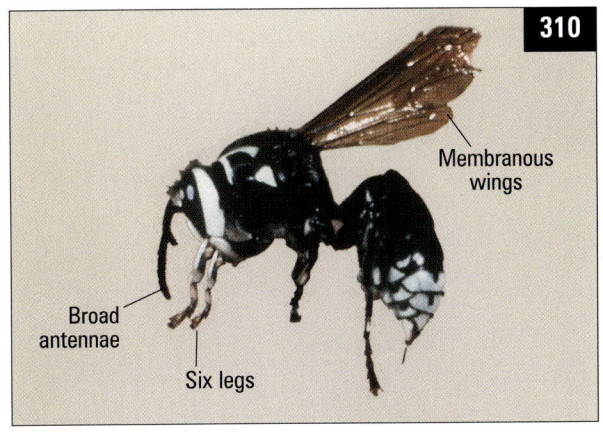

310 Vespid. Vespids belong to the order Hymenoptera. They have three body segments, six legs, and membranous wings.

HEMIPTERIDS

Hemipterids possess half membranous/half sclerotic wings. They overlap and are well demonstrated in triatome bugs (311, 312), while the membranous portion is vestigial in cimicids (bedbugs). Bedbugs (313, 314) include *Cimex lectularius* and *C. hemipterus*. *C. lectularius* is about the size of a small tick (5–7 mm), while *C. hemipterus* is slightly longer. Despite the name, bedbugs are rarely found in mattresses. Rather, they hide in cracks and behind peeling paint. At night, they emerge to feed, often leaving groups of three bites in a row (breakfast, lunch, and dinner). Treatment of the environment with chemical insecticides is the mainstay of treatment, as repellents are less effective than against mosquitoes and pyrethroid resistance is emerging (Curtis *et al.*, 2003).

Triatome reduviids are vectors for Chagas' disease. They can be recognized by their overlapping half-membranous wings that fail to cover the lateral portions of the abdomen. A tiger stripe pattern is often visible where the abdomen is exposed. Triatome feeding bites are typically painless, although they are also capable of delivering a painful defensive bite. Unilateral eyelid swelling (Romana's sign) is associated with triatome bugs. Chagas' disease can result in cardiomegaly or megacolon.

Wheel bugs (315, 316) are common throughout North America. Although they are not known to be disease vectors, they deliver a painful bite.

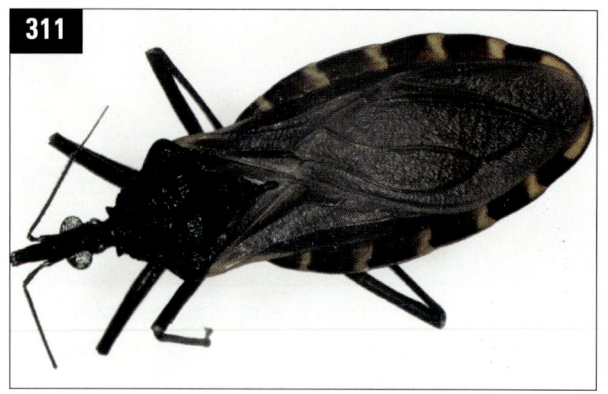

311 Triatome bug. Triatome bugs have overlapping wings with a proximal sclerotic portion and distal membranous portion. The abdomen protrudes beyond the overlapping wings.

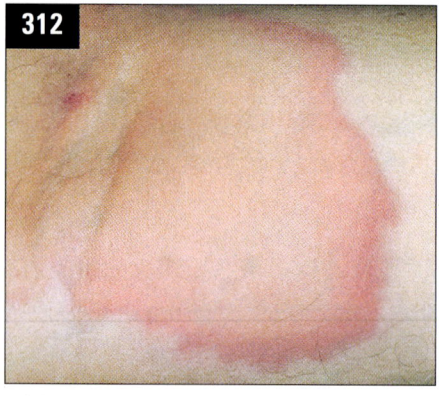

312 Triatome bite. Similar to bedbugs, triatome bugs inhabit cracks and crevices and feed by night. Patients who are bitten repeatedly may develop a high degree of immunity with marked erythema and edema at the site of the bite.

313 Bedbug (*Cimex*). Despite their name, bedbugs are often found behind peeling wallpaper or in cracks and crevices. They are about the size of a tick, red/brown in color and flattened. The wings are vestigial and only the sclerotic proximal portion remains.

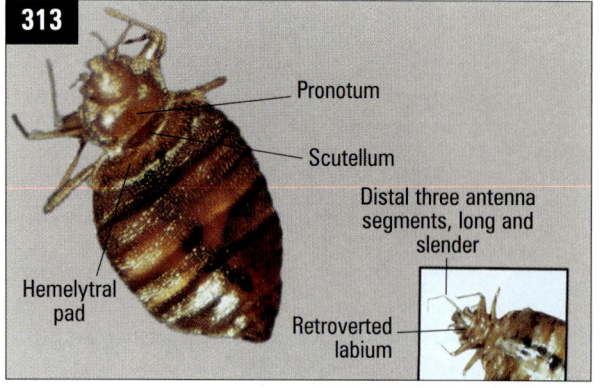

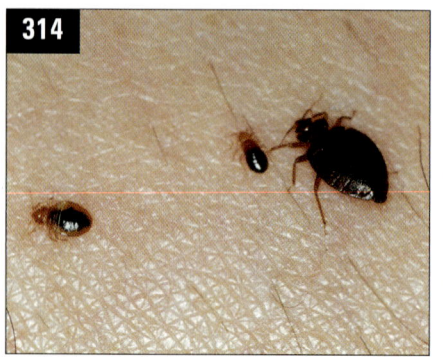

314 Bedbugs. Begbugs attach until they are engorged. They vary in size by age and maturity.

LEPIDOPTERIDS

Urticating hairs are common among caterpillars, cocoons, butterflies, and moths. The hairs are barbed and easily become embedded in the cornea, causing ophthalmia nodosa. Toxin-mediated reactions relate to histamine, kinins, and plasminogen activators in the hairs. Lesions may be papular or hemorrhagic, and symptoms include pain, itching, and urticaria. Gypsy moth caterpillars (*Lymantria dispar*) are common in the northeastern United States. Gypsy moth dermatitis results from direct contact with the caterpillar, or from hairs in clothesline-dried clothing. Tape stripping of skin lesions will demonstrate caterpillar hairs. *Megalopyge opercularis*, the puss caterpillar (317–319), is common in central Texas.

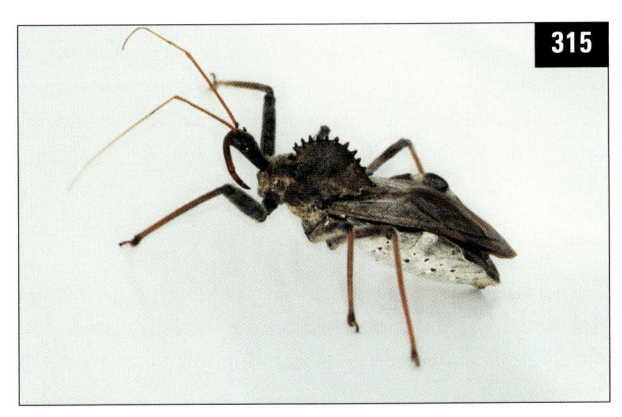

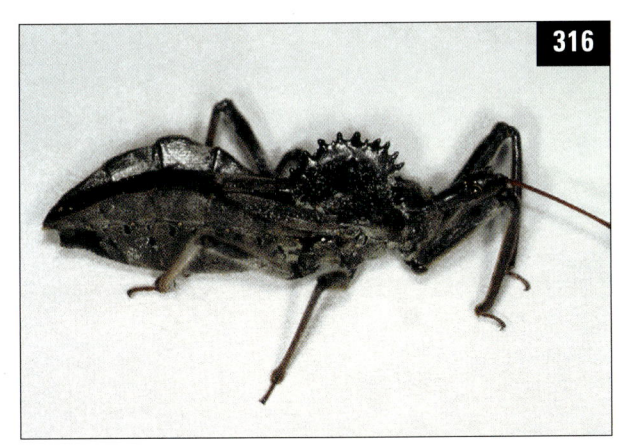

315 Wheel bug. When threatened, wheel bugs defend themselves with a very painful bite. It is reputed to be the most painful bite inflicted by any arthropod. Wheel bugs are not typically aggressive, and although they are quite common, bites are relatively infrequent.

316 Wheel bug. Wheel bugs are readily identified by the spoked wheel on the dorsal thorax.

317 *Megalopyge opercularis* (puss caterpillar). The wooly asp or puss caterpillar has rows of toxic hairs that inflict painful stings. The cocoons contain many hairs and are also capable of producing dermatitis.

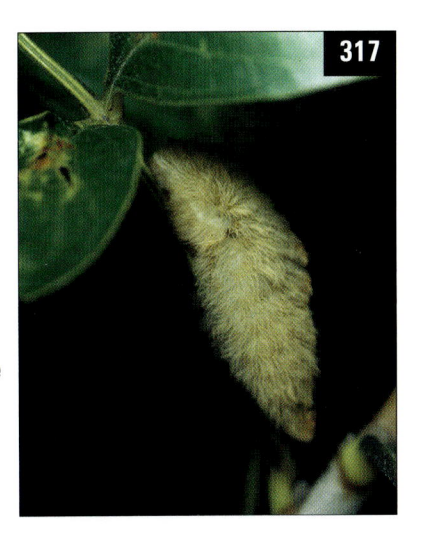

318 *Megalopyge opercularis* (puss caterpillar) reaction. The hemorrhagic train-track pattern of the sting corresponds to the pattern of hairs visible in figure **317**.

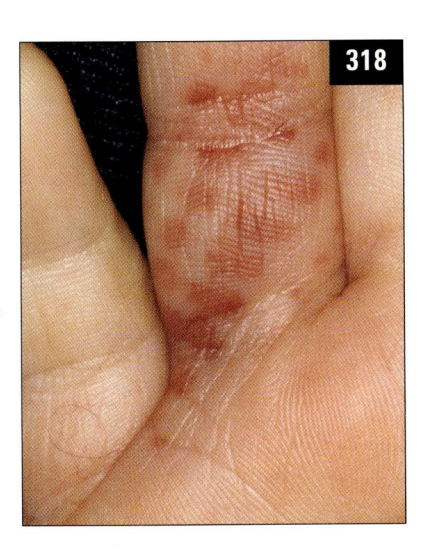

319 Megalopyge opercularis (puss caterpillar). Puss caterpillars are commonly found in oak trees. When the tree is trimmed, the falling caterpillars cause stings. Although the caterpillar itself may never be seen, the hemorrhagic pattern of the sting is diagnostic.

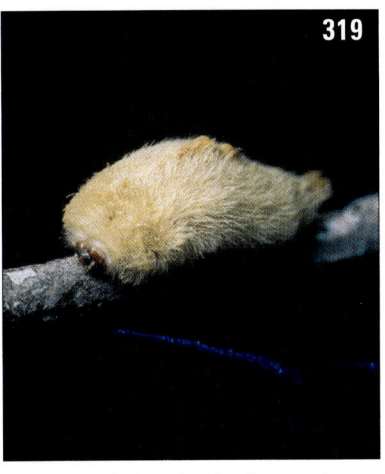

It produces a characteristic 'railroad track' pattern of hemorrhage. Saddleback caterpillars (*Sibine stimulea*) (320) are another important cause of caterpillar dermatitis in the United States.

COLEOPTERIDS

Blister beetles (321) and false blister beetles can produce blistering in humans. Cantharidin is the toxin responsible for the blisters. Cantharidin is also used medically for wart therapy. Adult beetles may contain up to 10% cantharidin by weight. Exposure to 'beetle juice' produces sizable blisters. *Paederus eximius*, or Rove beetles, are an important species in parts of Africa and Asia (Dursteler & Nyquist, 2004).

SIPHONAPTERIDS

Fleas (322–327) are ubiquitous pests in most parts of the world. The most common flea on dogs is *Ctenocephalides felis*, the cat flea. *Ctenocephalides*

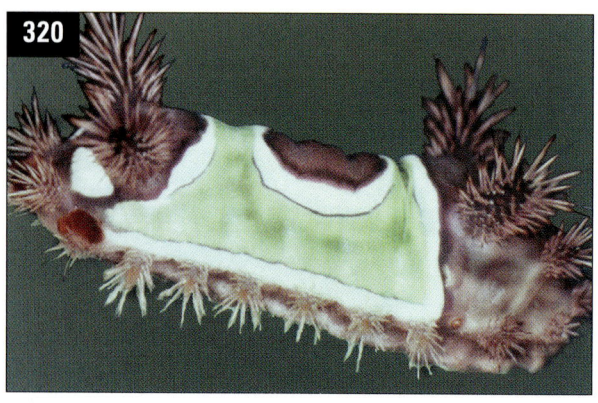

320 *Sibine stimulea* (saddleback caterpillar). The saddle of the saddleback caterpillars varies in color from shades of tan to bright green. The caterpillar is highly ornate and easily recognized.

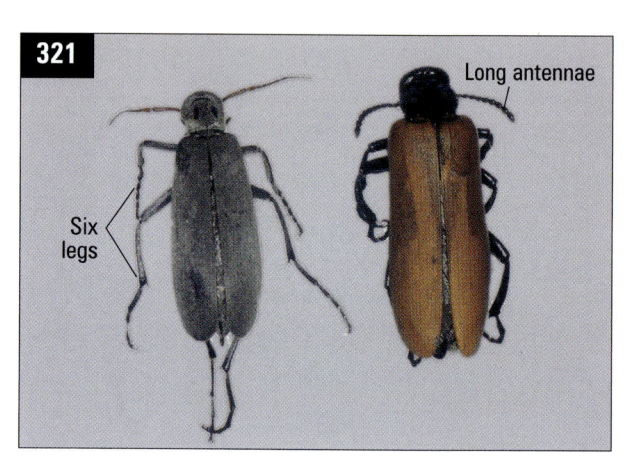

321 Blister beetles. Species of blister beetle vary from tan to brown to gray and may have stripes. All are capable of producing severe blistering reactions and are particularly hazardous if the eye is affected.

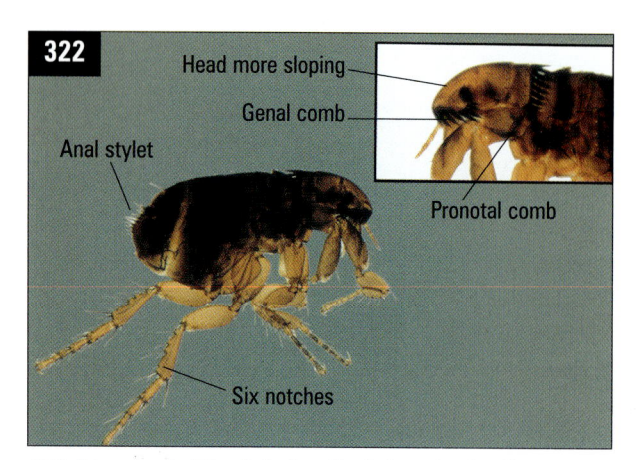

322 *Ctenocephalides felis* (cat flea), female. Cat fleas are the most common type of flea on dogs in most areas. Fleas have little host specificity and will gravitate to any warm body. In south Texas, they carry endemic typhus.

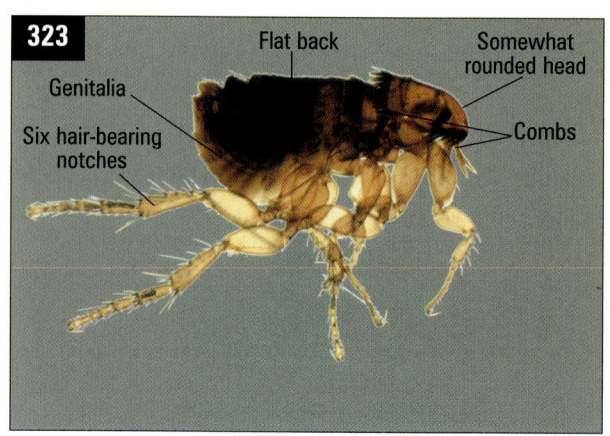

323 *Ctenocephalides felis* (cat flea), male. Fleas are well adapted for survival. The pupae can survive undisturbed for years, then emerge rapidly in response to the vibrations of footsteps.

Arthropods and Infestations

fleas are easily recognized by the ctenidia (combs). The pronotal comb resembles a mane of hair while the genal comb resembles a mustache. *C. canis*, the dog flea, has eight hair-bearing notches on the dorsal hind tibia, while *C. felis* has six. *Pulex irritans*, the human flea, is historically implicated as a plague vector, although the oriental rat flea is now implicated more commonly.

Flea pupae can lay dormant for years, but hatch rapidly in response to vibration. Bites are most common on the lower legs, where they present as intensely pruritic papulovesicles. Allergic patients tend to react to a wide range of fleas, rather than to a specific flea (Hudson *et al.*, 1960). Fleas are also important disease vectors, carrying plague, endemic typhus, brucellosis, melioidosis, and erysipeloid.

Tungiasis presents with papular necrotic lesions on the feet, especially adjacent to the great toenail, where the female sand flea embeds. The disease is common in warm coastal areas.

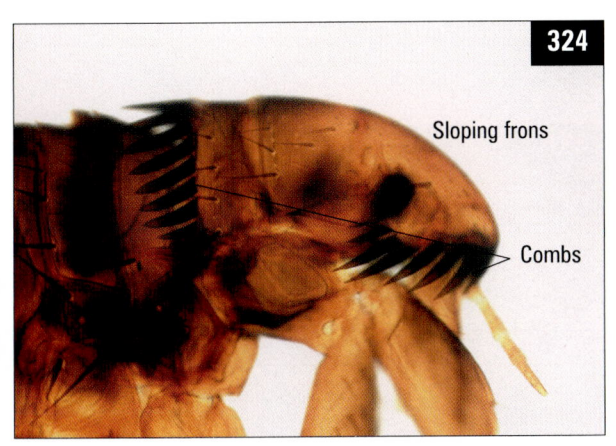

324 *Ctenocephalides felis* (cat flea). The genal and pronotal combs are clearly visible. They are characteristic of dog and cat fleas.

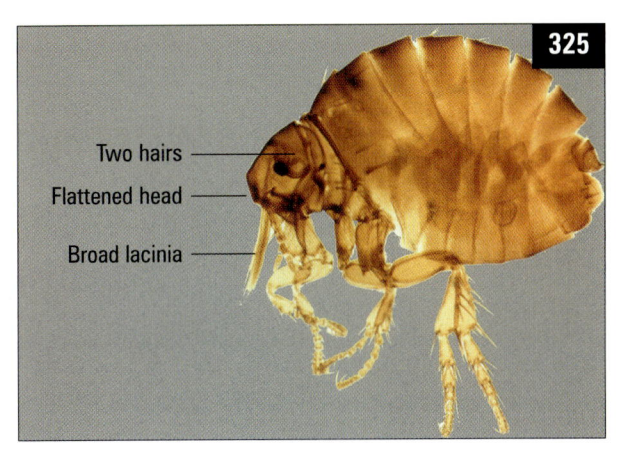

325 *Echidnophaga gallinacea*. The broad lacinia of this poultry flea allows it to 'stick tight' to its host. Like other fleas, it shows little host specificity and may be found on a wide variety of animals.

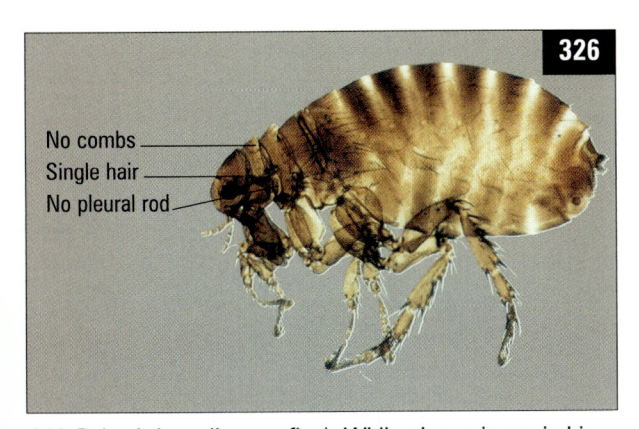

326 *Pulex irritans* (human flea). While plague is carried in nature by the rat flea, it is the human flea and pneumonic spread that accounted for the death of about one-third of Europe's population during the great plague epidemics.

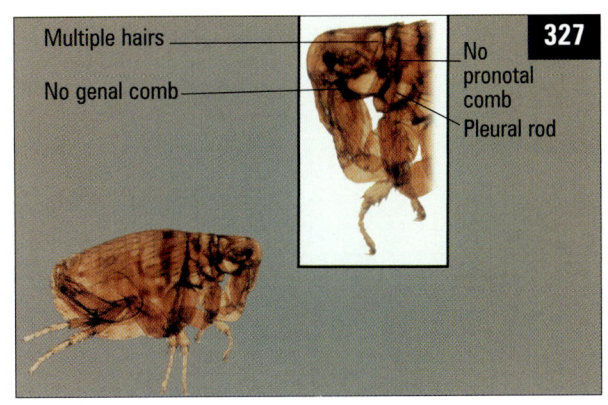

327 *Xenopsylla cheopis*. The oriental rat flea is the vector for endemic plague in nature. It is characterized by a pleural rod and lack of combs.

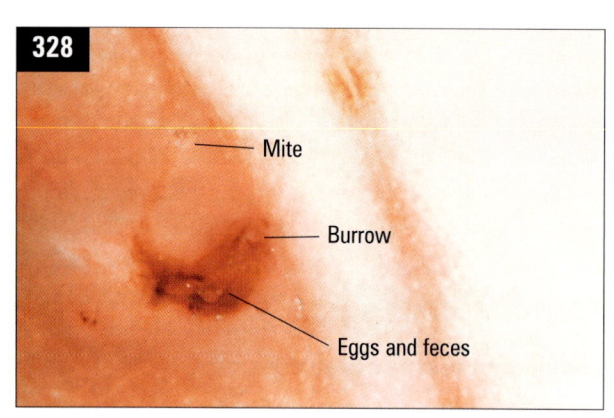

328 *Sarcoptes scabei* (human itch mite). (Courtesy of Jeff Meffert, MD.) Dermatoscopic examination easily demonstrates the anterior portion of the mite as a V-shaped structure within the burrow.

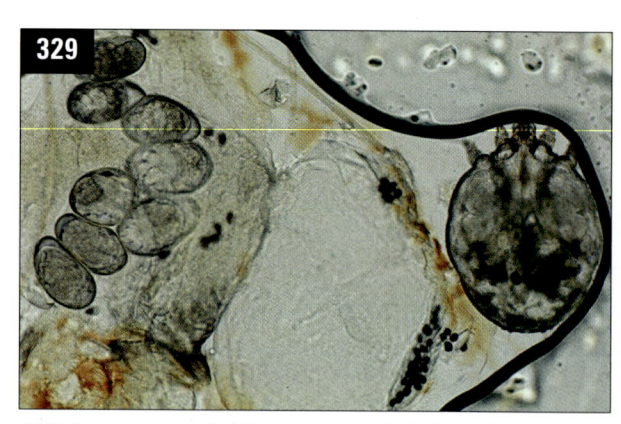

329 *Sarcoptes scabei* (human itch mite). Scraping demonstrate the female mite, ova, and fecal pellets. Any of these is diagnostic of the infestation.

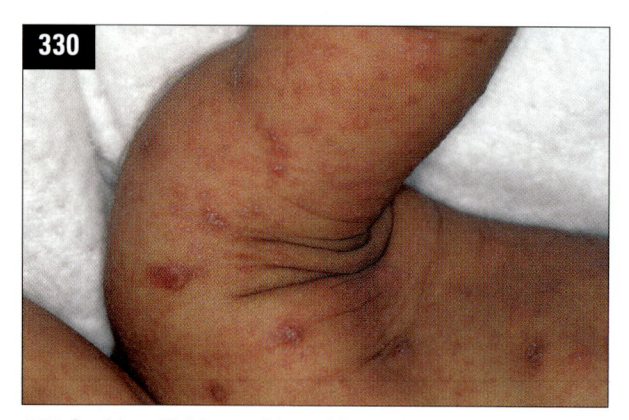

330 Scabies. Children with scabies exhibit severe pruritus and often excoriate themselves extensively. Mites and ova may be found under the nails.

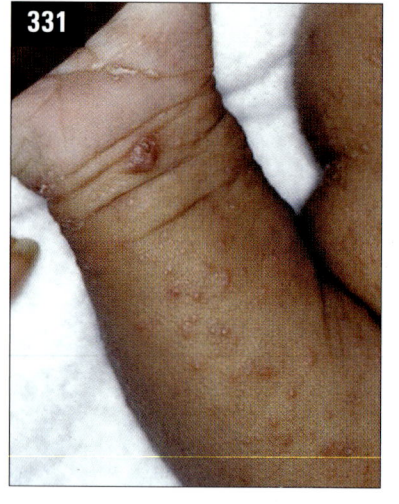

331 Scabies. Burrows are common on the wrist flexures as well as the webspaces, genitalia, and umbilicus.

ARACHNIDS

MITES
SCABIES

Sarcoptes scabei, the human itch mite (328–338), occurs at all ages. In the very young, the inflammatory response is often dramatic and secondary infection is common. In aging patients, the presentation is often atypical, with subtle excoriations and prurigo-like lesions. In children, scabies infestation may mimic Langerhans cell histiocytosis histologically and misdiagnosis has resulted in treatment with chemotherapy (Burch *et al.*, 2004).

Itch commonly occurs out of proportion to the physical findings. Pruritic nodules may occur in the genital region and on the breasts. All close physical contacts, such as sexual partners and family members, require treatment. Widespread epidemics may occur in nursing homes, daycare centers, prisons, and hospital wards. These epidemics are notoriously difficult to control. (Voss & Wallrauch, 1995; van Vliet *et al.*, 1998; Andersen *et al.*, 2000).

Permethrin is widely used to treat scabies infestations. Lindane has also been used. In many countries, benzyl benzoate and precipitated sulfur are commonly used. Ivermectin has been used off-label.

Arthropods and Infestations

332 Scabies. Scabies often produces acral pustules in young children and infants. Acropustulosis of infancy is a diagnosis of exclusion and should only be made after scabies has been thoroughly excluded by history and physical examination. If more than one individual is involved, scabies is more likely.

333 Scabies. Burrows can be subtle and are often best demonstrated in areas that are hard to reach. A drop of gentian violet or india ink can help demonstrate the burrows. Many skin marking pens contain gentian violet. After the area is painted, the excess dye is removed with an alcohol prep pad.

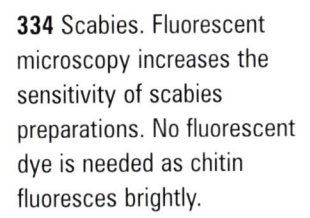

334 Scabies. Fluorescent microscopy increases the sensitivity of scabies preparations. No fluorescent dye is needed as chitin fluoresces brightly.

335 Scabies. Scabies nodules are common on the scrotum and persist for months, even after successful treatment of the infestation.

336 Scabies. In both males and females, scabies nodules may be numerous on the thighs and genitalia.

337 Scabies. The chitinous shell of the scabies ova is easily visible with the aid of a fluorescent microscope. The condenser can be lowered in routine light microscopy to increase the refractility of the chitin.

338 Scabies. The umbilicus is a common site for burrows and should always be examined when scabies is suspected.

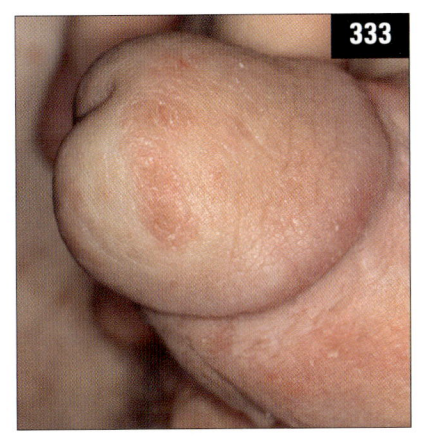

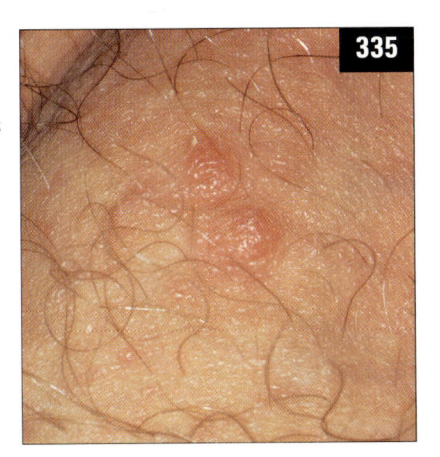

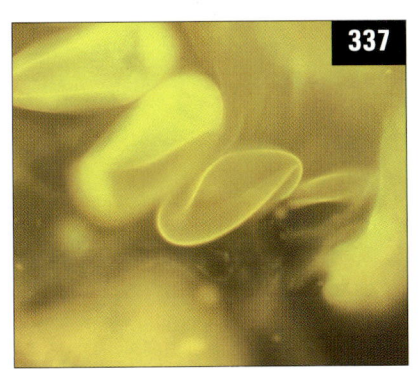

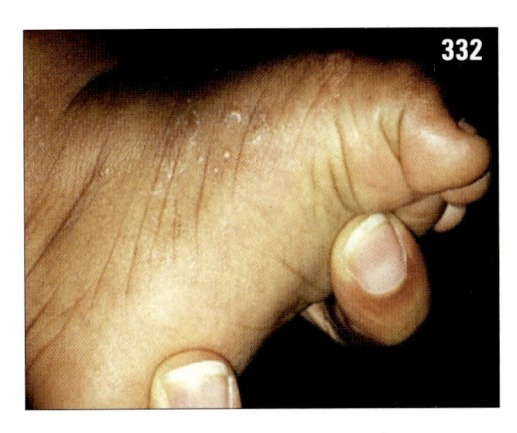

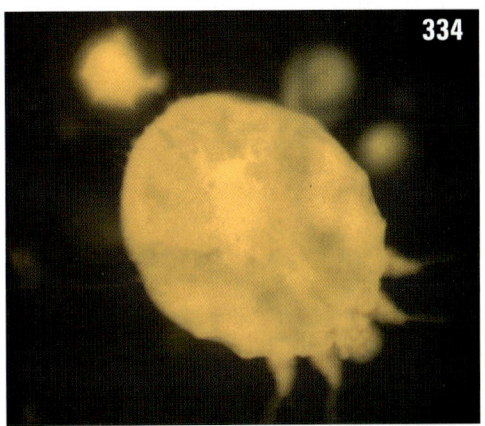

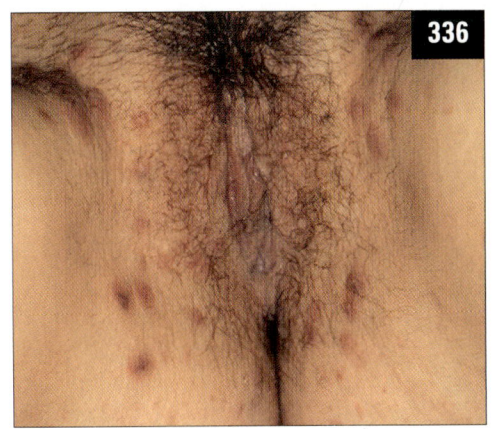

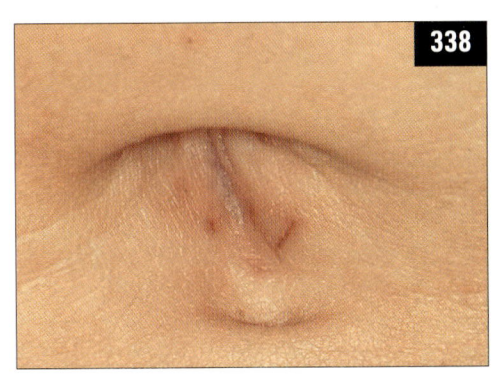

Demodex mites

Demodex mites (339–342) are normal inhabitants of human hair follicles. When they overpopulate, they can produce folliculitis (343) and acneiform lesions.

Zoonotic and environmental mites

Mites are ubiquitous, being found in everything from straw and flower bulbs to cheese. Cutaneous reactions to zoonotic and environmental mites (344–350) may manifest as papular, papulovesicular, bullous, urticarial, and morbilliform eruptions. Bullous lesions may be misdiagnosed as immunobullous disease. Chigger bites

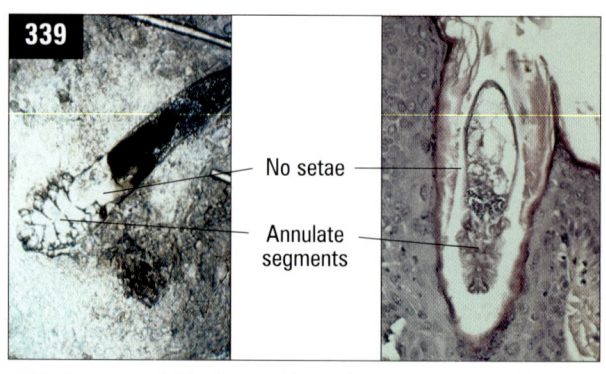

339 *Demodex folliculorum*. *Demodex* mites are readily transferred from mothers to their children, and humans become infested shortly after birth.

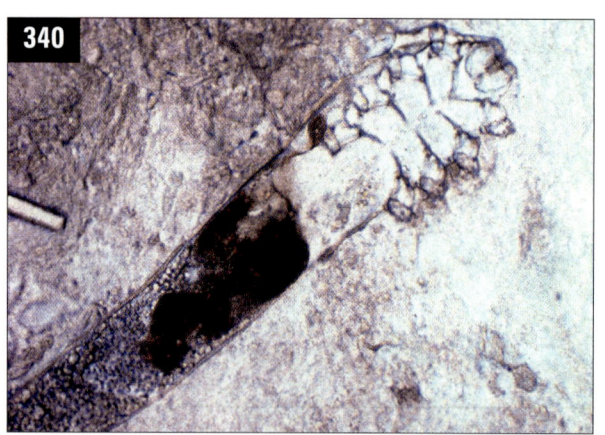

340 *Demodex folliculorum*. The mite is characterized by an elongated abdomen. The cephalothorax is small by comparison.

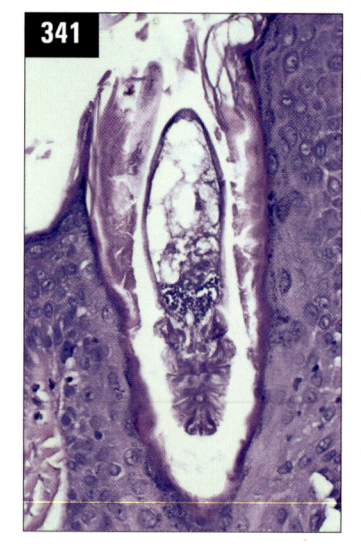

341 *Demodex folliculorum*. When present in histologic sections, *Demodex* mites are often associated with follicular inflammation. The mite itself or bacteria within mites may be the inciting antigen. It may not simply be a matter of having mites, it may be that 'sick' mites harbor bacteria that cause human disease.

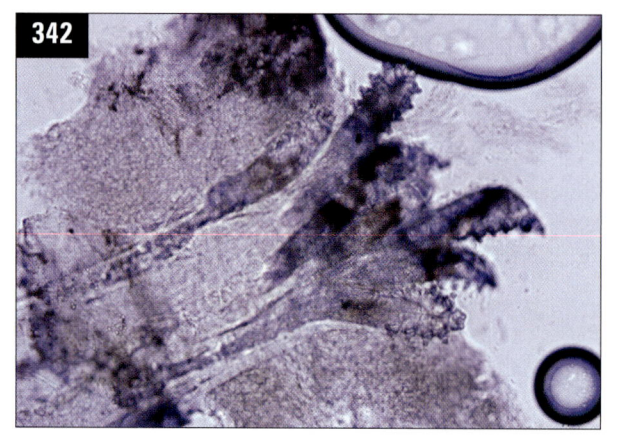

342 *Demodex folliculorum*. Adhesive stripping of the follicle demonstrates 'floral arrangements' of mites within follicular keratin.

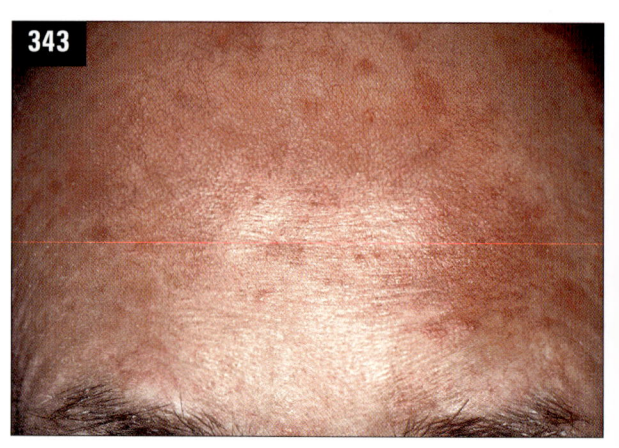

343 Folliculitis due to *Demodex folliculorum*. Demodectic folliculitis often responds best to topical sulfur preparations.

Arthropods and Infestations

344 Straw mite. Environmental mites are ubiquitous and commonly cause dermatitis.

345 Canine scabies. Canine scabies causes mange in dogs and pruritus in humans who have contact with the dog.

346 *Cheyletiella* mite. *Cheyletiella* mites cause 'walking dandruff' in dogs, cats, and rabbits. It may cause itch, rash, or a vesiculobullous reaction in humans.

347 Chigger mite. The larval chigger mite has only six legs, while the adult has eight, like other arachnids.

348 *Laelaps castroi* mite. Laelaps mites commonly infest rodents, although mites readily transfer between birds, rodents, and humans.

349 Northern fowl mite. Mite dermatitis may paradoxically increase after nests have been removed, as the mites look for another source of food.

350 Psoroptes mite. Animal scab mites are relatives of mange mites. They may produce human dermatitis in those who contact animals.

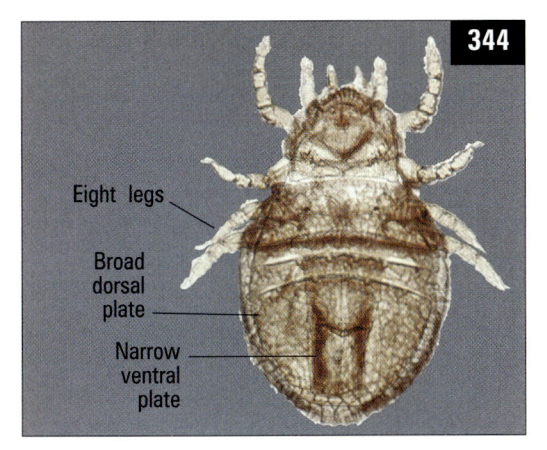

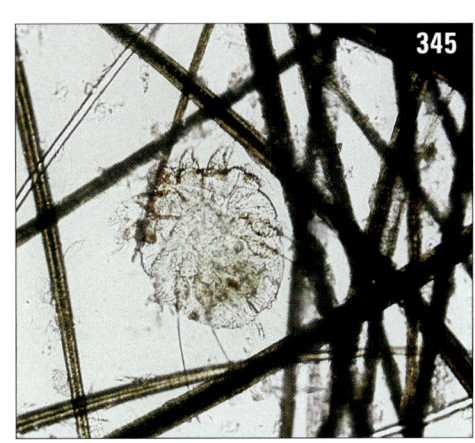

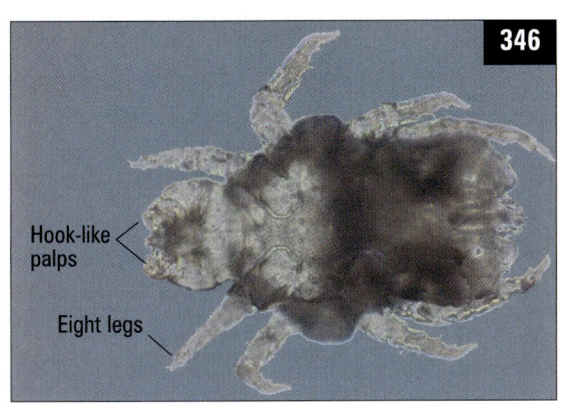

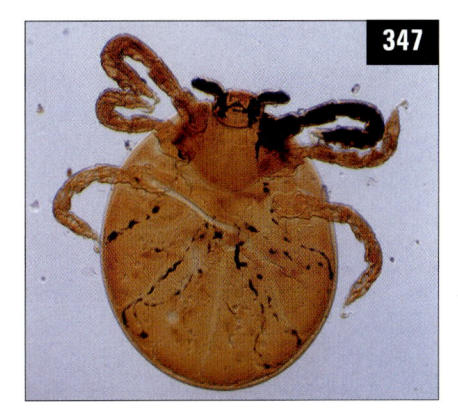

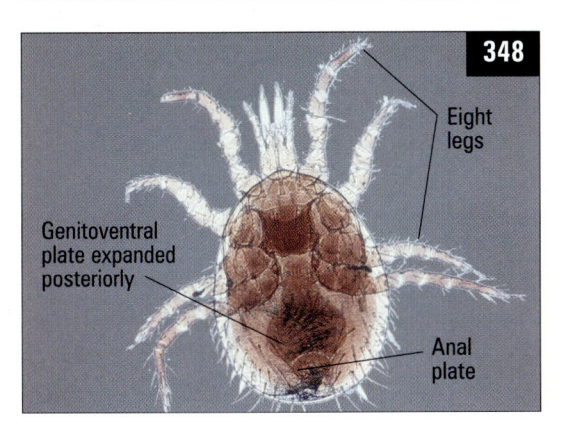

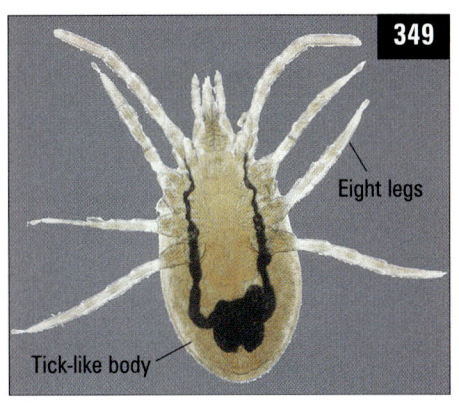

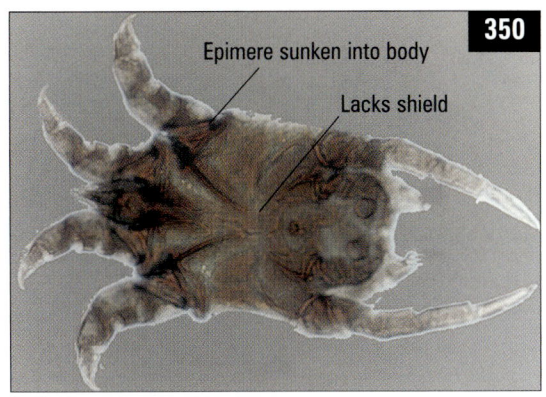

commonly affect the lower legs, but are also common along the elastic edges of jockey briefs and on the glans penis. In Asia, chiggers are important vectors of scrub typhus. House mouse mites transmit rickettsial pox in the United States, especially in New York city. Some mites bite and run, while others create a feeding tube and remain attached to the skin. Skin scrapings or potassium hydroxide (KOH) preparations may reveal the mite.

Cheyletiella mites are non-burrowing mites found on cats, rabbits, and dogs. In the animals, they produce 'walking dandruff'. When *Cheyletiella* is suspected, the animal should be evaluated by a veterinarian. Various adjunctive measures can be helpful in establishing the diagnosis. In one study, samples collected by vacuum cleaning were more helpful than tape impressions, hair pluckings, or skin scrapings (Saevik *et al.*, 2004).

TICKS

Dermacentor variabilis (351) and *D. andersoni* (352, 353) ticks both have brown legs and highly ornate dorsal plates. The scutum in the female is smaller, allowing the abdomen to engorge. *D. variabilis* is most common on the eastern seaboard, although it may be found throughout the United States, except the Rocky Mountain states. *D. andersoni*, in contrast, is generally confined to the Rocky Mountain states.

D. variabilis is the most important vector for Rocky Mountain spotted fever. Rocky Mountain spotted fever typically presents with fever and headache. Rash is commonly absent, especially in the early stages when antibiotic therapy must be initiated. The rash is petechial and acral in location. *D. andersoni* carries Rocky Mountain spotted fever (354) in the Rocky Mountain states. It also serves as a vector for Colorado tick fever, Q-fever, and tularemia. *Dermacentor* ticks are an important cause of tick paralysis, a rapidly progressive ascending paralysis. The ticks typically attach to the head and neck and may not be noticed in areas covered by hair. Removal of the tick results in prompt recovery. Because the tick is often not discovered, the associated death rate is about 10%, with the tick ultimately identified by the mortician or at the time of autopsy.

Ornithodoros ticks (355) carry borrelial relapsing fever. They are typical soft ticks that live in close association with a single host and take multiple small blood meals. In contrast to hard ticks, they lack a scutum (dorsal plate) and have retroverted mouthparts.

Amblyomma americanum (356) has a wide distribution, extending from Texas to New Jersey.

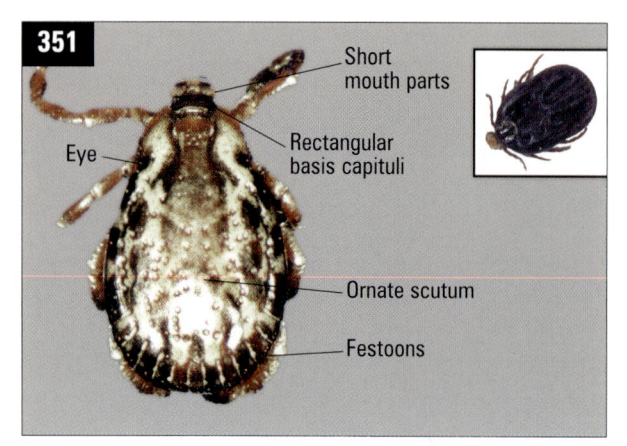

351 *Dermacentor variabilis* (engorged female). This tick is particularly common on the eastern seaboard of the United States and is the most common vector for Rocky Mountain spotted fever.

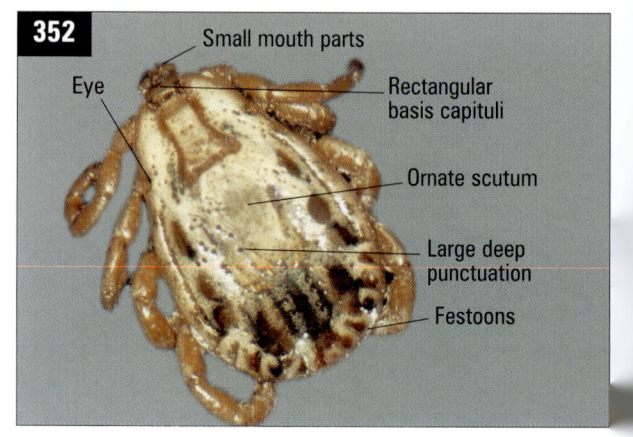

352 *Dermacentor andersoni*. This tick is found in the western United States and is also an important vector for Rocky Mountain spotted fever.

Arthropods and Infestations

Amblyomma ticks attach preferentially to the legs. The female is easily identified by the characteristic white dorsal spot on the scutum. This spot is responsible for the common name 'lone star tick' often applied to *A. americanum*. In males, inverted horseshoe-shaped markings are noted on the posterior portion of the hard dorsal plate. *Amblyomma* ticks are common in many parts of the world. In Africa, they carry tick typhus. In the southeastern United States, they carry *Ehrlichia chaffeensis*, the agent of human monocytic ehrlichiosis. They also appear to be a vector of southern Lyme disease.

Amblyomma ticks have been implicated in the transmission of Rocky Mountain spotted fever, Camp Bullis rickettsial fever, and tularemia.

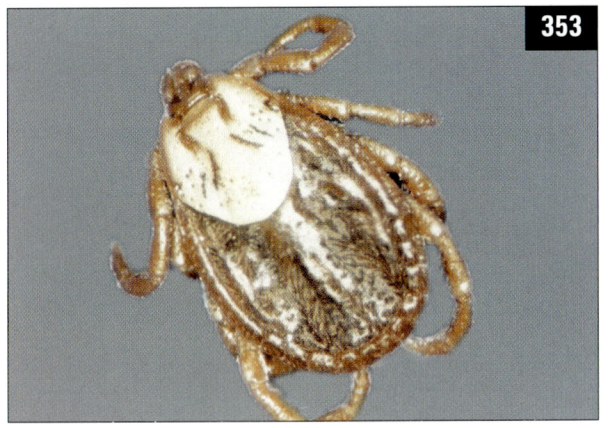

353 *Dermacentor andersoni* (female). The female has a small scutum (dorsal shield) allowing the abdomen to expand as the tick feeds.

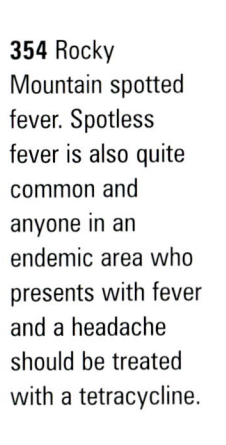

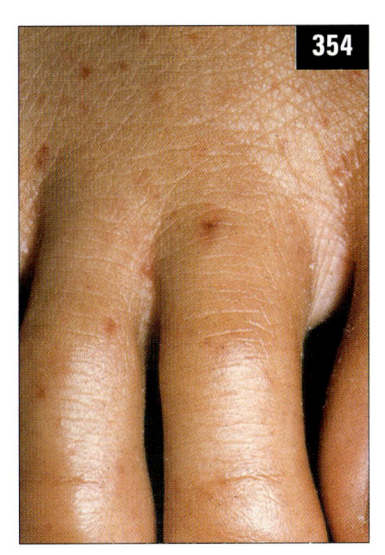

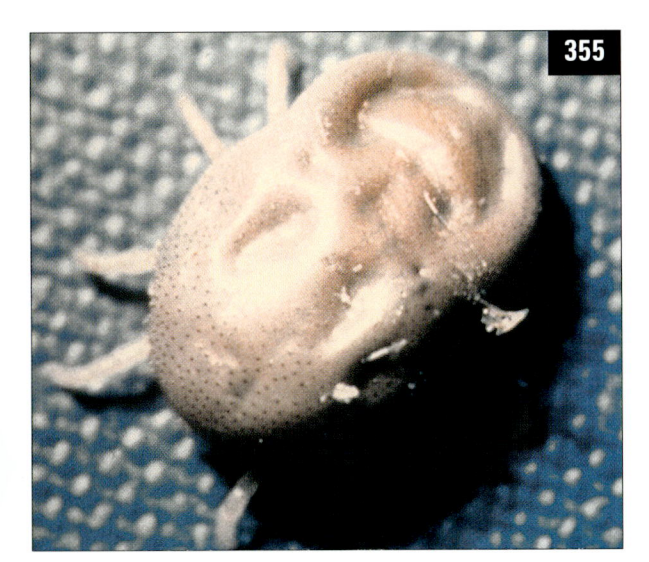

354 Rocky Mountain spotted fever. Spotless fever is also quite common and anyone in an endemic area who presents with fever and a headache should be treated with a tetracycline.

355 *Ornithodoros* tick. These are soft ticks with retroverted mouth parts. They lack the hard dorsal plate (scutum) characteristic of hard ticks. *Ornithodoros* ticks carry relapsing fever.

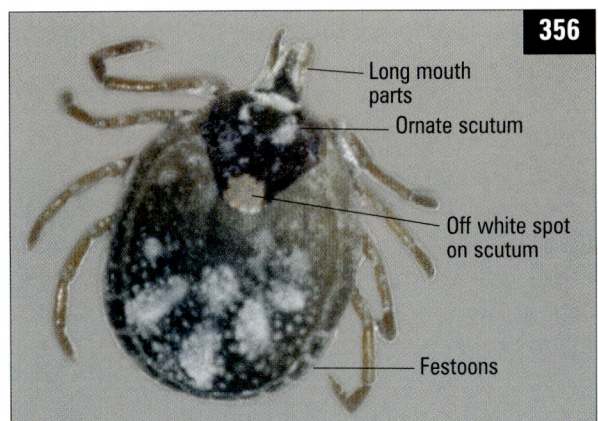

356 *Amblyomma americanum*. The female lone star tick has an ornate scutum with a single dot. Males have a larger ornate scutum with horshoe-shaped markings along the posterior margin. Both have long anterior mouth parts.

Rhipicephalus ticks (357) are common brown dog ticks. They are implicated in transmission of Rocky Mountain spotted fever, Mediterranean fever, canine ehrlichiosis, babesiosis, Congo–Crimean hemorrhagic fever, and canine visceral leishmaniasis (Coutinho *et al.*, 2005). Rickettsial diseases often present with a black eschar at the site of the tick bite (358).

Ixodes scapularis, the eastern black legged shoulder tick, is an important vector of Lyme disease. Adult females demonstrate a small inornate brown scutum. *Ixodes* (359–361) ticks also carry babesiosis and human anaplasmosis.

Localized tick bite reactions respond to corticosteroids topically or by intra-lesional injection. Most tick-borne diseases respond to tetracycline, and tetracyclines remain the drugs of choice for rickettsial disease, even in children. Tick control requires identification of sites of infestation, with removal of leaf debris and application of acaricides. Exclusion of animal hosts and bait stations that treat the host with an acaricide can be used effectively to reduce the incidence of arthropod-borne disease. Permethrin-treated clothing in combination with DEET or another repellent can also be highly effective. Some north African camel ticks are resistant to permethrin, and the agent triggers a pheromone-like response in the tick. Permethrin resistance has also been described in parts of Mexico (Foil *et al.*, 2004). A veterinarian should be consulted for advice concerning treatment of family pets or livestock. Agents such as topical fipronil, amitraz, and pyriproxyfen are available.

SPIDERS

Black and brown widow spiders are common throughout the world. The female *Latrodectus mactans* (362) is a large shiny black spider with a round abdomen bearing a red hourglass design. The male is much smaller. Latrotoxins are neurotoxins that produce abdominal pain and rigidity mimicking an acute surgical abdomen. The pain and rigidity respond to benzodiazepines and intravenous calcium gluconate. Antivenin can produce rapid relief of tetany and priapism, even after substantial delays in therapy (Hoover & Fortenberry, 2004).

Loxosceles spiders (363–365) are also found throughout the world. Although the brown recluse is the best known spider in this group, *L. laeta*, *L. rufescens*, *L. deserta*, and *L. arizonica* also cause

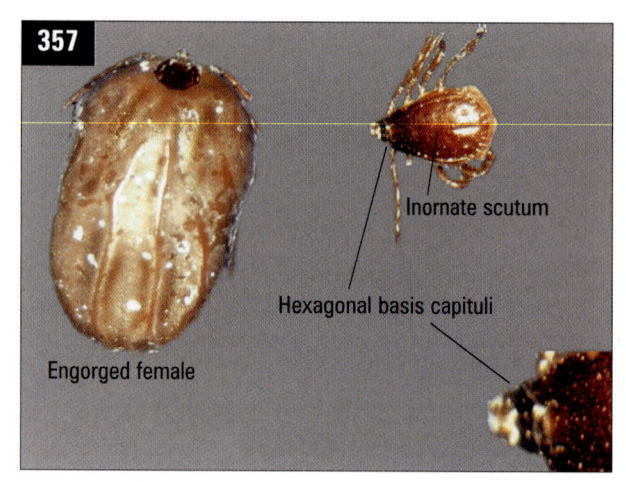

357 *Rhipicephalus* tick. Brown dog ticks have inornate dorsal plates. The mouth parts are relatively short and attached at a hexagonal base.

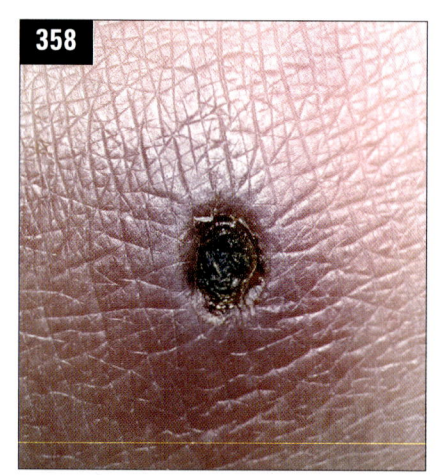

358 Rickettsial diseases often present with a black eschar at the site of the tick bite.

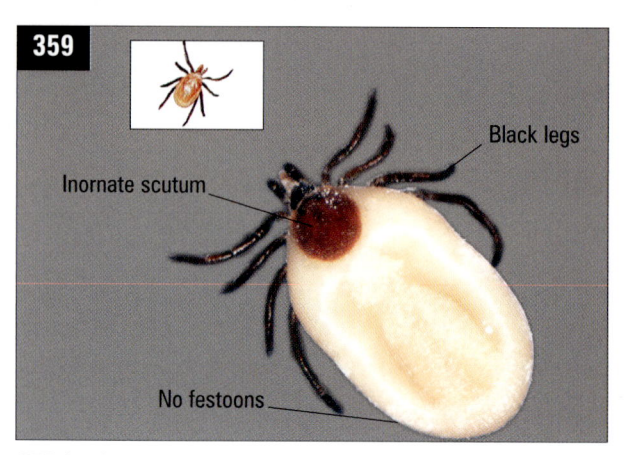

359 *Ixodes scapularis*. The female has a small inornate scutum. A prominent anterior anal groove is also characteristic.

Arthropods and Infestations

360 *Ixodes* ticks. Note the expansion of the abdomen in an engorged female tick.

361 *Ixodes* tick. An engorged female hard tick can be differentiated from a soft tick by the anterior mouth parts and the presence of a small scutum.

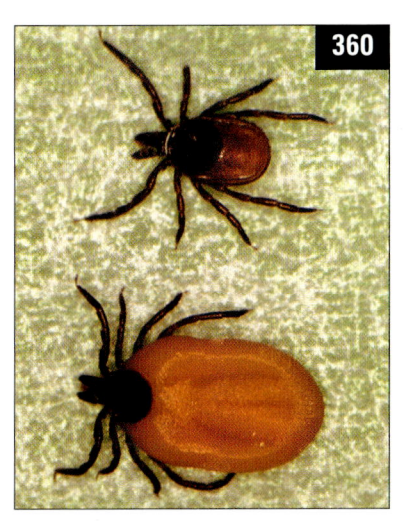

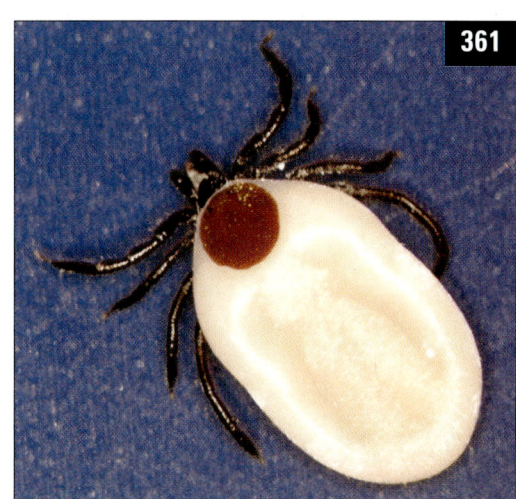

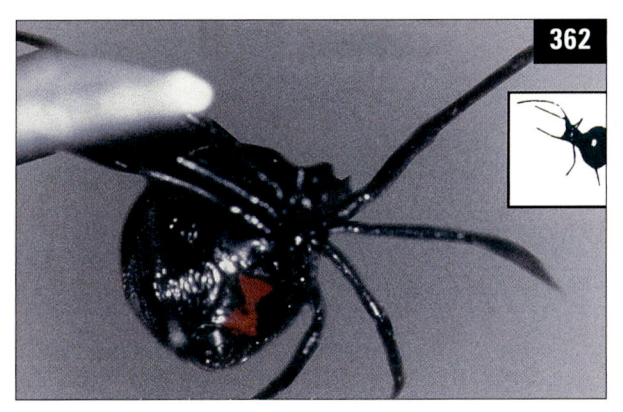

362 *Latrodectus mactans* (black widow spider). The female has a large glossy black body with an hourglass design on the ventral abdomen.

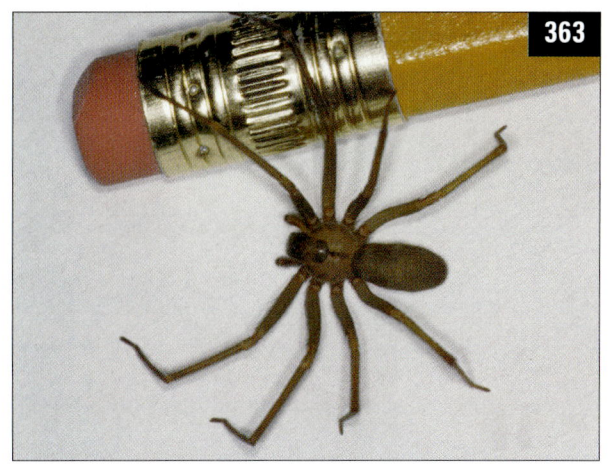

363 *Loxosceles* (brown recluse spider). Brown recluse spiders have a prominent violin case pattern on the thorax.

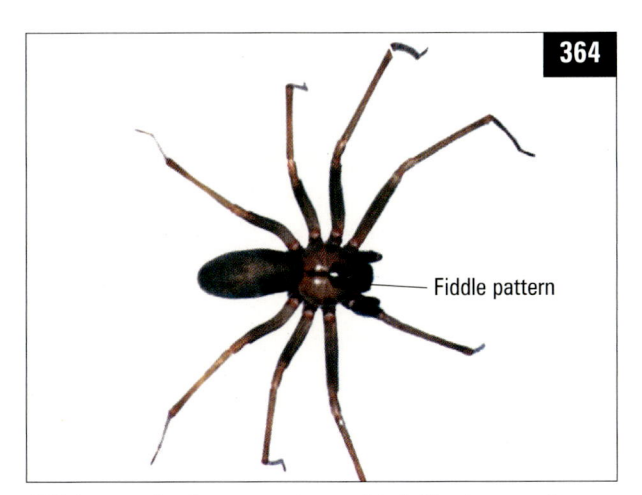

364 *Loxosceles* (brown recluse spider). The legs are long and delicate, and the abdomen is relatively small.

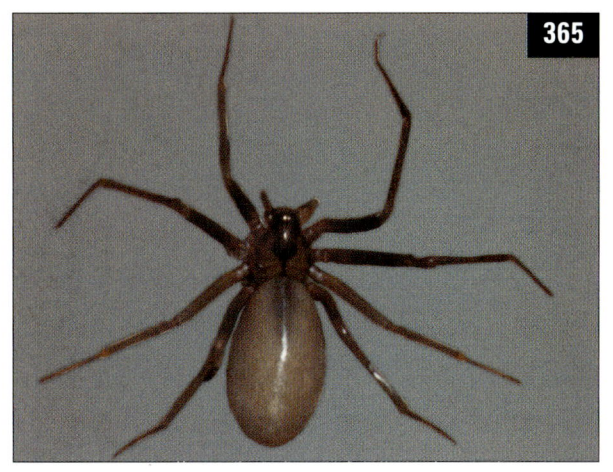

365 *Loxosceles* (brown recluse spider). Brown recluse spiders cause dermonecrotic reactions as well as disseminated intravascular coagulation.

skin necrosis. Brown recluse spiders are often found in woodpiles, in attics, and under radiators. They are not aggressive spiders, and houses may be heavily infested with not a single bite being reported. Dermonecrotic bite reactions (366, 367) commonly present as ulcerations, but may also appear as dry, necrotic eschars. Systemic reactions include hemolytic anemia and disseminated intravascular coagulation (Lane & Youse, 2004). The mainstay of treatment for brown spider bites is rest, ice, and elevation. Intradermal injection of polyclonal anti-*Loxosceles* Fab fragments has been shown to attenuate necrosis in an animal model up to 4 hours after envenomation, but such treatment is not readily available (Gomez *et al.*, 1999). The results with hyperbaric oxygen, dapsone, colchicine, triamcinolone, and prednisone have been generally disappointing (Elston, 2005; Elston *et al.*, 2005). Of these treatments, intra-lesional triamcinolone is the safest, and some anecdotal data support its use.

Tegenaria agrestis is a European funnel-web spider that has become common in houses in the Pacific northwest. In Europe, it is largely a rural spider, with *T. gigantea* and *T. domestica* predominating in human dwellings. *T. agrestis* venom has been implicated in local necrosis and central nervous system toxicity. Data on toxicity are stronger for Australian funnel-web spiders. Bites of Australian *Hadronyche*, *Atrax*, and *Missulenacan* spiders may produce severe pain and bleeding (Isbister & Gray, 2004). Severe systemic symptoms, including myocardial damage, may occur.

Tarantulas (368) are particularly common in the southwestern United States, although similar

366 Dermonecrotic brown recluse bite reaction. Those with milder cutaneous reactions may absorb more venom and may be at greater risk for systemic reactions.

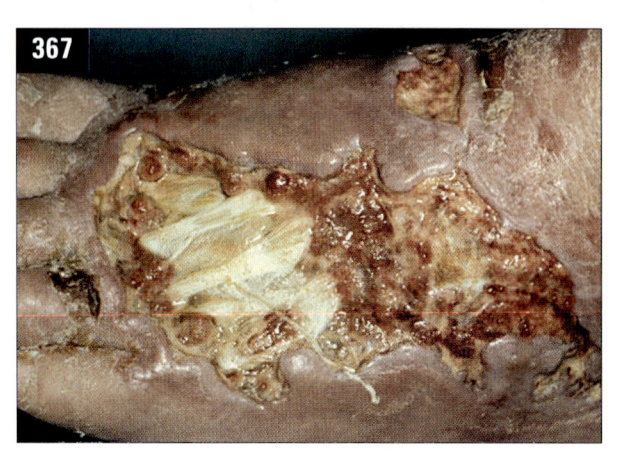

367 Dermonecrotic bite reaction. Severe reactions may expose bone or tendon. Rest, ice, and elevation are the mainstays of treatment, although some convincing anecdotal reports support the use of intralesional corticosteroids as well.

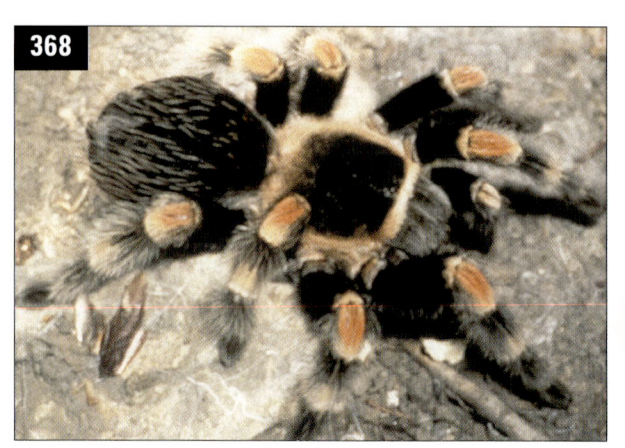

368 Tarantula. Tarantulas can cause contact urticaria. Many species flick barbed hairs into the eyes of an attacker.

spiders occur throughout the world. Many species possess urticating hairs in patches on the dorsal abdomen. The hairs are flicked at perceived attackers in a defensive fashion (Cooke et al., 1972). Urticating hairs are absent on most African and Asian species, but common in North American species. The hairs may embed in the cornea, producing ophthalmia nodosa similar to that seen with caterpillars and moths.

SCORPIONS

Scorpions vary widely in toxicity, with the most toxic species being found in Africa and south Asia. With less toxic species, pain and paresthesia predominate. *Centruroides vittatus* (369, 370) is common in Texas. *C. exilicauda* and *C. sculpturatus* (371) in Arizona are closely related species, occasionally implicated in more severe envenomations. *C. noxius*, *C. limpidus*, and *C.*

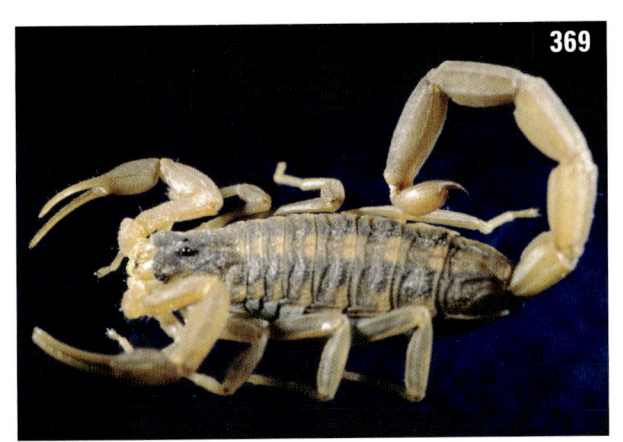

369 *Centruroides vittatus* scorpion. These scorpions are quite common in the southwest United States. They tend to hide under table tops and in shoes.

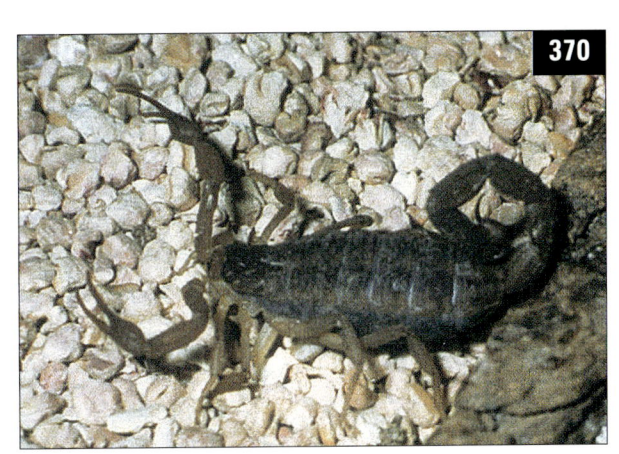

370 *Centruroides vittatus* scorpion. The sting is quite painful, but serious reactions are rare.

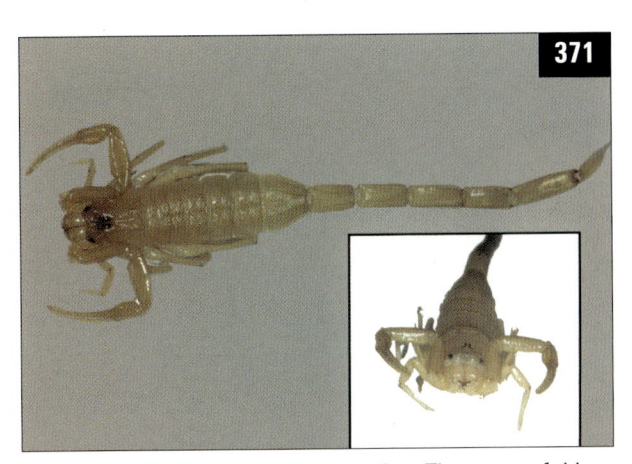

371 *Centruroides sculpturatus* scorpion. The range of this scorpion is expanding into the southwestern United States. It is the scorpion most often associated with severe reactions in the United States.

suffusus have also been reported to be toxic. Highly toxic Buthid scorpions include African species such as *Parabuthus granulatus*, *P. capensis*, *P. transvaalicus* (372), *Uroplectes lineatus*, and *Leiurus quinquestriatus*. *Androctonus australis* and *Buthus occitanus tunetanus* are found in Asia and north Africa. *Androctonus crassicauda* is another toxic Asian scorpion. In Brazil, *Tityus serrulatus* is an important toxic species. *Vaejovis* scorpions (373, 374) have been reported to cause dermonecrotic reactions.

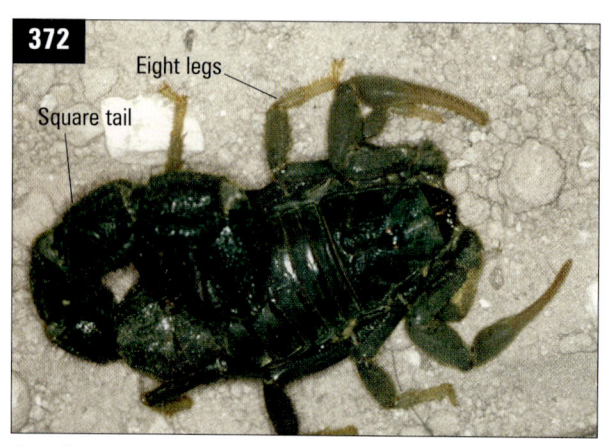

372 *Parabuthus transvaalicus*. An African scorpion often associated with serious envenomation.

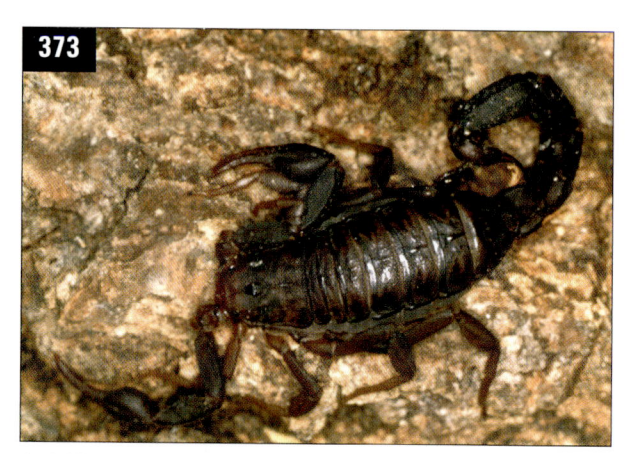

373 *Vaejovis* scorpion. These brown scorpions are found in the southeastern United States. They have been associated with dermonecrotic reactions resembling those of brown recluse spider bites.

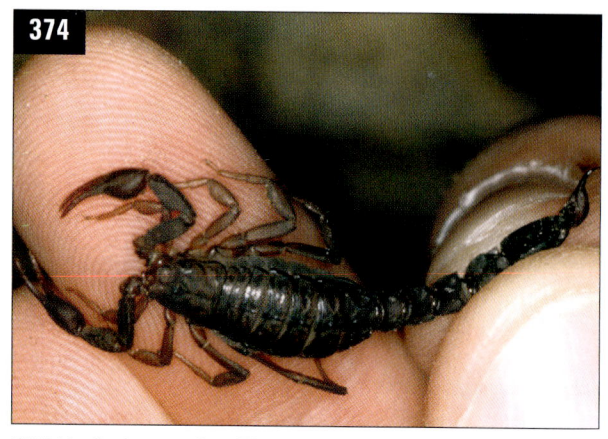

374 *Vaejovis* scorpion. These plain brown scorpions are fairly small and hide easily in bark.

Arthropods and Infestations

CENTIPEDES AND MILLIPEDES

Centipedes (375) inject a neurotoxic venom that produces swelling, pain, and paresthesia (376). Centipede ingestion can produce toxicity that ranges from coronary ischemia to rhabdomyolysis, proteinuria, and renal failure (Ozsarac *et al.*, 2004; Hasan & Hassan, 2005). Millipedes (377) secrete a noxious fluid that causes chemical burns. Millipede burns are particularly serious if they involve the eyes.

375 Centipede. Centipedes inject venom through anterior mouth parts. Children may mistake large centipedes for snakes and report that they have suffered a snake bite. The centipede bite has a characteristic chevron shape which helps differentiate it. Edema is generally far less than with a snake bite and systemic symptoms are generally mild.

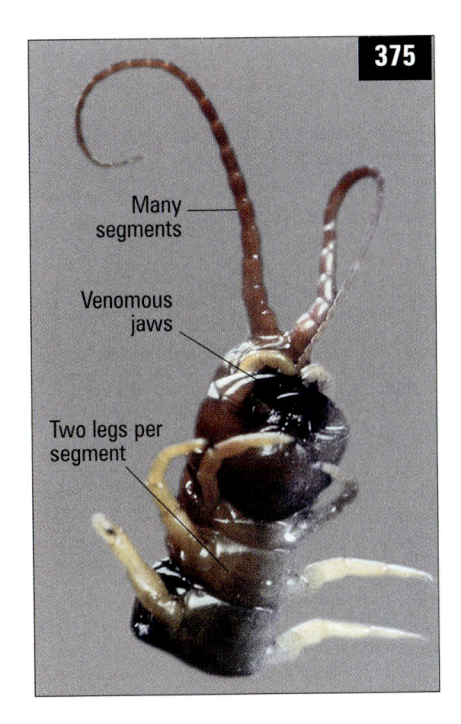

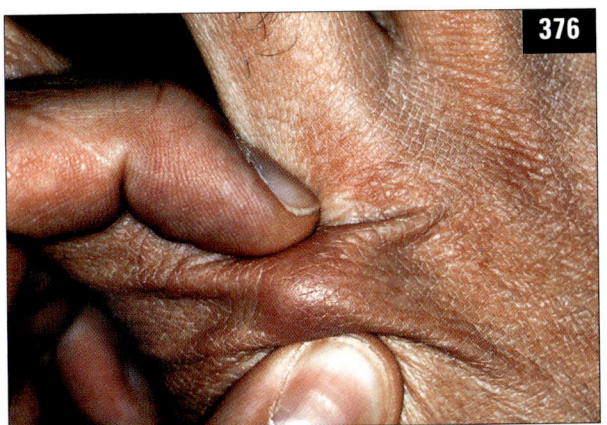

376 Centipede bite. Edema following a bite from the centipede pictured in figure **375**.

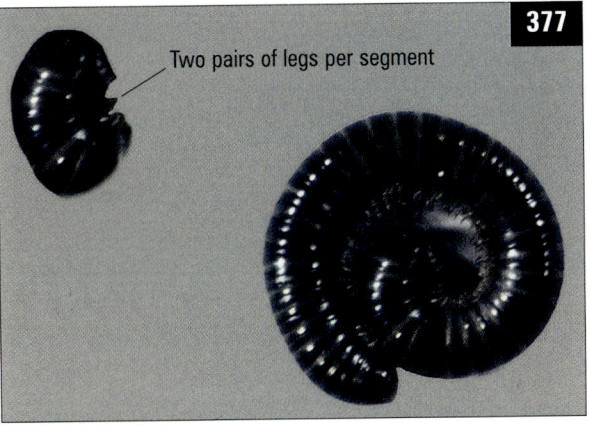

377 Millipede. Millipedes can exude caustic fluid resulting in arcuate burns. Millipedes in clothing have resulted in burns mistaken for child abuse.

REFERENCES

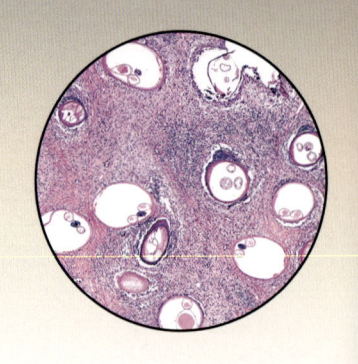

CHAPTER 1 BACTERIAL INFECTIONS

Akesson P, Moritz L, Truedsson M, Christensson B, von Pawel-Rammingen U (2006). IdeS, a highly specific immunoglobulin G (IgG)-cleaving enzyme from *Streptococcus pyogenes*, is inhibited by specific IgG antibodies generated during infection. *Infection and Immunity* **74**(1):497–503.

Anan TJ, Culik DA (1989). *Neisseria gonorrhoeae* dissemination and gonococcal meningitis. *J Am Board Family Prac* **2**(2):123–125.

Bhatia A, Brodell RT (1999). 'Hot tub folliculitis'. Test the waters – and the patient – for *Pseudomonas*. *Postgrad Med* **106**(4):43–46.

Blacksell SD, Bryant NJ, Paris DH, Doust JA, Sakoda Y, Day NP (2007). Scrub typhus serologic testing with the indirect immunofluorescence method as a diagnostic gold standard: a lack of consensus leads to a lot of confusion. *Clin Infect Dis* **44**(3):391–401.

Byrnes JM (2006). Necrotizing fasciitis: a common problem in Darwin. *Int J Lower Extremity Wounds* **5**(4):271–276.

Centers for Disease Control and Prevention (CDC) (2004). Fatal cases of Rocky Mountain spotted fever in family clusters – three states, 2003. *MMWR* **53**(19):407–410.

Chapman AS, Murphy SM, Demma LJ, et al. (2006a). Rocky Mountain spotted fever in the United States, 1997–2002. *Vector Borne and Zoonotic Dis* **6**(2):170–178.

Chapman AS, Bakken JS, Folk SM, et al. (2006b). Tickborne Rickettsial Diseases Working Group; CDC. Diagnosis and management of tickborne rickettsial diseases: Rocky Mountain spotted fever, ehrlichioses, and anaplasmosis: United States: a practical guide for physicians and other health-care and public health professionals. *MMWR Recommendations and Reports* **55**(RR-4):1–27.

Elston DM (2007). Community-acquired methicillin-resistant *Staphylococcus aureus*. *J Am Acad Derm* **56**(1):1–16.

Falagas ME, Bliziotis IA, Fragoulis KN (2007). Oral rifampin for eradication of *Staphylococcus aureus* carriage from healthy and sick populations: a systematic review of the evidence from comparative trials. *Am J Infect Control* **35**(2):106–114.

Feder HM Jr, Abeles M, Bernstein M, Whitaker-Worth D, Grant-Kels JM (2006). Diagnosis, treatment, and prognosis of erythema migrans and Lyme arthritis. *Clinics in Dermatol* **24**(6):509–520.

Fleisher G, Heeger P, Topf P (1983). *Hemophilus influenzae* cellulitis. *Am J Emerg Med* **1**(3):274–277.

Friedlander AM (1999). Clinical aspects, diagnosis and treatment of anthrax. *J Appl Microbiol* **87**(2):303.

Giordano PA, Elston D, Akinlade BK, et al. (2006). Cefdinir *vs.* cephalexin for mild to moderate uncomplicated skin and skin structure infections in adolescents and adults. *Curr Med Res Opin* **22**(12):2419–2428.

Golger A, Ching S, Goldsmith CH, Pennie RA, Bain JR (2007). Mortality in patients with necrotizing fasciitis. *Plastic and Reconstructive Surg* **119**(6):1803–1807.

Gucluer H, Ergun T, Demircay Z (1999). Ecthyma gangrenosum. *Int J Dermatol* **38**(4):299–302.

Holdiness MR (2002). Management of cutaneous erythrasma. *Drugs* **62**(8):1131–1141.

Iredell J, Whitby M, Blacklock Z (1992). *Mycobacterium marinum* infection: epidemiology and presentation in Queensland 1971–1990. *Med J Aus* **157**(9):596–598.

Klempner MS, Styrt B (1988). Prevention of recurrent staphylococcal skin infections with low-dose oral clindamycin therapy. *JAMA* **260**(18):2682–2685.

Ladhani S (2001). Recent developments in staphylococcal scalded skin syndrome. *Clin Microbiol Infect* **7**(6):301–307.

Longshaw CM, Wright JD, Farrell AM, Holland KT (2002). *Kytococcus sedentarius*, the organism associated with pitted keratolysis, produces two keratin-degrading enzymes. *J Appl Microbiol* **93**(5):810–816.

Low N, Broutet N, Adu-Sarkodie Y, Barton P, Hossain M, Hawkes S (2006). Global control of sexually transmitted infections. *Lancet* **368**(9551):2001–2016.

Macfie J, Harvey J (1977). The treatment of acute superficial abscesses: a prospective clinical trial. *Br J Surg* **64**(4):264–266.

Marra CM, Colina AP, Godornes C, *et al.* (2006). Antibiotic selection may contribute to increases in macrolide-resistant *Treponema pallidum*. *J Infect Dis* **194**(12):1771–1773.

McGinley-Smith DE, Tsao SS (2003). Dermatoses from ticks. *J Am Acad Dermatol* **49**(3):363–392.

Meislin HW, Lerner SA, Graves MH, *et al.* (1977). Cutaneous abscesses. Anaerobic and aerobic bacteriology and outpatient management. *Ann Int Med* **87**(2):145–149.

Meislin HW (1986). Pathogen identification of abscesses and cellulitis. *Ann Emerg Med* **15**(3):329–332.

Melski JW, Reed KD, Mitchell PD, Barth GD (1993). Primary and secondary erythema migrans in central Wisconsin. *Arch Dermatol* **129**(6):709–716.

Nagi KS, Joshi R, Thakur RK (1996). Cardiac manifestations of Lyme disease: a review. *Can J Cardiol* **12**(5):503–506.

Nordstrom KM, McGinley KJ, Cappiello L, Zechman JM, Leyden JJ (1987). Pitted keratolysis. The role of *Micrococcus sedentarius*. *Arch Dermatol* **123**(10):1320–1325.

Perez-Roth E, Lopez-Aguilar C, Alcoba-Florez J, Mendez-Alvarez S (2006). High-level mupirocin resistance within methicillin-resistant *Staphylococcus aureus* pandemic lineages. *Antimicrobial Agents and Chemotherapy* **50**(9):3207–3211.

Ramos-e-Silva M, Pereira AL (2005). Life-threatening eruptions due to infectious agents. *Clin Dermatol* **23**(2):148–156.

Raoult D, Woodward T, Dumler JS (2004). The history of epidemic typhus. *Infect Dis Clin N Am* **18**(1):127–140.

Raz R, Miron D, Colodner R, Staler Z, Samara Z, Keness Y (1996). A 1-year trial of nasal mupirocin in the prevention of recurrent staphylococcal nasal colonization and skin infection. *Arch Internal Med* **156**(10):1109–1112.

Rittenhouse S, Biswas S, Broskey J, *et al.* (2006). Selection of retapamulin, a novel pleuromutilin for topical use. *Antimicrobial Agents and Chemotherapy* **50**(11):3882–3885.

Rozmajzl PJ, Houhamdi L, Jiang J, Raoult D, Richards AL (2006). Validation of a *Rickettsia prowazekii*-specific quantitative real-time PCR cassette and DNA extraction protocols using experimentally infected lice. *Ann NY Acad Sci* **1078**:617–619.

Sigurdsson AF, Gudmundsson S (1989). The etiology of bacterial cellulitis as determined by fine-needle aspiration. *Scand J Infect Dis* **21**(5):537–542.

Silpapojakul K, Chayakul P, Krisanapan S, Silpapojakul K (1993). Murine typhus in Thailand: clinical features, diagnosis and treatment. *Quart J Med* **86**(1):43–47.

Simon MS, Cody RL (1992). Cellulitis after axillary lymph node dissection for carcinoma of the breast. *Am J Med* **93**(5):543–548.

Singh AE, Romanowski B (1999). Syphilis: review with emphasis on clinical, epidemiologic, and some biologic features. *Clin Microbiol Rev* **12**(2):187–209.

Sorensen RW (1989). Lyme disease: neurologic manifestations. *Comprehensive Therapy* **15**(7):16–22.Steere AC, Schoen RT, Taylor E (1987). The clinical evolution of Lyme arthritis. *Ann Internal Med* **107**(5):725–731.

Van Seymortier P, Verellen K, De Jonge I (2004). *Mycobacterium marinum* causing tenosynovitis. 'Fish tank finger'. *Acta Orthopaedica Belgica* **70**(3):279–282.

Weinstein L, Le Frock J (1971). Does antimicrobial therapy of streptococcal pharyngitis or pyoderma alter the risk of glomerulonephritis? *J Infect Dis* **124**(2):229–231.

Wenner KA, Kenner JR (2004). Anthrax. *Dermatol Clin* **22**(3):247–256.

Windsor JJ (2001). Cat-scratch disease: epidemiology, aetiology and treatment. *Br J Biomed Sci* **58**(2):101–110.

CHAPTER 2 FUNGAL INFECTIONS

Adams JS, Godin MS, Tsogas N (2002). Pathology quiz case: disseminated blastomycosis. *Arch Otolaryngol Head Neck Surg* **128**:853–854.

Adams SP (2002). Dermacase. Erosio interdigitalis blastomycetica. *Can Fam Physician* **48**:271, 277.

Anderson DJ, Schmidt C, Goodman J, Pomeroy C (1992). Cryptococcal disease presenting as cellulitis. *Clin Infect Dis* **14**:666–672.

Arsura EL, Kilgore WB, Ratnayake SN (1998). Erythema nodosum in pregnant patients with coccidioidomycosis. *Clin Infect Dis* **27**:1201–1203.

Baumgardner DJ, Knavel EM, Steber D, Swain GR (2006). Geographic distribution of human blastomycosis cases in Milwaukee, Wisconsin, USA: association with urban watersheds. *Mycopathologia* **161**:275–282.

Borman AM, Campbell CK, Fraser M, Johnson EM (2007). Analysis of the dermatophyte species isolated in the British Isles between 1980 and 2005 and review of worldwide dermatophyte trends over the last three decades. *Med Mycol* **45**(2):131–141.

Bradley VR, Patterson CC, Scarborough DA (2006). Verrucous facial plaques – blastomycosis. *Arch Dermatol* **142**:385–390.

Bradsher RW, Chapman SW, Pappas PG (2003). Blastomycosis. *Infect Dis Clin North Am* **17**:21–40.

References

Bromel C, Sykes JE (2005). Epidemiology, diagnosis, and treatment of blastomycosis in dogs and cats. *Clin Tech Small Anim Pract* **20**:233–239.

Brook I (2002). Secondary bacterial infections complicating skin lesions. *J Med Microbiol* **51**:808–812.

Bullpitt P, Weedon D (1978). Sporotrichosis: a review of 39 cases. *Pathology* **10**:249–256.

Centers for Disease Control (CDC) (1993). Coccidioidomycosis: United States, 1991–1992. *MMWR* **42**:21–24.

Chayakulkeeree M, Ghannoum MA, Perfect JR (2006). Zygomycosis: the re-emerging fungal infection. *Eur J Clin Microbiol Infect Dis* **25**:215–229.

Chiller TM, Gagliani JN, Stevens, DA (2003). Coccidioidomycosis. *Infect Dis Clin N Am* **17**:41–57.

Cohen PR, Bank DE, Silvers DN, Grossman ME (1990). Cutaneous lesions of disseminated histoplasmosis in human immunodeficiency virus-infected patients. *J Am Acad Dermatol* **23**:422–428.

Conces DJ Jr (1996). Histoplasmosis. *Semin Roentgenol* **31**:14–27.

Crespo-Erchiga V, Florencio VD (2006). *Malassezia* yeasts and pityriasis versicolor. *Curr Opin Infect Dis* **19**:139–147.

Crum NF (2005). Disseminated coccidioidomycosis with cutaneous lesions clinically mimicking mycosis fungoides. *Int J Dermatol* **44**:958–960.

Crum-Cianflone NF, Truett AA, Teneza-Mora N, et al. (2006). Unusual presentations of coccidioidomycosis: a case series and review of the literature. *Medicine* (Baltimore) **85**:263–277.

Dalmau J, Pimentel CL, Alegre M, et al. (2006). Treatment of protothecosis with voriconazole. *J Am Acad Dermatol* **55**:S122–123.

Daniel CR 3rd, Gupta AK, Daniel MP, Daniel CM (1997). Two feet-one hand syndrome: a retrospective multicenter survey. *Int J Dermatol* **36**:658–660.

Daniel CR 3rd, Norton LA, Scher RK (1992). The spectrum of nail disease in patients with human immunodeficiency virus infection. *J Am Acad Dermatol* **27**:93–97.

Davies SF, Sarosi GA (1997). Epidemiological and clinical features of pulmonary blastomycosis. *Semin Respir Infect* **12**:206–218.

DiCaudo DJ, Connolly SM (2001). Interstitial granulomatous dermatitis associated with pulmonary coccidioidomycosis. *J Am Acad Dermatol* **45**:840–845.

DiCaudo DJ, Yiannias JA, Laman SD, Warschaw KE (2006). The exanthem of acute pulmonary coccidioidomycosis: clinical and histopathologic features of 3 cases and review of the literature. *Arch Dermatol* **142**:744–746.

Dignani MC, Anaissie E (2004). Human fusariosis. *Clin Microbiol Infect* **1**:67–75.

Driezen S (1984). Oral candidiasis. *Am J Med* **77**:28–33.

Foster KW, Ghannoum MA, Elewski BE (2004). Epidemiologic surveillance of cutaneous fungal infection in the United States from 1999 to 2002. *J Am Acad Dermatol* **50**:748–752.

Frater JL, Hall GS, Procop GW (2001). Histologic features of zygomycosis: emphasis on perineural invasion and fungal morphology. *Arch Pathol Lab Med* **125**:375–378.

Gupta AK, Lynch LE (2004). Onychomycosis: review of recurrence rates, poor prognostic factors, and strategies to prevent disease recurrence. *Cutis* **74**:10–15.

Hall J, Perry VE (1998). Tinea nigra palmaris: differentiation from malignant melanoma or junctional nevi. *Cutis* **62**:45–46.

Hardman S, Stephenson I, Jenkins DR, Wiselka MJ, Johnson EM (2005). Disseminated *Sporothrix schenckii* in a patient with AIDS. *J Infect* **51**:e73–77.

High WA, Fitzpatrick JE (2007). Topical antifungal agents. In: *Fitzpatrick's Dermatology in General Medicine*. K Wolff et al. (eds). 7th edn. McGraw-Hill, New York.

High WA (2007). Onychomycosis. In: *Uncomplicated Skin and Soft-Tissue Infections*. DM Elston, R Scher (eds). Professional Communications West Inslip, New York.

Hussein MR, Rashad UM (2005). Rhinosporidiosis in Egypt: a case report and review of literature. *Mycopathologia* **159**:205–207.

Imwidthaya P, Poungvarin N (2000). Cryptococcosis in AIDS. *Postgrad Med J* **76**:85–88.

Janniger CK (1992). Majocchi's granuloma. *Cutis* **50**:267–268.

Kantrow SM, Boyd AS (2003). Protothecosis. *Dermatol Clin* **21**:249–255.

Kauffman CA (2002). Management of histoplasmosis. *Expert Opin Pharmacother* **3**:1067–1072.

Koga T, Matsuda T, Matsumoto T, Furue M (2003). Therapeutic approaches to subcutaneous mycoses. *Am J Clin Dermatol* **4**:537–543.

Kostman JR, DiNubile MJ (1993). Nodular lymphangitis: a distinctive but often unrecognized syndrome. *Ann Intern Med* **118**:883–888.

Kumari R, Laxmisha C, Thappa DM (2005). Disseminated cutaneous rhinosporidiosis. *Dermatol Online J* **11**:19.

La Touché CJ (1967). Scrotal dermatophytosis. An insufficiently documented aspect of tinea cruris. *Br J Dermatol* **79**:339–344.

Lemos LB, Guo M, Baliga M (2000). Blastomycosis: organ involvement and etiologic diagnosis. *Ann Diagn Pathol* **4**:391–406.

Lesueur BW, Warschaw K, Fredrikson L (2002). Necrotizing cellulitis caused by *Apophysomyces elegans* at a patch test site. *Am J Contact Dermat* **13**:140–142.

Lin SJ, Schranz J, Teutsch SM (2001). Aspergillus case-fatality rate: systematic review of the literature. *Clin Infect Dis* **32**:358–366.

Litvintseva AP, Kestenbaum L, Vilgalys R, Mitchell TG (2005). Comparative analysis of environmental and clinical populations of *Cryptococcus neoformans*. *J Clin Microbiol* **43**:556–564.

Lottenberg R, Waldman RH, Ajello L, Hoff GL, Bigler W, Zellner SR (1979). Pulmonary histoplasmosis associated with exploration of a bat cave. *Am J Epidemiol* **110**:156–161.

Lupi O, Tyring SK, McGinnis MR (2005). Tropical dermatology: fungal tropical diseases. *J Am Acad Dermatol* **53**:931–951.

Mays SR, Bogle MA, Bodey GP (2006). Cutaneous fungal infections in the oncology patient: recognition and management. *Am J Clin Dermatol* **7**:31–43.

Mendoza L, Vilela R, Rosa PS, Fernandes Belone AF (2005). *Lacazia loboi* and *Rhinosporidium seeberi*: a genomic perspective. *Rev Iberoam Micol* **22**:213–216.

Miller SD, David-Bajar K (2004). Images in clinical medicine. A brilliant case of erythrasma. *N Engl J Med* **351**:1666.

Morris-Jones R (2002). Sporotrichosis. *Clin Exp Dermatol* **27**:427–431.

Murakawa GJ, Kerschmann R, Berger T (1996). Cutaneous *Cryptococcus* infection and AIDS: report of 12 cases and review of the literature. *Arch Dermatol* **132**:545–548.

O'Donnell B, Powell F, Hone R, O'Loughlin S (1990). Kerion: clinical spectrum in nine cases. *Ir J Med Sci* **159**:14–18.

Oklota CA, Brodell RT (2004). Uncovering tinea incognito. Topical corticosteroids can mask typical features of ringworm. *Postgrad Med* **116**:65–66.

Olofinlade O, Cacciarelli A (2000). Treatment of the wrong disease with the right medication: a case of generalized leishmaniasis involving the liver and the gastrointestinal tract. *Am J Gastroenterol* **95**:1377.

Park DW, Sohn JW, Cheong HJ, et al. (2006). Combination therapy of disseminated coccidioidomycosis with caspofungin and fluconazole. *BMC Infect Dis* **6**:26.

Perez C, Colella MT, Olaizola C, et al. (2005). Tinea nigra: report of twelve cases in Venezuela. *Mycopathologia* **160**:235–238.

Reisberger EM, Abels C, Landthaler M, Szeimies RM (2003). Histopathological diagnosis of onychomycosis by periodic acid Schiff-stained nail clippings. *Br J Dermatol* **148**:749–754.

Roberts BJ, Friedlander SF (2005). Tinea capitis: a treatment update. *Pediatr Ann* **34**:191–200.

Rodriguez G, Barrera GP (1997). The asteroid body of lobomycosis. *Mycopathologia* **136**:71–74.

Rosenstein NE, Emery KW, Werner SB, et al. (2001). Risk factors for severe pulmonary and disseminated coccidioidomycosis. *Clin Infect Dis* **32**:708–715.

Saag MS, Graybill RJ, Larsen RA, et al. (2000). Practice guidelines for the management of cryptococcal disease. Infectious Diseases Society of America. *Clin Infect Dis* **30**:710–718.

Sampathkumar P, Paya CV (2001). *Fusarium* infection after solid-organ transplantation. *Clin Infect Dis* **32**:1237–1240.

Sayegh-Carreno R, Abramovits-Ackerman W, Giron GP (1989). Therapy of tinea nigra plantaris. *Int J Dermatol* **28**:46–48.

van Burik JA, Colven R, Spach DH (1998). Cutaneous aspergillosis. *J Clin Microbiol* **36**:3115–3121.

Vijaikumar M, Thappa DM, Karthikeyan K, Jayanthi S (2002). Verrucous lesion of the palm. *Postgrad Med J* **78**:302,305–306.

Weinberg JM, Koestenblatt EK, Jennings MB (2005). Utility of histopathologic analysis in the evaluation of onychomycosis. *J Am Podiatr Med Assoc* **95**:258–263.

Weinberg JM, Koestenblatt EK, Tutrone WD, Tishler HR, Najarian L (2003). Comparison of diagnostic methods in the evaluation of onychomycosis. *J Am Acad Dermatol* **49**:193–197.

Wheat LJ (2006). Improvements in diagnosis of histoplasmosis. *Expert Opin Biol Ther* **6**:1207–1221.

Williams JV, Eichenfield LF, Burke BL, Barnes-Eley M, Friedlander SF (2005). Prevalence of scalp scaling in prepubertal children. *Pediatrics* **115**:e1–6.

CHAPTER 3 VIRAL DISEASES

Anderson MJ, Jones SE, Minson AC (1985). Diagnosis of human parvovirus infection by dot-blot hybridization using cloned viral DNA. *J Med Virol* **15**(2):163–172.

Andersson JP (1991). Clinical aspects on Epstein–Barr virus infection. *Scand J Infect Dis Suppl* **80**: 94–104.

Ashley RL, Militoni J, Lee F, Nahmias A, Corey L (1988). Comparison of Western blot (immunoblot) and glycoprotein G-specific immunodot enzyme assay for detecting antibodies to herpes simplex virus types 1 and 2 in human sera. *J Clin Microbiol* **26**(4):662–667.

Bailey RE (1994). Diagnosis and treatment of infectious mononucleosis. *Am Fam Phys* **49**(4): 879–888.

Baldanti F, Biron KK, Gerna G (1998). Interpreting human cytomegalovirus antiviral drug susceptibility testing: the role of mixed virus populations. *J Infect Dis* **177**(3): 823–824.

Ballanger F, Barbarot S, Mollat C, et al. (2006). Two giant orf lesions in a heart/lung transplant patient. *Eur J Dermatol* **16**(3): 284–286.

References

Bell AT, Fortune B, Sheeler R (2006). Clinical inquiries. What test is the best for diagnosing infectious mononucleosis? *J Fam Pract* **55**(9):799–802.

Berretta M, Cinelli R, Martellotta F, Spina M, Vaccher E, Tirelli U (2003). Therapeutic approaches to AIDS-related malignancies. *Oncogene* **22**(42):6646–6659.

Blatt J, Kastner O, Hodes DS (1978). Cutaneous vesicles in congenital cytomegalovirus infection. *J Pediatr* **92**(3):509.

Bosch FX, Manos MM, Munoz N, et al. (1995). Prevalence of human papillomavirus in cervical cancer: a worldwide perspective. International biological study on cervical cancer (IBSCC) Study Group. *J Natl Cancer Inst* **87**(11):796–802.

Bourboulia D, Whitby D, Boshoff C, et al. (1998). Serologic evidence for mother-to-child transmission of Kaposi sarcoma-associated herpesvirus infection. *JAMA* **280**(1):31–32.

Bowden JB, Hebert AA, Rapini RP (1989). Dermal hematopoiesis in neonates: report of five cases. *J Am Acad Dermatol* **20**(6):1104–1110.

Bowsher D (1997). The management of postherpetic neuralgia. *Postgrad Med J* **73**(864):623–629.

Brandt O, Abeck D, Gianotti R, Burgdorf W (2006). Gianotti–Crosti syndrome. *J Am Acad Dermatol* **54**(1):136–145.

Broliden K, Tolfvenstam T, Norbeck O (2006). Clinical aspects of parvovirus B19 infection. *J Intern Med* **260**(4):285–304.

Brown J, Janniger CK, Schwartz RA, Silverberg NB (2006). Childhood molluscum contagiosum. *Int J Dermatol* **45**(2):93–99.

Buttner M, Rziha HJ (2002). Parapoxviruses: from the lesion to the viral genome. *J Vet Med B Infect Dis Vet Public Health* **49**(1):7–16.

Chorba T, Coccia P, Holman RC, et al. (1986). The role of parvovirus B19 in aplastic crisis and erythema infectiosum (fifth disease). *J Infect Dis* **154**(3):383–393.

Colsky AS, Jegasothy SM, Leonardi C, Kirsner RS, Kerdel FA (1998). Diagnosis and treatment of a case of cutaneous cytomegalovirus infection with a dramatic clinical presentation. *J Am Acad Dermatol* **38**(2 Pt 2):349–351.

Corey L, Adams HG, Brown ZA, Holmes KK (1983). Genital herpes simplex virus infections: clinical manifestations, course, and complications. *Ann Intern Med* **98**(6):958–972.

Cotton DW, Cooper C, Barrett DF, Leppard BJ (1987). Severe atypical molluscum contagiosum infection in an immunocompromised host. *Br J Dermatol* **116**(6):871–876.

Dal Pozzo F, Andrei G, Lebeau I, et al. (2007). In vitro evaluation of the anti-orf virus activity of alkoxyalkyl esters of CDV, cCDV and (S)-HPMPA. *Antiviral Res* **75**(1):52–57.

De Clercq E, Naesens L, De Bolle L, Schols D, Zhang Y, Neyts J (2001). Antiviral agents active against human herpesviruses HHV-6, HHV-7 and HHV-8. *Rev Med Virol* **11**(6):381–395.

De Clercq E, Neyts J (2004). Therapeutic potential of nucleoside/nucleotide analogues against poxvirus infections. *Rev Med Virol* **14**(5):289–300.

Degraeve C, De Coninck A, Senneseael J, Roseeuw D (1999). Recurrent contagious ecthyma (Orf) in an immunocompromised host successfully treated with cryotherapy. *Dermatology* **198**(2):162–163.

Dellamonica P, Bernard E, Ortonne JP, Defontaine A (1983). The Orf nodule. *Sem Hop* **59**(32):2233–2238.

Drago F, Rebora A (1999). The new herpesviruses: emerging pathogens of dermatological interest. *Arch Dermatol* **135**(1):71–75.

Ebell MH (2004). Epstein–Barr virus infectious mononucleosis. *Am Fam Physician* **70**(7):1279–1287.

Erbagci Z, Erbagci I, Almila Tuncel A (2005). Rapid improvement of human orf (ecthyma contagiosum) with topical imiquimod cream: report of four complicated cases. *J Dermatolog Treat* **16**(5–6):353–356.

Fazel N, Wilczynski S, Lowe L, Su LD (1999). Clinical, histopathologic, and molecular aspects of cutaneous human papillomavirus infections. *Dermatol Clin* **17**(3):521–536, viii.

Helm K, Lane AT, Orosz J, Metlay L (1990). Systemic cytomegalovirus in a patient with the keratitis, ichthyosis, and deafness (KID) syndrome. *Pediatr Dermatol* **7**(1):54–56.

Hofmann B, Schuppe HC, Adams O, Lenard HG, Lehmann P, Ruzicka T (1997). Gianotti–Crosti syndrome associated with Epstein–Barr virus infection. *Pediatr Dermatol* **14**(4):273–277.

Homsy J, Meyer M, Tateno M, Clarkson S, Levy JA (1989). The Fc and not CD4 receptor mediates antibody enhancement of HIV infection in human cells. *Science* **244**(4910):1357–1360.

Huerter CJ, Alvarez L, Stinson R (1991). Orf: case report and literature review. *Cleve Clin J Med* **58**(6):531–534.

Inglis S, Shaw A, Koenig S (2006). Chapter 11: HPV vaccines: Commercial Research & Development. *Vaccine* **24** Suppl 3: S99–S105.

Jemsek J, Greenberg SB, Taber L, Harvey D, Gershon A, Couch RB (1983). Herpes zoster-associated encephalitis: clinicopathologic report of 12 cases and review of the literature. *Medicine* (Baltimore) **62**(2):81–97.

References

Kedes DH, Ganem D (1997). Sensitivity of Kaposi's sarcoma-associated herpesvirus replication to antiviral drugs. Implications for potential therapy. *J Clin Invest* **99**(9):2082–2086.

Kimberlin DW, Lin CY, Jacobs RF, et al. (2001). Safety and efficacy of high-dose intravenous acyclovir in the management of neonatal herpes simplex virus infections. *Pediatrics* **108**(2):230–238.

Kirkham C, Harris S, Grzybowski S (2005). Evidence-based prenatal care: Part I. General prenatal care and counseling issues. *Am Fam Physician* **71**(7):1307–1316.

Kodner CM, Nasraty S (2004). Management of genital warts. *Am Fam Phys* **70**(12):2335–2342.

Lederman ER, Green GM, DeGroot HE, et al. (2007). Progressive ORF virus infection in a patient with lymphoma: successful treatment using imiquimod. *Clin Infect Dis* **44**(11):e100–103.

Lee JY (1989). Cytomegalovirus infection involving the skin in immunocompromised hosts. A clinicopathologic study. *Am J Clin Pathol* **92**(1):96–100.

Lesher JL Jr (1988). Cytomegalovirus infections and the skin. *J Am Acad Dermatol* **18**(6):1333–1338.

Levy JA (1997). Three new human herpesviruses (HHV6, 7, and 8). *Lancet* **349**(9051):558–563.

Lin P, Torres G, Tyring SK (2003). Changing paradigms in dermatology: antivirals in dermatology. *Clin Dermatol* **21**(5):426–446.

Mancini AJ (1998). Exanthems in childhood: an update. *Pediatr Ann* **27**(3):163–170.

Mancini AJ, Shani-Adir A (2003). Other viral diseases. In: *Dermatology*. JL Bolognia, J Jorizzo, R Rapini (eds). Harcourt, London, Chapter 1, pp.1255–1270.

McCrary ML, Severson J, Tyring SK (1999). Varicella zoster virus. *J Am Acad Dermatol* **41**(1):1–14; quiz 15–16.

Meyers JD (1991). Prevention and treatment of cytomegalovirus infection. *Ann Rev Med* **42**:179–187.

Mitka M (2006). FDA approves shingles vaccine: herpes zoster vaccine targets older adults. *JAMA* **296**(2):157–158.

Morrow RA, Friedrich D, Meier A, Corey L (2005). Use of 'biokit HSV-2 Rapid Assay' to improve the positive predictive value of Focus HerpeSelect HSV-2 ELISA. *BMC Infect Dis* **5**:84.

Mortimer PP, Humphries RK, Moore JG, Purcell RH, Young NS (1983). A human parvovirus-like virus inhibits haematopoietic colony formation *in vitro*. *Nature* **302**(5907):426–429.

Mosquera MM, de Ory F, Gallardo V, et al. (2005). Evaluation of diagnostic markers for measles virus infection in the context of an outbreak in Spain. *J Clin Microbiol* **43**(10):5117–5121.

Naesens L, Stephens CE, Andrei G, et al. (2006). Antiviral properties of new arylsulfone derivatives with activity against human betaherpesviruses. *Antiviral Res* **72**(1):60–67.

Nahass GT, Goldstein BA, Zhu WY, Serfling U, Penneys NS, Leonardi CL (1992). Comparison of Tzanck smear, viral culture, and DNA diagnostic methods in detection of herpes simplex and varicella-zoster infection. *JAMA* **268**(18):2541–2544.

Nahmias AJ, Lee FK, Beckman-Nahmias S (1990). Sero-epidemiological and -sociological patterns of herpes simplex virus infection in the world. *Scand J Infect Dis Suppl* **69**:19–36.

Ohkuma M (1990). Molluscum contagiosum treated with iodine solution and salicylic acid plaster. *Int J Dermatol* **29**(6):443–445.

Porter CD, Blake NW, Archard LC, Muhlemann MF, Rosedale N, Cream JJ (1989). Molluscum contagiosum virus types in genital and non-genital lesions. *Br J Dermatol* **120**(1):37–41.

Resnick SD (1997). New aspects of exanthematous diseases of childhood. *Dermatol Clin* **15**(2):257–266.

Ricci G, Patrizi A, Neri I, Specchia F, Tosti G, Masi M (2003). Gianotti–Crosti syndrome and allergic background. *Acta Derm Venereol* **83**(3):202–205.

Ross AH (1962). Modification of chicken pox in family contacts by administration of gamma globulin. *N Engl J Med* **267**:369–376.

Sandler A, Snedeker JD (1987). Cytomegalovirus infection in an infant presenting with cutaneous vasculitis. *Pediatr Infect Dis J* **6**(4):422–423.

Schmidt E, Weissbrich B, Brocker EB, Fleischer K, Goebeler M, Stich A (2006). Orf followed by erythema multiforme. *J Eur Acad Dermatol Venereol* **20**(5):612–613.

Schmidt NJ, Gallo D, Devlin V, Woodie JD, Emmons RW (1980). Direct immunofluorescence staining for detection of herpes simplex and varicella-zoster virus antigens in vesicular lesions and certain tissue specimens. *J Clin Microbiol* **12**(5):651–655.

Snoeck R, Andrei G, De Clercq E (1998). Specific therapies for human papilloma virus infections. *Curr Opin Infect Dis* **11**(6):733–737.

Solomon AR, Rasmussen JE, Varani J, Pierson CL (1984). The Tzanck smear in the diagnosis of cutaneous herpes simplex. *JAMA* **251**(5):633–635.

Spear JB, Kessler HA, Dworin A, Semel J (1988). Erythema nodosum associated with acute cytomegalovirus mononucleosis in an adult. *Arch Intern Med* **148**(2):323–324.

Speck LM, Tyring SK (2006). Vaccines for the prevention of human papillomavirus infections. *Skin Therapy Lett* **11**(6):1–3.

Staras SA, Dollard SC, Radford KW, Flanders WD, Pass RF, Cannon MJ (2006). Seroprevalence of cytomegalovirus infection in the United States, 1988–1994. *Clin Infect Dis* **43**(9):1143–1151.

Tan ST, Blake GB, Chambers S (1991). Recurrent orf in an immunocompromised host. *Br J Plast Surg* **44**(6):465–467.

Thomas JR 3rd, Doyle JA (1981). The therapeutic uses of topical vitamin A acid. *J Am Acad Dermatol* **4**(5):505–513.

Thompson CH (1998). Immunoreactive proteins of molluscum contagiosum virus types 1, 1v, and 2. *J Infect Dis* **178**(4):1230–1231.

Tirelli U, Bernardi D, Spina M, Vaccher E (2002). AIDS-related tumors: integrating antiviral and anticancer therapy. *Crit Rev Oncol Hematol* **41**(3):299–315.

Tokimasa S, Hara J, Osugi Y, *et al.* (2002). Ganciclovir is effective for prophylaxis and treatment of human herpesvirus-6 in allogeneic stem cell transplantation. *Bone Marrow Transplant* **29**(7):595–598.

Whitley R (2006). New approaches to the therapy of HSV infections. *Herpes* **13**(2):53–55.

Wikstrom A (1995). Clinical and serological manifestations of genital human papillomavirus infection. *Acta Derm Venereol* (Stockh) Suppl **193**:1–85.

Wildly P (1973). Herpes: history and classification. In: *The Herpesviruses*. AS Kaplan (ed). Academic Press, New York.

Yeung-Yue KA, Brentjens MH, Lee PC, Tyring SK (2002a). Herpes simplex viruses 1 and 2. *Dermatol Clin* **20**(2):249–266.

Yeung-Yue KA, Brentjens MH, Lee PC, Tyring SK (2002b). The management of herpes simplex virus infections. *Curr Opin Infect Dis* **15**(2):115–122.

Young NS, Brown KE (2004). Parvovirus B19. *N Engl J Med* **350**(6):586–597.

zur Hausen H (1996). Papillomavirus infections: a major cause of human cancers. *Biochim Biophys Acta* **1288**(2):F55–78.

CHAPTER 4 TROPICAL AND EXOTIC INFECTIOUS DISEASES

Albanese G, Venturi C, Galbiati G (2001). Treatment of larva migrans cutanea (creeping eruption): a comparison between albendazole and traditional therapy. *Int J Dermatol* **40**(1):67–71.

Albuquerque CF, da Silva SH, Camargo ZP (2005). Improvement of the specificity of an enzyme-linked immunosorbent assay for diagnosis of paracoccidioidomycosis. *J Clin Microbiol* **43**(4):1944–1946.

Aliagaoglu C, Atasoy M, Karakuzu A, Cayir K, Melikoglu M (2006). Rapidly developing giant sized lupus vulgaris on the chest associated with bilateral scrofuloderma on the neck. *J Dermatol* **33**(7):481–485.

Al-Karawi KS, Al-Amro Al-Akloby OM, Mugharbel RM (2004). Ectopic cutaneous schistosomiasis. *Int J Dermatol* **43**(7):550–551.

Amer M (1994). Cutaneous schistosomiasis. *Dermatol Clin* **12**(4):713–717.

Amsbaugh S, Huiras E, Wang NS, Wever A, Warren S (2006). Bacillary angiomatosis associated with pseudoepitheliomatous hyperplasia. *Am J Dermatopathol* **28**(1):32–35.

Andraca R, Edson RS, Kern EB (1993). Rhinoscleroma: a growing concern in the United States? Mayo Clinic experience. *Mayo Clin Proc* **68**(12):1151–1157.

Ansart S, Perez L, Jaureguiberry S, Danis M, Bricaire F, Caumes E (2007). Spectrum of dermatoses in 165 travelers returning from the tropics with skin diseases. *Am J Trop Med Hyg* **76**(1):184–186.

Aram H, Leibovici V (1987). Ultrasound-induced hyperthermia in the treatment of cutaneous leishmaniasis. *Cutis* **40**(4):350–353.

Awadzi K, Opoku NO, Addy ET, Quartey BT (1995). The chemotherapy of onchocerciasis. XIX: The clinical and laboratory tolerance of high dose ivermectin. *Trop Med Parasitol* **46**(2):131–137.

Batista AC, Soares CT, Lara VS (2005). Failure of nitric oxide production by macrophages and decrease in CD4+ T cells in oral paracoccidioidomycosis: possible mechanisms that permit local fungal multiplication. *Rev Inst Med Trop Sao Paulo* **47**(5):267–273.

Ben-Youssef R, Baron P, Edson F, Raghavan R, Okechukwu O (2005). *Stronglyoides stercoralis* infection from pancreas allograft: case report. *Transplantation* **80**(7):997–998.

Bern C, Adler-Moore J, Berenguer J, *et al.* (2006). Liposomal amphotericin B for the treatment of visceral leishmaniasis. *Clin Infect Dis* **43**(7):917–924.

Bhardwaj P, Mahajan V (2003). Lupus vulgaris. *Indian Pediatr* **40**(9):902–903.

Boer A, Blodorn-Schlicht N, Wiebels D, Steinkraus V, Falk TM (2006). Unusual histopathological features of cutaneous leishmaniasis identified by polymerase chain reaction specific for *Leishmania* on paraffin-embedded skin biopsies. *Br J Dermatol* **155**(4):815–819.

Boggino HE, Borkowski J, Xiao SY (2001). Polypoid intranasal mass in a 32-year-old woman. *Arch Pathol Lab Med* **125**:159–160.

Bonatti H, Mendez J, Guerrero I, *et al.* (2006). Disseminated *Bartonella* infection following liver transplantation. *Transpl Int* **19**(8):683–687.

References

Britton WJ, Lockwood DN (2004). Leprosy. *Lancet* 363(9416):1209–1219.

Burns RA, Roy JS, Woods C, Padhye AA, Warnock DW (2000). Report of the first human case of lobomycosis in the United States. *J Clin Microbiol* 38(3):1283–1285.

Camargo ZP, Baruzzi RG, Maeda SM, Floriano MC (1998). Antigenic relationship between *Loboa loboi* and *Paracoccidioides brasiliensis* as shown by serological methods. *Med Mycol* 36(6):413–417.

Cardo LJ (2006). *Leishmania*: risk to the blood supply. *Transfusion* 46(9):1641–1645.

da Silva SH, Colombo AL, Blotta MH, Queiroz-Telles F, Lopes JD, de Camargo ZP (2005). Diagnosis of neuroparacoccidioidomycosis by detection of circulating antigen and antibody in cerebrospinal fluid. *J Clin Microbiol* 43(9):4680–4683.

Davis-Reed L, Theis JH (2000). Cutaneous schistosomiasis: report of a case and review of the literature. *J Am Acad Dermatol* 42(4):678–680.

de Almeida SM (2005). Central nervous system paracoccidioidomycosis: an overview. *Braz J Infect Dis* 9(2):126–133.

De Palma L, Marinelli M, Pavan M, Manso E, Ranaldi R (2006). A rare European case of Madura foot due to actinomycetes. *Joint, Bone, Spine* 73:321–324.

De Vries GA, Laarman JJ (1975). A case of Lobo's disease in the dolphin *Somalia guianensis*. *Aquat Mamm* 1:105–114.

Doenhoff MJ, Pica-Mattoccia L (2006). Praziquantel for the treatment of schistosomiasis: its use for control in areas with endemic disease and prospects for drug resistance. *Expert Rev Anti Infect Ther* 4(2):199–210.

Dourmishev AL, Dourmishev LA, Schwartz RA (2005). Ivermectin: pharmacology and application in dermatology. *Int J Dermatol* 44(12):981–988.

EL Haq IA, Fahal AH, Gasim ET (1996). Fine needle aspiration cytology of mycetoma. *Acta Cytol* 40(3):461–464.

Elsayed S, Kuhn SM, Barber D, Church DL, Adams S, Kasper R (2004). Human case of lobomycosis. *Emerg Infect Dis* 10(4):715–718.

Elsner E, Thewes M, Worret WI (1997). Cutaneous larva migrans detected by epiluminescent microscopy. *Acta Derm Venereol* 77(6):487–488.

Esterre P, Andriantsimahavandy A, Ramarcel ER, Pecarrere JL (1996). Forty years of chromoblastomycosis in Madagascar: a review. *Am J Trop Med Hyg* 55(1):45–47.

Fahal AH, Suliman SH (1994). The clinical presentation of mycetoma. *Sudan Med J* 32:46–65.

Fernández-Vozmediano JM, Armario Hita JC, González Cabrerizo A (2004). Rhinoscleroma in three siblings. *Pediatr Dermatol* 21(2):134–138.

Fischer M, Chrusciak Talhari A, Reinel D, Talhari S (2002). [Sucessful treatment with clofazimine and itraconazole in a 46-year-old patient after 32 years duration of disease.] *Hautarzt* 53(10):677–681.

Foreman EB, Abraham PJ, Garland JL (2006). Not your typical strongyloides infection: a literature review and case study. *South Med J* 99(8):847–852.

Gardon J, Boussinesq M, Kamgno J, Gardon-Wendel N, Demanga N, Duke BO (2002). Effects of standard and high doses of ivermectin on adult worms of *Onchocerca volvulus*: a randomised controlled trial. *Lancet* 360(9328):203–210.

Gardon J, Gardon-Wendel N, Demanga N, Kamgno J, Chippaux JP, Boussinesq M (1997). Serious reactions after mass treatment of onchocerciasis with ivermectin in an area endemic for *Loa loa* infection. *Lancet* 350(9070):18–22.

Goldman L (1979). Pre-Columbian rhinoscleroma. *Arch Dermatol* 115(1):106–107.

Gupta SK, Nigam S, Mandal AK, Kumar V (2006). S-100 as a useful auxiliary diagnostic aid in tuberculoid leprosy. *J Cutan Pathol* 33(7):482–486.

Hall LR, Pearlman E (1999). Pathogenesis of onchocercal keratitis (river blindness). *Clin Microbiol Rev* 12(3):445–453.

Hartzell JD, Zapor M, Peng S, Straight T (2004). Leprosy: a case series and review. *South Med J* 97(12):1252–1256.

Herr RA, Tarcha EJ, Taborda PR, Taylor JW, Ajello L, Mendoza L (2001). Phylogenetic analysis of *Lacazia loboi* places this previously uncharacterized pathogen within the dimorphic *Onygenales*. *J Clin Microbiol* 39(1):309–314.

Herwaldt BL (1999). Leishmaniasis. *Lancet* 354(9185):1191–1199.

Heukelbach J, Wilcke T, Meier A, Saboia Moura RC, Feldmeier H (2003). A longitudinal study on cutaneous larva migrans in an impoverished Brazilian township. *Travel Med Infect Dis* 1(4):213–218.

Iijima S, Takase T, Otsuka F (1995). Treatment of chromomycosis with oral high-dose amphotericin B. *Arch Dermatol* 131(4):399–401.

Iyengar P, Laughlin S, Keshavjee S, Chamberlain DW (2005). Rhinoscleroma of the larynx. *Histopathology* 47:215–226.

Jardim MR, Antunes SL, Simons B, et al. (2005). Role of PGL-I antibody detection in the diagnosis of pure neural leprosy. *Lepr Rev* 76(3):232–240.

Johnston FH, Morris PS, Speare R, et al. (2005). Strongyloidiasis: a review of the evidence for Australian practitioners. *Aust J Rural Health* 13(4):247–254.

Jung AC, Paauw DS (1998). Diagnosing HIV-related disease: using the CD4 count as a guide. *J Gen Intern Med* **13**(2):131–136.

Kallestrup P, Zinyama R, Gomo E, et al. (2006). Schistosomiasis and HIV in rural Zimbabwe: efficacy of treatment of schistosomiasis in individuals with HIV coinfection. *Clin Infect Dis* **42**(12):1781–1789.

Kaminagakura E, Bonan PR, Lopes MA, Almeida OP, Scully C (2006). Cytokeratin expression in pseudoepitheliomatous hyperplasia of oral paracoccidioidomycosis. *Med Mycol* **44**(5):399–404.

Kang TJ, Yeum CE, Kim BC, You EY, Chae GT (2004). Differential production of interleukin-10 and interleukin-12 in mononuclear cells from leprosy patients with a Toll-like receptor 2 mutation. *Immunology* **112**(4):674–680.

Kenner BM, Rosen T (2006). Cutaneous amebiasis in a child and review of the literature. *Pediatr Dermatol* **23**(3):231–234.

Kreitzer T, Saoud A (2006). Bacillary angiomatosis following the use of long-term methotrexate therapy: a case report. *W V Med J* **102**(1):317–318.

Kullavanijaya P, Wongwaisayawan H (1993). Outbreak of cercarial dermatitis in Thailand. *Int J Dermatol* **32**(2):113–115.

Kumar B, Muralidhar S (1999). Cutaneous tuberculosis: a twenty-year prospective study. *Int J Tuberc Lung Dis* **3**(6):494–500.

Kumar B, Rai R, Kaur I, Sahoo B, Muralidhar S, Radotra BD (2001). Childhood cutaneous tuberculosis: a study over 25 years from northern India. *Int J Dermatol* **40**(1):26–32.

Kwon IH, Kim HS, Lee JH, et al. (2003). A serologically diagnosed human case of cutaneous larva migrans caused by *Ancylostoma caninum*. *Korean J Parasitol* **41**(4):233–237.

Lam CS, Tong MK, Chan KM, Siu YP (2006). Disseminated strongyloidiasis: a retrospective study of clinical course and outcome. *Eur J Clin Microbiol Infect Dis* **25**(1):14–18.

Lane JE, Walsh DS, Meyers WM, Klassen-Fischer MK, Kent DE, Cohen DJ (2006). Borderline tuberculoid leprosy in a woman from the state of Georgia with armadillo exposure. *J Am Acad Dermatol* **55**(4):714–716.

Lawrence DN, Ajello L (1986). Lobomycosis in western Brazil: report of a clinical trial with ketoconazole. *Am J Trop Med Hyg* **35**(1):162–166.

Lee NH, Choi EH, Lee WS, Ahn SK (2000). Tuberculosis cellulitis. *Clin Exp Dermatol* **25**:222–223.

Leman JA, Small G, Wilks D, Tidman MJ (2001). Localized papular cutaneous schistosomiasis: two cases in travellers. *Clin Exp Dermatol* **26**(1):50–52.

Libraty DH, Byrd TF (1996). Cutaneous miliary tuberculosis in the AIDS era: case report and review. *Clin Infect Dis* **23**(4):706–710.

Lupi O, Tyring SK, McGinnis MR (2005). Tropical dermatology: fungal tropical diseases. *J Am Acad Dermatol* **53**:931–951.

Magana M, Magana ML, Alcantara A, Perez-Martin MA (2004). Histopathology of cutaneous amebiasis. *Am J Dermatopathol* **26**(4):280–284.

Maiti PK, Ray A, Bandyopadhyay S (2002). Epidemiological aspects of mycetoma from a retrospective study of 264 cases in West Bengal. *Trop Med Int Health* **7**:788–792.

Malik AN, John L, Bruceson AD, Lockwood DN (2006). Changing pattern of visceral leishmaniasis, United Kingdom, 1985–2004. *Emerg Infect Dis* **12**(8):1257–1259.

Mamoni RL, Blotta MH (2005). Kinetics of cytokines and chemokines gene expression distinguishes *Paracoccidioides brasiliensis* infection from disease. *Cytokine* **32**(1):20–29.

Marciano-Cabral F, Cabral G (2003). *Acanthamoeba* spp. as agents of disease in humans. *Clin Microbiol Rev* **16**(2):273–307.

Matz H, Berger S, Gat A, Brenner S (2003). Bilharziasis cutanea tarda: a rare presentation of schistosomiasis. *J Am Acad Dermatol* **49**(5):961–962.

McGinnis MR (1996). Mycetoma. *Dermatol Clin* **14**(1):97–104.

McKee PH, Wright E, Hutt MS (1983). Vulval schistosomiasis. *Clin Exp Dermatol* **8**(2):189–194.

Meghari S, Rolain JM, Grau GE, et al. (2006). Antiangiogenic effect of erythromycin: an *in vitro* model of *Bartonella quintana* infection. *J Infect Dis* **193**(3):380–386.

Mlika RB, Tounsi J, Fenniche S, Hajlaoui K, Marrak H, Mokhtar I (2006). Childhood cutaneous tuberculosis: a 20-year retrospective study in Tunis. *Dermatol Online J* **12**(3):11.

Mueller M, Balasegaram M, Koummuki Y, Ritmeijer K, Santana MR, Davidson R (2006). A comparison of liposomal amphotericin B with sodium stibogluconate for the treatment of visceral leishmaniasis in pregnancy in Sudan. *J Antimicrob Chemother* **58**(4):811–815.

Murakawa GJ, McCalmont T, Altman J, et al. (1995). Disseminated acanthamebiasis in patients with AIDS. A report of five cases and a review of the literature. *Arch Dermatol* **131**(11):1291–1296.

Negi SS, Basir SF, Gupta S, Pasha ST, Khare S, Lal S (2005). Comparative study of PCR, smear examination, and culture for diagnosis of cutaneous tuberculosis. *J Commun Dis* **37**(2):83–92.

References

Negroni R, Tobon A, Bustamante B, Shikanai-Yasuda MA, Patino H, Restrepo A (2005). Posaconazole treatment of refractory eumycetoma and chromoblastomycosis. *Rev Inst Med Trop Sao Paulo* **47**(6):339–346.

Nguyen JC, Murphy ME, Nutman TB, *et al.* (2005). Cutaneous onchocerciasis in an American traveler. *Int J Dermatol* **44**(2):125–128.

Nogueira MG, Andrade GM, Tonelli E (2006). Clinical evolution of paracoccidioidomycosis in 38 children and teenagers. *Mycopathologia* **161**(2):73–81.

Norton SA (2006). Dolphin-to-human transmission of lobomycosis? *J Am Acad Dermatol* **55**(4):723–724.

Okulicz JF, Stibich AS, Elston DM, Schwartz RA (2004). Cutaneous onchocercoma. *Int J Dermatol* **43**(3):170–172.

O'Quinn JC, Dushin R (2005). Cutaneous larva migrans: case report with current recommendations for treatment. *J Am Podiatr Med Assoc* **95**(3):291–294.

Paige CF, Scholl DT, Truman RW (2002). Prevalence and incidence density of *Mycobacterium leprae* and *Trypanosoma cruzi* infections within a population of wild nine-banded armadillos. *Am J Trop Med Hyg* **67**(5):528–532.

Paul C, Pialeux G, Dupont B, *et al.* (1993). Infection due to *Klebsiella rhinoscleromatis* in two patients infected with human immunodeficiency virus. *Clin Infect Dis* **16**(3):441–442.

Payet B, Chaumentin G, Boyer M, Amaranto P, Lemonon-Meric C, Lucht F (2006). Prolonged latent schistosomiasis diagnosed 38 years after infestation in a HIV patient. *Scand J Infect Dis* **38**(6–7):572–575.

Poirriez J, Breuillard F, Francois N, *et al.* (2000). A case of chromomycosis treated by a combination of cryotherapy, shaving, oral 5-fluorocytosine, and oral amphotericin B. *Am J Trop Med Hyg* **63**(1–2):61–63.

Potter B, Rindfleisch K, Kraus CK (2005). Management of active tuberculosis. *Am Fam Physician* **72**(11):2225–2232.

Pritzker AS, Kim BK, Agrawal D, Southern PM Jr, Pandya AG (2004). Fatal granulomatous amebic encephalitis caused by *Balamuthia mandrillaris* presenting as a skin lesion. *J Am Acad Dermatol* **50**(2 Suppl):S38–41.

Rai VM, Shenoi SD, Gowrinath K (2005). Tuberculous gluteal abscess coexisting with scrofuloderma and tubercular lymphadenitis. *Dermatol Online J* **11**(3):14.

Reich A, Kobierzycka M, Cislo M, Schwartz RA, Szepietowski JC (2006). Psoriasiform lupus vulgaris with 30 years duration. *Scand J Infect Dis* **38**(6–7):556–558.

Reif JS, Mazzoil MS, McCulloch SD, *et al.* (2006). Lobomycosis in Atlantic bottlenose dolphins from the Indian River Lagoon, Florida. *J Am Vet Med Assoc* **228**(1):104–108.

Rigopoulos D, Paparizos V, Katsambas A (2004). Cutaneous markers of HIV infection. *Clin Dermatol* **22**(6):487–498.

Ritmeijer K, Dejenie A, Assefa Y, *et al.* (2006). A comparison of miltefosine and sodium stibogluconate for treatment of visceral leishmaniasis in an Ethiopian population with high prevalence of HIV infection. *Clin Infect Dis* **43**(3):357–364.

Robbins JB, Riedel BD, Jones T, Boyd AS (2004). Nasal tumor in a Peruvian man. *Am J Dermatopathol* **26**(3):248, 254.

Rosenberg AS, Morgan MB (2001). Disseminated acanthamoebiasis presenting as lobular panniculitis with necrotizing vasculitis in a patient with AIDS. *J Cutan Pathol* **28**(6):307–313.

Rowland K, Guthmann R, Jamieson B, Malloy D (2006). How should we manage a patient with a positive PPD and prior BCG vaccination? *J Fam Pract* **55**(8):718–720.

Sadeghian G, Nilforoushzadeh MA (2006). Effect of combination therapy with systemic glucantime and pentoxifylline in the treatment of cutaneous leishmaniasis. *Int J Dermatol* **45**(7):819–821.

Saha S, Dhar A, Karak AK (2006). Mycetoma sans sinuses. *Indian J Dermatol Venereol Leprol* **72**(2):143–144.

Saha M, Shipley D, McBride S, Kennedy C, Vega-Lopez F (2006). Atypical cutaneous leishmaniasis in two patients receiving low-dose methotrexate. *Br J Dermatol* **155**(4):830–833.

Sangüeza OP, Fleet SL, Requena L (2000). Update on the histologic findings of cutaneous infections. In: *Advances in Dermatology*, Volume 16. Mosby, St. Louis, pp. 361–423.

Sangüeza OP, Sangüeza JM, Stiller MJ, Sangüeza P (1993). Mucocutaneous leishmaniasis: a clinicopathologic classification. *J Am Acad Dermatol* **28**(6):927–932.

Schlupen EM, Schirren CG, Hoegl L, Schaller M, Volkenandt M (1997). Molecular diagnosis of deep nodular bacillary angiomatosis and monitoring of therapeutic success. *Br J Dermatol* **136**(5):747–751.

Schwartz RA, Nychay SG, Janniger CK, Lambert WC (1997). Bacillary angiomatosis: presentation of six patients, some with unusual features. *Br J Dermatol* **136**:60–65.

Sehgal VN, Wagh SA (1990). The history of cutaneous tuberculosis. *Int J Dermatol* **29**(9):666–668.

Sethuraman G, Kaur J, Nag HL, Khaitan BK, Sharma VK, Singh MK (2006). Symmetrical scrofuloderma with tuberculosis verrucosa cutis. *Clin Exp Dermatol* **31**(3):475–477.

Setia MS, Steinmaus C, Ho CS, Rutherford GW (2006). The role of BCG in the prevention of leprosy: a meta-analysis. *Lancet Infect Dis* **6**(3):162–170.

Sindermann H, Engel J (2006). Development of miltefosine as an oral treatment for leishmaniasis. *Trans R Soc Trop Med Hyg* **100**(Suppl 1):S17–20.

Sinha S, Kannan S, Nagaraju B, Sengupta U, Gupte MD (2004). Utility of serodiagnostic tests for leprosy: a study in an endemic population in South India. *Lepr Rev* **75**(3):266–273.

Slater LN, Welch DF, Min KW (1992). *Rochalimaea henselae* causes bacillary angiomatosis and peliosis hepatis. *Arch Intern Med* **152**(3):602–606.

Soto J, Berman J (2006). Treatment of New World cutaneous leishmaniasis with miltefosine. *Trans R Soc Trop Med Hyg* **100**(Suppl 1):S34–40.

Spach DH, Koehler JE (1998). *Bartonella*-associated infections. *Infect Dis Clin North Am* **12**(1):137–155.

Stavropoulos PG, Papakonstantinou AM, Petropoulou H, Kontochristopoulos G, Katsambas A (2006). Cryotherapy as an adjunct to systemic antimonials for cutaneous leishmaniasis in children. *J Eur Acad Dermatol Venereol* **20**(6):765–766.

Steinberg JP, Galindo RL, Kraus ES, Ghanem KG (2002). Disseminated acanthamebiasis in a renal transplant recipient with osteomyelitis and cutaneous lesions: case report and literature review. *Clin Infect Dis* **35**(5):e43–49.

Stingl P (1997). Onchocerciasis: clinical presentation and host parasite interactions in patients of southern Sudan. *Int J Dermatol* **36**(1):23–28.

van Doorn HR, Koelewijn R, Hofwegen H, *et al.* (2007). Use of enzyme-linked immunosorbent assay and dipstick assay for detection of *Strongyloides stercoralis* infection in humans. *J Clin Microbiol* **45**(2):438–442.

Vemuganti GK, Pasricha G, Sharma S, Garg P (2005). Granulomatous inflammation in *Acanthamoeba* keratitis: an immunohistochemical study of five cases and review of literature. *Indian J Med Microbiol* **23**(4):231–238.

Veraldi S, Arancio L (2006). Giant bullous cutaneous larva migrans. *Clin Exp Dermatol* **31**(4):613–614.

Veraldi S, Bottini S, Carrera C, Gianotti R (2005). Cutaneous larva migrans with folliculitis: a new clinical presentation of this infestation. *J Eur Acad Dermatol Venereol* **19**(5):628–630.

Verma G, Kanawaty D, Hyland R (2005). Rhinoscleroma causing upper airway obstruction. *Can Respir J* **12**(1):43–45.

Villahermosa LG, Fajardo TT Jr, Abalos RM, *et al.* (2004). Parallel assessment of 24 monthly doses of rifampin, ofloxacin, and minocycline versus 2 years of World Health Organization multidrug therapy for multibacillary leprosy. *Am J Trop Med Hyg* **70**(2):197–200.

Visbal G, San-Blas G, Murgich J, Franco H (2005). *Paracoccidioides brasiliensis*, paracoccidioidomycosis, and antifungal antibiotics. *Curr Drug Targets Infect Disord* **5**(3):211–226.

Walker SL, Whittam L, Vega-Lopez F, Lockwood DN (2006). Milia complicating successfully treated cutaneous leishmaniasis in three children. *Br J Dermatol* **155**(4):860–861.

Warren K, Goldstein E, Hung VS, Koehler JE, Richardson W (1998). Use of retinal biopsy to diagnose *Bartonella* (formerly *Rochalimaea*) *henselae* retinitis in an HIV-infected patient. *Arch Ophthalmol* **116**(7):937–940.

Wathen PI (1996). Hansen's disease. *South Med J* **89**(7):647–652.

WHO (a). http://www.who.int/en/

WHO (b). http://www.who.int/lep/mdt/regimens/en/index.html

Willard RJ, Jeffcoat AM, Benson PM, Walsh DS (2005). Cutaneous leishmaniasis in soldiers from Fort Campbell, Kentucky returning from Operation Iraqi Freedom highlights diagnostic and therapeutic options. *J Am Acad Dermatol* **52**(6):977–987.

Wolfe MS, Petersen JL, Neafie RC, Connor DH, Purtilo DT (1974). Onchocerciasis presenting with swelling of limb. *Am J Trop Med Hyg* **23**(3):361–368.

Zaias N, Taplin D, Rebell G (1969). Mycetoma. *Arch Dermatol* **99**(2):215–225.

Zouhair K, Akhdari N, Nejjam F, Ouazzani T, Lakhdar H (2007). Cutaneous tuberculosis in Morocco. *Int J Infect Dis* **11**(3):209–212.

CHAPTER 5 ARTHROPODS AND INFESTATIONS

Andersen BM, Haugen H, Rasch M, Heldal Haugen A, Tageson A (2000). Outbreak of scabies in Norwegian nursing homes and home care patients: control and prevention. *J Hospital Infect* **45**:160–164.

Borkhardt A, Wilda M, Fuchs U, Gortner L, Reiss I (2003). Congenital leukaemia after heavy abuse of permethrin during pregnancy. *Arch Dis Child Fetal Neonatal Ed* **88**(5):F436–437.

Burch JM, Krol A, Weston WL (2004). Sarcoptes scabiei infestation misdiagnosed and treated as Langerhans cell histiocytosis. *Pediatr Dermatol*;**21**(1):58–62.

Cilek JE, Petersen JL, Hallmon CE (2004). Comparative efficacy of IR3535 and DEET as repellents against adult *Aedes aegypti* and *Culex quinquefasciatus*. *J Am Mosq Control Assoc* **20**(3):299–304.

Cooke JA, Roth VD, Miller F (1972). The urticating hairs of Theraphosid spiders. *Am Museum Novitates* **2498**:1–43.

References

Coutinho MT, Bueno LL, Sterzik A, et al. (2005). Participation of *Rhipicephalus sanguineus* (Acari: Ixodidae) in the epidemiology of canine visceral leishmaniasis. *Vet Parasitol* **128**(1–2):149–155.

Curtis CF, Jana-Kara B, Maxwell CA (2003). Insecticide treated nets: impact on vector populations and relevance of initial intensity of transmission and pyrethroid resistance. *J Vector Borne Dis* **40**(1–2):1–8.

Dursteler BB, Nyquist RA (2004). Outbreak of rove beetle pustular contact dermatitis in Pakistan among deployed US personnel. *Mil Med* **169**(1):57–60.

Elston DM (2005). Life-threatening stings, bites, infestations, and parasitic diseases. *Clin Dermatol* **23**:164–170.

Elston DM, Miller SD, Young RJ, et al. (2005). Comparison of colchicine, dapsone, triamcinolone, and diphenhydramine therapy for the treatment of brown recluse spider envenomation. A double blind, controlled study in a rabbit model. *Arch Dermatol* **141**:595–597.

Foil LD, Coleman P, Eisler M, et al. (2004). Factors that influence the prevalence of acaricide resistance and tick-borne diseases. *Vet Parasitol* **125**(1–2):163–181.

Gomez HF, Miller MJ, Trachy JW, Marks RM, Warren JS (1999). Intradermal anti-loxosceles Fab fragments attenuate dermonecrotic arachnidism. *Academic Emerg Med* **6**:1195–1202.

Hasan S, Hassan K (2005). Proteinuria associated with centipede bite. *Pediatr Nephrol* **20**(4):550–551.

Hoover NG, Fortenberry JD (2004). Use of antivenin to treat priapism after a black widow spider bite. *Pediatrics* **114**(1):e128–129.

Hudson BW, Feingold BF, Kartman L (1960). Allergy to flea bites. *Exper Parasitol* **9**:264–270.

Isbister GK, Gray MR (2004). Bites by Australian mygalomorph spiders (Araneae, Mygalomorphae), including funnel-web spiders (Atracinae) and mouse spiders (Actinopodidae: *Missulena* spp.). *Toxicon* **43**(2):133–140.

Ko CJ, Elston DM (2004). Pediculosis. *J Am Acad Dermatol* **50**:1–12.

Lane DR, Youse JS (2004). Coombs-positive hemolytic anemia secondary to brown recluse spider bite: a review of the literature and discussion of treatment. *Cutis* **74**(6):341–347.

Menegaux F, Baruchel A, Bertrand Y, et al. (2006). Household exposure to pesticides and risk of childhood acute leukaemia. *Occup Environ Med* **63**(2):131–134.

Naucke TJ, Kropke R, Benner G, et al. (2007). Field evaluation of the efficacy of proprietary repellent formulations with IR3535(R) and Picaridin against *Aedes aegypti*. *Parasitol Res* **101**(1):169–177.

Ozsarac M, Karcioglu O, Ayrik C, Somuncu F, Gumrukcu S (2004). Acute coronary ischemia following centipede envenomation: case report and review of the literature. *Wilderness Environ Med* **15**(2):109–112.

Oude Elberink JN, De Monchy JG, Van Der Heide S, Guyatt GH, Dubois AE (2002). Venom immunotherapy improves health-related quality of life in patients allergic to yellow jacket venom. *J Allergy Clin Immunol* **110**(1):174–182.

Ross EA, Savage KA, Utley LJ, Tebbett IR (2004). Insect repellent [correction of repallant] interactions: sunscreens enhance DEET (N,N-diethyl-m-toluamide) absorption. *Drug Metab Dispos* **32**(8):783–785.

Saevik BK, Bredal W, Ulstein TL (2004). *Cheyletiella* infestation in the dog: observations on diagnostic methods and clinical signs. *J Small Anim Pract* **45**(10):495–500.

van Vliet JA, Samson M, van Steenbergen JE (1998). Causes of spread and return of scabies in health care institutes; literature analysis of 44 epidemics. *Nederlands Tijdschrift voor Geneeskunde* **142**:354–357.

Voss A, Wallrauch C (1995). Occupational scabies in healthcare workers. *Infect Contr Hosp Epidemiol* **16**:4.

ILLUSTRATED GLOSSARY

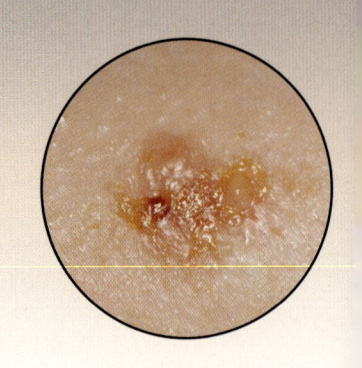

HISTORY AND PHYSICAL EXAMINATION

In the practice of dermatology, the classic approach to history and physical examination is inverted. That is to say, the physician generally begins with a physical examination based on the chief complaint. A directed history and review of systems is then based on the physical findings. Important historical elements include time and site of onset, evolution, modifying factors (therapy, sunlight, temperature, occupation), associated symptoms and their intensity, as well as family history and exposures. A detailed drug history and history of medication allergy should be sought.

HOW TO EXAMINE THE SKIN

Adequate illumination is imperative. It may be appropriate to examine the entire skin surface, especially in critically ill patients who cannot indicate the sites of involvement. The conjunctiva and oral and genital mucosa may also demonstrate important findings. A light source positioned obliquely to the lesions may reveal important morphological information that is lost with direct lighting. Closer inspection of individual lesions is often helpful and is facilitated by the use of a hand lens or magnifying loupes. Palpation of lesional skin can provide information on temperature, consistency, and depth of tissue involvement, and may be critical to determine the adequate depth of a biopsy specimen. Examination of the regional lymph nodes is valuable in many settings.

Four aspects of the lesion(s) should be recorded:
- Morphology.
- Shape.
- Distribution.
- Color.

MORPHOLOGY

Most skin lesions have a characteristic morphology which, once defined, will narrow the differential diagnosis. The following list describes the features of the common primary lesions:
- Macule – a flat, non-palpable lesion (378) distinguished from adjacent, normal skin by a change in color.
- Papule – a small, solid and raised lesion less than 5 mm in diameter (379).
- Nodule – a larger, raised lesion greater than 5 mm in diameter.
- Plaque – a flat-topped lesion with a diameter considerably greater than its height (380).
- Wheal – a transient swelling of the skin of any size, often associated with surrounding, localized erythema (the flare) (381).
- Vesicle – a blister less than 5 mm in diameter (382).
- Bulla – a blister greater than 5 mm in diameter.
- Pustule – a visible accumulation of pus, therefore white, yellow, or green in color (383).
- Erosion – an area of skin from which the epidermis alone has been lost (384).
- Ulcer – an area of skin from which the epidermis and part of the dermis has been lost (385).
- Fissure – a cleft-shaped ulcer (386).
- Telangiectasia – a visibly-dilated, small, dermal blood vessel (387).
- Comedone – accumulation of keratin and sebum lodged in a dilated pilosebaceous orifice (388).

A primary lesion can be associated with additional, superimposed features:
- Scale – a flake of keratinized epidermal cells lying on the skin surface (389).

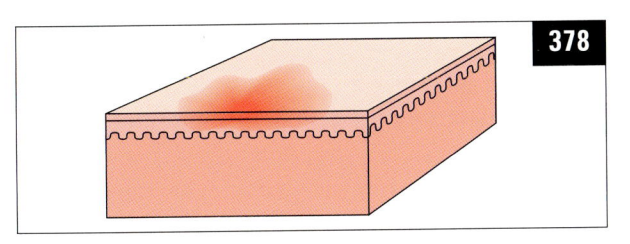

Illustrated Glossary

378 Macule.

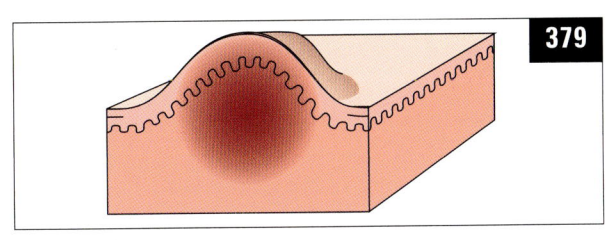

379 Papule.

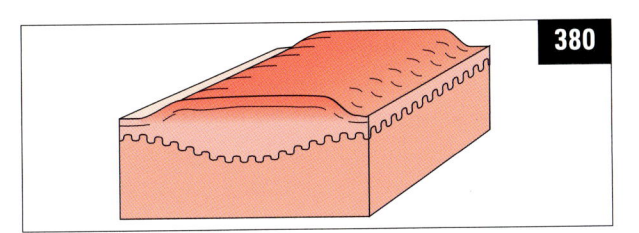

380 Plaque.

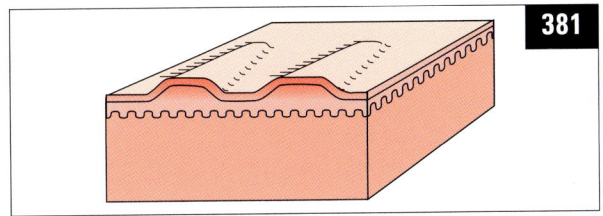

381 Wheal.

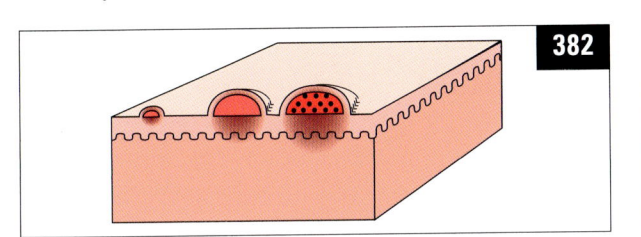

382 Vesicle.

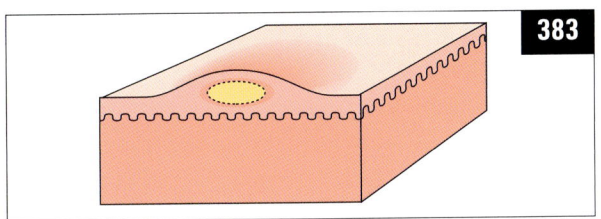

383 Pustule.

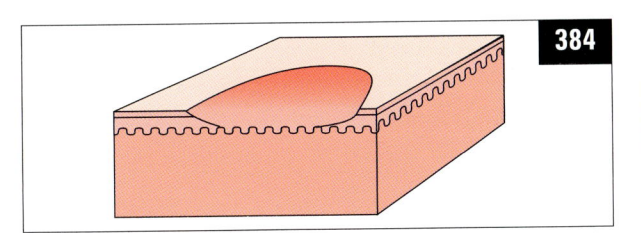

384 Erosion.

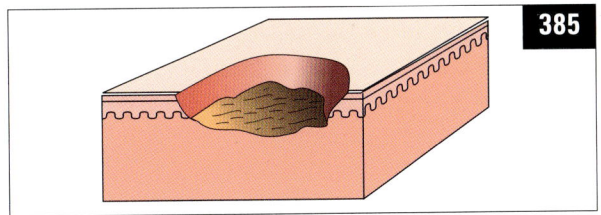

385 Ulcer.

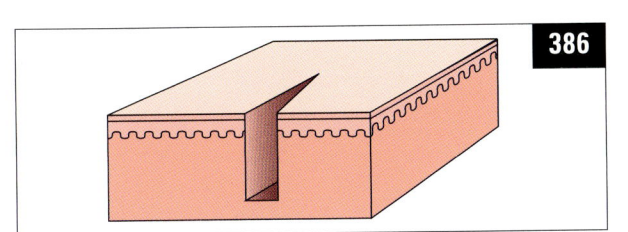

386 Fissure.

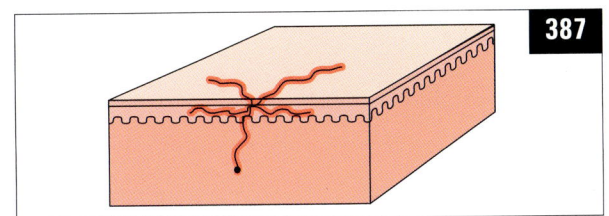

387 Telangiectasia.

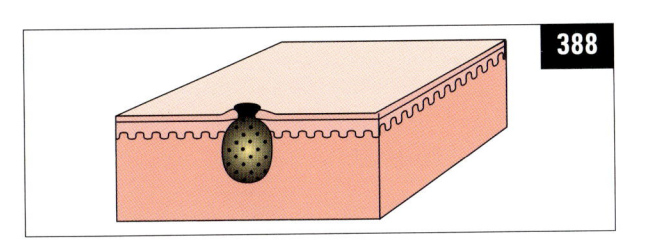

388 Comedone.

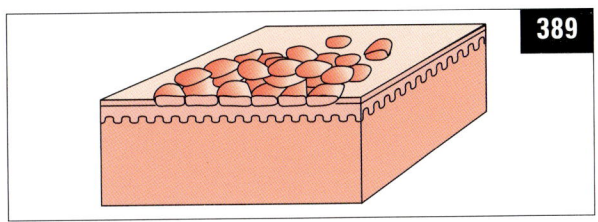

389 Scale.

- Crust – dried serous or sanguineous exudate (**390**).
- Hyperkeratosis – an area of thickened stratum corneum (**391**).
- Atrophy – thinning of the skin due to the partial loss of one or more of the tissue layers of the skin (epidermis, dermis, subcutis) (**392**).
- Sclerosis – hardening of the skin due to dermal pathological change (often an expansion of collagenous elements) characterized by induration.
- Lichenification – thickened skin with increased markings usually due to prolonged scratching (**393**).
- Umbilicated – shaped like the umbilicus (**394**).
- Exudate – material escaped from blood vessels with a high content of protein, cells, or cellular debris (**395**).
- Warty – horny excrescence (**396**).
- Excoriation – scratch or abrasion of the skin (**397**).

SHAPE

The shape of an individual lesion has a clinical significance as certain dermatoses consist of lesions possessing a characteristic shape. The following list defines the nomenclature for the commonly observed shapes or patterns:

- Linear (**398**).
- Annular describes a ring-shaped lesion (**399**).
- Target describes a lesion consisting of concentric rings.
- Polycyclic describes a pattern of interlocking rings.
- Arcuate describes lesions that are arc shaped.
- Serpiginous describes a linear lesion which is wavy in shape (**400**).
- Whorled is used to describe lesions which follow the developmental lines of Blaschko and demonstrate a curved or spiral pattern (**401**).
- Digitate refers to lesions which are finger-like in shape.
- Zosteriform means resembling herpes zoster (see pp. 66, 67).

DISTRIBUTION

The majority of skin diseases have a characteristic distribution or a predilection for certain sites. Other dermatoses vary in extent of involvement according to their severity. The recognition of particular configurations is important diagnostically, while defining the extent of involvement is useful for prognostic and therapeutic reasons. Discrete lesions occurring in a localized area are called grouped (**402**) while multiple lesions distributed over a wide area of skin are called scattered (**403**).

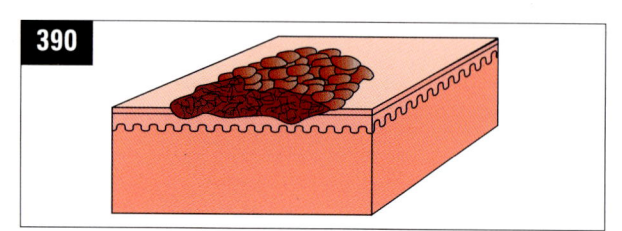

390 Crust.

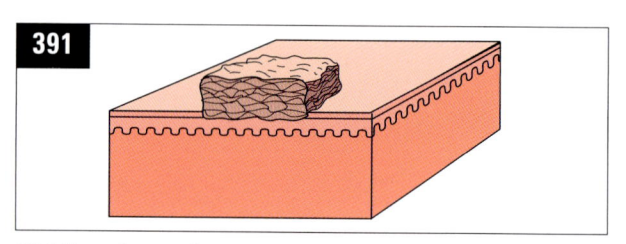

391 Hyperkeratosis.

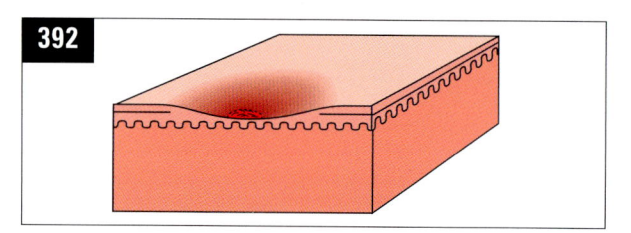

392 Atrophy.

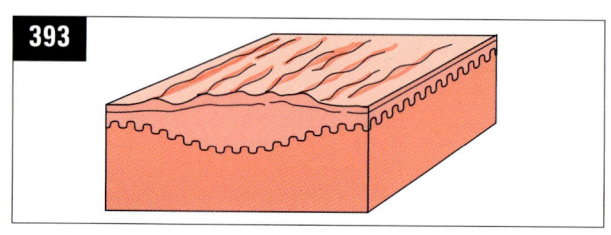

393 Lichenification.

Illustrated Glossary

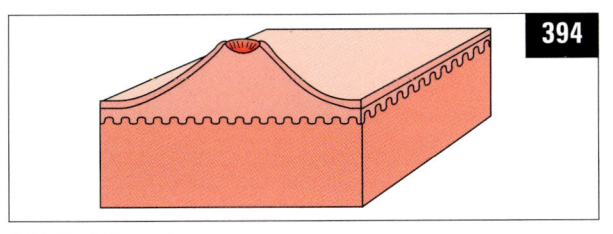

394 Umbilicated.

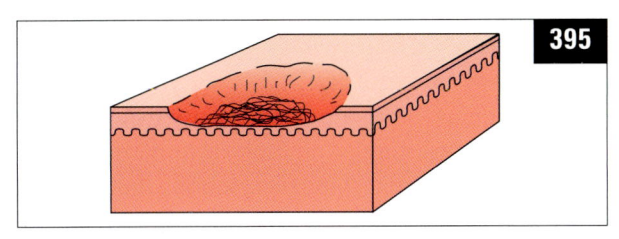

395 Exudate.

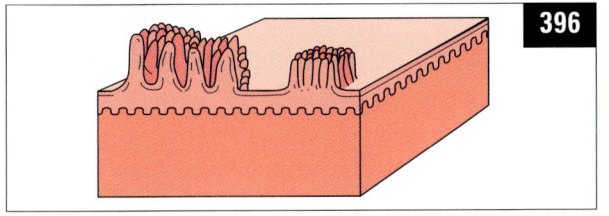

396 Warty.

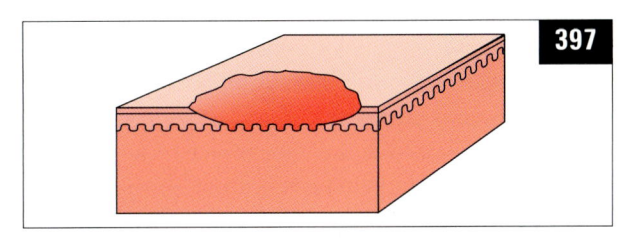

397 Excoriation.

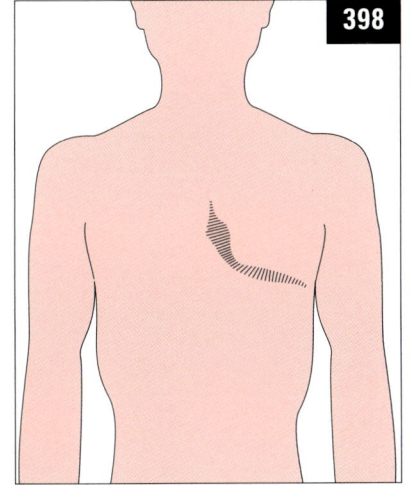

398 Linear lesion.

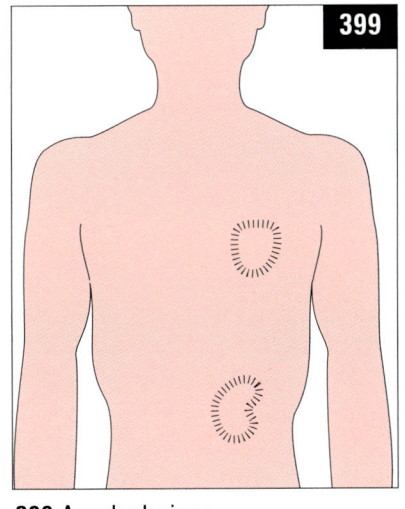

399 Annular lesions.

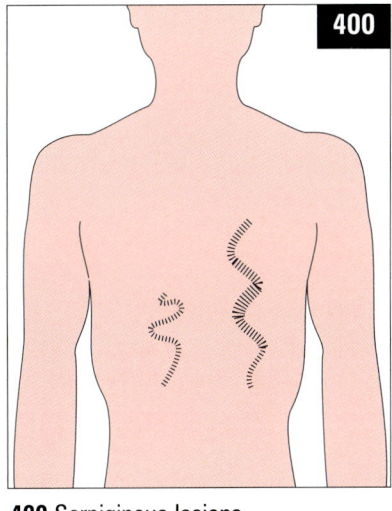

400 Serpiginous lesions.

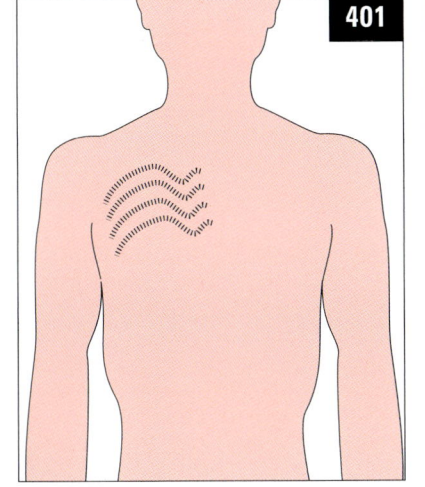

401 Whorled lesions.

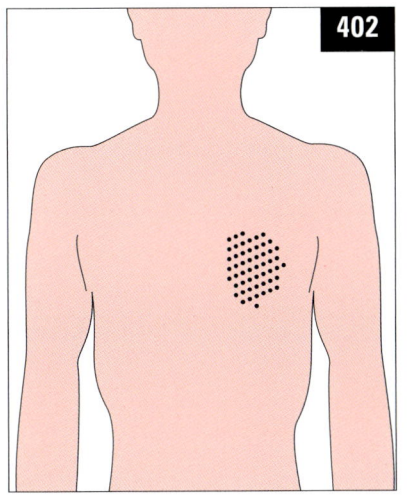

402 Grouped lesions.

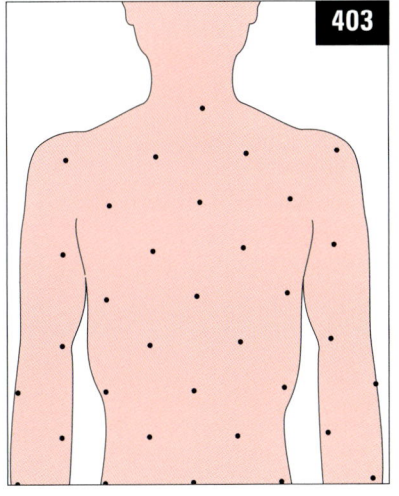

403 Scattered lesions.

There are terms which define widespread distributions more exactly:
- Exanthem refers to a predominantly truncal eruption consisting of multiple, symmetrical, erythematous, maculopapular lesions. Such dermatoses (called exanthematous) can be further described as being either *morbilliform* (meaning measles-like, comprised of blotchy, pink, slightly elevated lesions) or *scarlatiniform* (meaning scarlet fever-like, comprised of tiny erythematous papules).
- Confluent describes the appearance of a coalescence of individual lesions to form a large area of involvement.
- Erythroderma implies that a particular dermatosis involves more than 90% of the body surface area and that the involvement is confluent.

The distribution of lesions can also be described according to regional involvement, the recognition of which can help pinpoint a diagnosis:
- Centrifugal – mostly affecting the extremities, e.g. granuloma annulare.
- Centripetal – mostly affecting the trunk, e.g. pemphigus vulgaris.
- Centrifacial – mostly involving the forehead, nose, and chin, e.g. rosacea.
- Palmoplantar – affecting the palms and soles, e.g. palmoplantar pustulosis.
- Flexural – involving the flexural skin, e.g. erythrasma.
- Extensor – involving the extensor skin, e.g. plaque psoriasis.
- Dermatomal – affecting the skin of one or more dermatomes, e.g. shingles (herpes zoster).
- Periorbital – distributed around the eyes, e.g. syringomata.
- Perioral – distributed around the mouth, e.g. perioral dermatitis.
- Light-exposed – involving the skin routinely exposed to sunlight, e.g. chronic actinic dermatitis.

COLOR
Cutaneous lesions can be flesh-colored, demonstrate a change in pigmentation (hyper- or hypopigmentation), or be characterized by redness. Erythema is redness due to microvascular dilatation which can be blanched by pressure. Purpura is a darker cutaneous redness due to erythrocyte extravasation; purpura cannot be blanched by pressure.

FORMULATING A DIFFERENTIAL DIAGNOSIS
It is generally best to begin with a physical examination based on a brief history of the chief complaint. A more thorough directed history is then obtained as noted above. The initial differential diagnosis is based on the physical examination, then refined based on history. It can be further refined by integrating the results of laboratory tests or biopsy.

Note: this Glossary is based on material from the Manson Publishing title by RJG Rycroft, SJ Robertson, SH Wakelin (2009). *A Colour Handbook of Dermatology*, 2nd edn, London.

INDEX

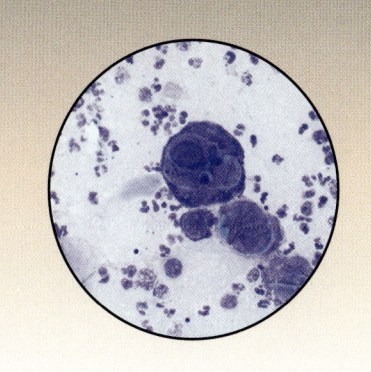

abscess 12, 13
acanthamebiasis 94
acrodermatitis chronic atrophicans (ACA) 30
Actinomyces 19, 90
actinomycetoma 90–1
acute miliary tuberculosis 86
acyclovir 64–5, 68
Aedes aegypti 104
Aeromonas hydrophila 18, 22
Aguiar–Pupo stomatitis 93
albendazole 101
Allescheria boydii 90
allylamines, oral 36
aluminium chloride 19
Amblyomma americanum 116–17
amebiasis 94–5
aminoglycosides 22
amocarzine 98
amphotericin B 50, 51, 52, 53, 55, 59, 93, 97
anaphylaxis 106
Ancylostoma braziliense 101
Androctonus spp. 122
angiomatosis, bacillary 85–6
anthrax, cutaneous 19
antistreptolysin O titer 14
arachnids 112–22
arthritis, Lyme disease 30
aspergillosis 55–6
Aspergillus 22
asteroid bodies, extracellular 50
Atrax 120
atrophy 138
azithromycin 24, 94

bacillary angiomatosis 85–6
bacille Calmette–Guérin (BCG) vaccine 86, 88
Balamuthia mandrillaris 95
Bartonella henselae 24, 85
Bartonella quintana 85

bedbugs 108
beetles 110
benzoyl peroxide 19
betamethasone 41
Blastomyces dermatitidis 52
blastomycosis
    North American 52
    South American 52, 93
blister beetle 110
blueberry muffin lesions 70
booklouse 104
Borrelia burgdorferi 30
bullae 136
    cellulitis 16
    impetigo 10, 11
    insect bites 105
    tinea pedis 43
bullous 'id' reaction 45
Buthus occitanus tunetanus 122

calcineurin inhibitors 40, 41
Calymmatobacterium granulomatis 24
Camp Bullis rickettsial fever 117
Candida 20, 22
candidiasis 46–7
cantharidin 82
capsofungin 53
carbuncle 11–12
caterpillars 109–10
cat-scratch disease 24, 25
cefixime 27
ceftriaxone 24, 27
cellulitis 16–17
centipedes 123
Centuroides spp. 121, 122
cephalexin 10
cephalosporins 10, 23
cercarial dermatitis 99, 100
Chagas' disease 108
chancre, syphilis 30, 31
chancroid 24, 25

Cheyletiella mites 115, 116
chickenpox 65
chigger bites 104, 105, 114–16
chloramphenicol 23, 28, 29, 84
chlorazole black E stain 40, 41
chloroquine 95
chlortetracycline 84
chromoblastomycosis 50, 91
chronic lymphocytic leukemia (CLL) 104, 105
ciclopiroxolamine 47
cidofovir 71, 83
Cimex (bedbugs) spp. 108
ciprofloxacin 11, 19, 24
Cladophialophora carrionii 91
Cladosporium 50
clarithromycin 20
clindamycin 12, 19
clofazimine 88, 92
clotrimazole 19, 41
Coccidioides immitis 52
coleopterids 110
Colorado tick fever 116
comedone 136, 137
complement fixation test 27–8
condylomata acuminata 76–7
corticosteroids, use in tinea corporis 38, 40, 41
Corynebacterium spp. 19, 20
crab louse 102, 103
crust 138
cryptococcosis 54–5
Cryptococcus neoformans 54
Ctenocephalides canis 111
Ctenocephalides felis 110–11
Culex quinquefasciatus 104
cutaneous barrier, impairment 9
cutaneous horn 75
cutaneous larva migrans 101
cytomegalovirus infection 70–1

dapsone 88

Index

Darling's disease (histoplasmosis) 50–1
dehydroemetine 95
Demodex mites 114
Dermacentor spp. 116
dermatitis
    cercarial 99, 100
    impetiginized 9
Dermatophilus congolensis 19
dermatophyte infections 34–44
    nosology 34
dermonecrotic bite reactions 120
dicloxacillin 10, 12
N,N-diethyl-3-methylbenzamide (DEET) 104, 118
dolphins 92
Donovan bodies 24
doxycycline 19, 28, 29

Echidnophaga gallinacea 111
ecthyma 20–1
ecthyma gangrenosum 22
ectothrix 35
eczema, impetiginized 9
eczema herpeticum 62–3
Ehrlichia chaffeensis 117
endospores 53
endothrix 35
Entamoeba histolytica 95–6
enzyme immunoassay (ELISA) 27, 88
epidermodysplasia veruciformis 78–9
epinephrine 106
Epstein–Barr virus (EPV) 68–9
erosio interdigitalis blastomycetica 47
erosion 136, 137
erysipelas 14–15
erythema chronicum migrans 30, 31
erythema infectiosum 73–4
erythema multiforme 62, 64
erythrasma 20–1, 42
erythromycin 18, 19, 20, 24
eschars, black 19, 55, 118
Escherichia coli 22
ethambutol 88
exantham subitum infection 71
excoriation 138, 139
exudate 138, 139

false blister beetle 110
famciclovir 64, 68
fifth disease, *see* erythema infectiosum

fire ant stings 106–7
fish tank granuloma 29
fissure 136, 137
Fite–Faraco stain 88, 89
flea bites 104, 110–11
fleas, cat/rat 27
fluconazole 53, 55, 59, 93
5-flucytosine 94
fluorescent treponemal antibody absorption (FTA-ABS) 32
fluoroquinolones 84
folliculitis
    Demodex mite infection 114
    fungal 40, 41
    staphylococcal 10, 11
Fonsecaea spp. 50, 91
Forchheimer's sign 80
foscarnet 71
Fournier's gangrene 17, 18
fungal hyphae 41, 49, 58
fungal infections
    deep 50–8
    superficial 34–49
furuncle 11–12, 13
fusarium 22
Fusarium spp. 55–6
fusidic acid cream 20

ganciclovir 71
genital lesions
    herpes simplex 60, 62
    molluscum contagiosum 80–1
    warts 74–8
gentamycin 22
Gianotti–Crosti syndrome 69
Giemsa staining 85
glomerulonephritis, post-staphylococcal 10
'glove and socks' syndrome, purpuric 74
Gomori methenamine-silver (GMS) 50, 90, 92, 94
gonococcemia, disseminated 26
gonorrhea 26–7
granuloma inguinale 24–5
griseofulvin 36
Grocott-methenamine silver 86
gypsy moth caterpillars 109

Hadronyche 120
Haemophilus ducreyi 24
Haemophilus influenzae, cellulitis 16–17
Hansen's disease, *see* leprosy
head lice 102–4

hematoxylin and eosin staining 84, 92
Hemipterids 108–9
herpes gladiatorum 62
herpes simplex infection 60–5
herpes zoster (shingles) 66–7
highly active antiretroviral therapy (HAART) 73
histoplasmosis 50–1
history 136
HIV/AIDS infection
    histoplasmosis 51
    Kaposi's sarcoma 72–3
    molluscum contagiosum 82
hookworm infection 101
Hortaea werneckii 48
'hot tub' folliculitis 10, 11
house mouse mites 116
human herpesvirus
    type 5 (HHV-5/cytomegalovirus) 71–2
    type 8 (HHV-8) 71–2
human papillomavirus (HPV) 74–8
    strains 77–8
hyalohyphomycosis 55–6
hymenopterid stings 106–7
hyperhidrosis 19
hyperkeratosis 138

icthyosis 70
imidazoles, topical 47
imiquimod 83
immunocompromised states
    acanthamebiasis 94
    coccidioidomycosis 52
    fusariosis 56
    herpes simplex infection 61, 62
    histoplasmosis 51
    molluscum contagiosum 81, 82
    onychomycosis 46
    see also HIV/AIDS infection
immunoglobulins, intravenous 71, 74
impetigo 8–11
indirect immunofluorescence assay (IFA) 27
infectious mononucleosis 68–9
insect bites 104–5
insecticides, chemical 104, 108, 118
interferon 71
intertrigo, candidal 46–7
iodoquinol 95
isoniazid 88
itraconazole 51, 52, 56, 59, 93, 94, 97

Index

ivermectin 98, 101, 104
Ixodes ticks 30, 118, 119

Jarisch–Herxheimer reaction 32
'jock itch', *see* tinea cruris

Kaposi's sarcoma 71–3
keratohyalin 83
keratolysis, pitted 19
kerion, tinea capitis 34, 35, 36
ketoconazole 59, 93, 97
'kissing' ulcers 25
Koplik spots 78
Kytococcus sedentarius 19

Lacazia loboi 92
lactic acid 82
Lactrodectus mactans 118, 119
Laelaps castroi 115
'larva currens' 100
larva migrans, cutaneous 101
leishmaniasis 96–7
Leishmania spp. 96
Leiurus quinquestriatus 122
Lepidopterids 109–10
leprosy 88–9
levofloxacin 27
lice 102–4
lichenification 138
lindane 104
Loa loa 98
lobomycosis 55, 92
'lone star' tick 117
Loxosceles spiders 118–20
lues maligna 32
lupus vulgaris 86, 87
Lymantria dispar (Gypsy moth) 109
Lyme disease 30, 31, 118
lymphadenopathy
 occipital 34–5
 rubella infection 80
lymphadenosis benigna cutis (lymphocytoma cutis) 30

maculae ceruleae 104
macule 136, 137
Madurella spp. 90
Majocchi's granuloma 40, 41
malaria 104
Malassezia 48
malathion 104
Mansonella perstans 98
Mayan culture 84
measles infection 78–9

mefloquine 97
Megalopyge opercularis 109–10
meglumine antimonate 96
meningococcemia 23
methicillin-resistant *Staphylococcus aureus* (MRSA) 10, 12, 13
metronidazole 95
miconazole 19, 20
Micrococcus sedentarius, *see Kytococcus sedentarius*
microhemagglutination assay 32
Mikulicz cells 84
milker's nodule 82–3
millipedes 123
minocycline 29, 88
Missulenacan 120
mites 112–16
molluscum contagiosum 80–2
molluscum contagiosum virus (MCV) 82
Montenegro skin test 96
mosquitoes 104
moths 109–10
Mucorales 56
mucormycosis 56–8
mupirocin 10, 19, 20
mycetoma 90–1
Mycobacterium leprae 88
Mycobacterium maninum 29
Mycobacterium tuberculosis 86

necrotizing fasciitis 17–18
Neisseria gonorrhoeae 26
Neisseria meningitidis 22, 23
newborns, herpes simplex infection 62
Nocardia 90
Northern fowl mite 115
nystatin 47

ofloxacin 27, 88
onchocerciasis 98–9
onchocercoma 98, 99
onychodystrophy 46
onychomycosis 44–6
oral candidiasis 47
orf 92–3
Orientia tsutsugamushi 28
Ornithodoros ticks 116, 117

Paederus eximius (Rove beetle) 110
papular acrodermatitis of childhood (Gianotti–Crosti syndrome) 69
papule 136, 137

Parabuthus spp. 122
Paracoccidioides brasiliensis 93
paracoccidioidomycosis 93
parvovirus B19 infection 73–4
Pastia's lines 14
pediculosis 102–4
Pediculus humanus capitis 102
Pediculus humanus humanus 102
penciclovir 64
penicillin
 intravenous 23
 oral 18
 pencillinase-resistant 10
penicillin G 32
pentamidine 94, 95, 97
pentoxifylline 96–7
Peptostreptococcus 18
peri-anal streptococcal disease 18
periodic acid-Schiff (PAS) staining 46, 50, 54, 84, 92, 94
perleche 47
permethrin 104, 118
Petrellidium boydii 90
phaeohyphomycosis 56, 57
Phialophora 50
physical examination 136
piperacillin 22
pitted keratolysis 19
pityriasis versicolor 48–9
Pityrosporum 48
plaques
 definition 136, 137
 erysipelas 14, 15
plasma cells 84, 85
polymerase chain reaction (PCR) testing 68, 87, 96
post-herpetic neuralgia (PHN) 68
potassium hydroxide (KOH) examination 36, 40, 44, 46, 47
poxvirus infection 80–3
praziquantel 100
Prototheca wickerhamii 59
protothecosis 59
pseudoepitheliomatous hyperplasia 83, 85
Pseudomonas aeruginosa septicemia 22
Pseudomonas infections 10
'pseudonit' 103
psocids 104
Psoroptes mite 115
Pthirus pubis (crab louse) 102, 103
Pulex irritans 111
purpuric 'glove and socks' syndrome 74

puss caterpillar 109–10
pustules 8, 136, 137
pyrazinamide 88
pyrethrins 104

Q-fever 116

rapid plasma reagent (RPR) 32
retapamulin 10, 12, 20
Rhinocladiella spp. 50, 91
rhinoscleroma 84–5
rhinosporidiosis 58–9
Rhinosporidium seeberi 58
Rhipicephalus ticks 118
Rhizopus 56
Rickettsia spp. 27
rickettsial diseases 116, 117, 118
Rickettsia rickettsii 28–9
rifampin 12, 23, 28, 84, 88, 94
'ringworm', see tinea corporis
Ritter's disease (staphylococcal scalded skin syndrome) 12–13
Rocky Mountain spotted fever 28–9, 116, 117
Romana's sign 108
'rose gardener's disease' 50
rubella infection 80
Russell bodies 84, 85

S-100 staining 88
Sabouraud's fungal medium 47, 48
saddleback caterpillar 110
salicylic acid 48, 78, 82
sandflies 96
'San Joaquin Valley Fever' 52
Sarcoptes scabei 112–13
scabies 112–13
    canine 115
scale 136, 137
scarlet fever 14
Schistosoma spp. 99, 100
schistosomiasis 99–100
sclerosis 138
sclerotic bodies 91
scorpions, bites 121–2
scrofuloderma 87
scrub typhus 28
Serratia marcescens 22
shingles (herpes zoster) 66–7
Sibine stimulea 110
Simulium spp. 98
siphonapterids 110–11
skin lesions
    distribution 138, 139
    morphology 136–8
    shape 138, 139

'slapped cheek' rash 73
sodium stibogluconate 97
spherules 53, 58
spider bites 118–21
sporangia 59
Sporothrix schenckii 50
'sporotrichoid spread' 29, 50
sporotrichosis 50, 51
staphylococcal scalded skin syndrome (SSSS) 12–13
Staphylococcus aureus 10, 11, 12, 22
    methicillin-resistant (MRSA) 10, 12, 13
Starry silver stain 87
Stevens–Johnson syndrome 83
stings, hymenopterid 106–7
'strawberry' tongue 14
straw mite 115
Streptococcus pyogenes 10, 14, 16, 17–18
Streptomyces 90
Strongyloides stercoralis 100–1
strongyloidiasis 100–1
sulfonamides 93
supersaturated potassium iodide (SSKI) 50
suramin 98
Swartz–Lamkin stain 49
swimmer's itch (cercarial dermatitis) 99
syphilis (lues) 30–3

'tape stripping' 48, 49
tarantulas 120–1
Tegenaria spp. 120
telangiectasia 136, 137
terbinafine 46, 93, 97
tetracycline 84
thiabendazole 101
ticks 29, 116–18, 119
tinea barbae 38
tinea capitis 34–6
tinea corporis 36–41
tinea cruris 42
tinea facei 38–9
tinea incognito 41
tinea manum 44, 45
tinea nigra 48–9
tinea pedis 42–4
tinea unguium 44
Tityus serrulatus 122
toluidine blue staining 46
Treponema pallidum 30, 32, 33
triamcinolone, intralesional 120
Triatome reduviids 108

triazoles, oral 36
trichomycosis axillaris 20
Trichophyton rubrum 42
Trichophyton tonsurans 34
Trichophyton violaceum 34
trimethoprim-sulfamethoxazole 24, 29, 84
trophozoites 94, 95
Tsutsugamushi fever (scrub typhus) 28
tuberculosis, cutaneous 86–8
tularemia 116, 117
tungiasis 111
typhus 27–8
Tzanck smears 64, 68

ulcer 136, 137
umbilicated lesions 138, 139
Uroplectes lineatus 122
urticaria, papular 104, 105
urticating hairs 109, 121

vaccines
    BCG 86, 88
    human papillomavirus 78
    varicella zoster virus 68
Vaejovis spp. 122
valacyclovir 64–5, 68
varicella, primary 65
varicella zoster immune globulin 68
varicella zoster virus infection 65–8
venom immunotherapy 106
vesicles 8, 136, 137
vespids 107
Vibrio vulnificus 18
vitamin A 78, 82
voriconazole 56, 58

Warthin–Starry staining 24
warts 74–8
warty lesions 138, 139
wasps 106
Western blot 64
wheal 136, 137
wheel bug 109
Whitefield's ointment 20
whitlow, herpetic 62
Wood's lamp 20, 21, 42
Wright–Giemsa staining 25

Ziehl–Neelsen stain 87